MW01519971

Public Health Intervention for the COVID-19 Pandemic

From Virus to Vaccine

World Scientific Series in Global Health Economics and Public Policy

ISSN: 2010-2089

Series Editor-in-Chief: Peter Berman *(The University of British Columbia, Canada & Harvard University, USA)*

The World Scientific Series in Global Health Economics and Public Policy, under the leadership of Professor Peter Berman, a renowned healthcare economist, public policy specialist and researcher in this field, seeks to fill this gap. It strives to publish high-quality scientific works, including monographs, edited volumes, references, handbooks, etc., which address subjects of primary scientific importance on the global scale, as related to international economic policies in healthcare, social capital and healthcare economics in different global markets, etc. The titles in this series appeal to researchers, graduate students, policy makers, practitioners and commercial businesses, dealing with healthcare economics worldwide.

Published:

More information on this series can also be found at
https://www.worldscientific.com/series/wssghepp

(Continued at end of book)

World Scientific Series in Global Health Economics and Public Policy – Vol. 9

Public Health Intervention for the COVID-19 Pandemic

From Virus to Vaccine

Edited by

David Patrick
The University of British Columbia, Canada
BC Centre for Disease Control, Canada

Ariana Saatchi
The University of British Columbia, Canada

World Scientific

NEW JERSEY · LONDON · SINGAPORE · BEIJING · SHANGHAI · HONG KONG · TAIPEI · CHENNAI · TOKYO

Published by

World Scientific Publishing Co. Pte. Ltd.

5 Toh Tuck Link, Singapore 596224

USA office: 27 Warren Street, Suite 401-402, Hackensack, NJ 07601

UK office: 57 Shelton Street, Covent Garden, London WC2H 9HE

Library of Congress Control Number: 2022006014

British Library Cataloguing-in-Publication Data
A catalogue record for this book is available from the British Library.

World Scientific Series in Global Health Economics and Public Policy — Vol. 9
PUBLIC HEALTH INTERVENTION FOR THE COVID-19 PANDEMIC
From Virus to Vaccine

ISBN 978-981-124-971-6 (hardcover)
ISBN 978-981-124-972-3 (ebook for institutions)
ISBN 978-981-124-973-0 (ebook for individuals)

For any available supplementary material, please visit
https://www.worldscientific.com/worldscibooks/10.1142/12654#t=suppl

Desk Editors: Aanand Jayaraman/Yulin Jiang

Typeset by Stallion Press
Email: enquiries@stallionpress.com

About the Editors

We are a group of public health professionals and scholars who share the goal of learning from the COVID-19 Pandemic in order to better counter future health threats and the endemic health and social landscapes that complicate our response.

David Patrick is an Infectious Disease Physician, Epidemiologist and Professor of Public Health with a 30-year focus on responding to epidemics. His work at the BC Centre for Disease Control and elsewhere has spanned HIV, vaccine-preventable diseases, SARS, pandemic H1N1, antimicrobial resistance and COVID-19. In January of 2021, his graduate class in Control of Communicable Diseases at the UBC School of Population and Public Health agreed that we were living one of the greatest case studies in the field. Together, we formed a vision to create a compendium of new learning on how to contain and mitigate the effects of the pathogen and the pandemic.

Ariana Saatchi is a PhD Candidate with the UBC Faculty of Pharmaceutical Sciences. She has a strong interest in antimicrobial stewardship and infectious diseases and has played a key role in coordinating and arranging the contributions to this volume.

About the Chapter Contributors and Series Editor

Each chapter is a contribution from one or more graduate level scholars in collaboration with faculty subject matter experts. Contributors ranged in attendance from three continents and drafted these chapters as the pandemic unfolded. Subject matter experts were all active in the public health, research or clinical response to the pandemic. More information on these authors is provided chapter by chapter.

The editors wish to express our deep thanks to every chapter author. While working hard to deal with a pandemic in your own lives and careers, you were nonetheless enthused about contributing. This project could never have been launched without your diverse skills, experiences, and efforts.

We especially wish to recognize Dr. Ali Okhowat for his excellent synthesis of introductory and concluding chapters. Okhowat is a family physician and public health physician in training. He was previously co-founder and Co-Lead of the World Health Organization (WHO) Innovation Hub and served as a Health Emergency Officer at its Headquarters in Geneva and the Eastern Mediterranean Regional Office in Cairo. He is currently the Co-Lead of the Enhanced Skills Program in Global Health at the University of British Columbia.

We also thank our series editor, who saw the wisdom of including a volume on COVID-19 interventions within a broad series on the pandemic. Peter Berman is a Health Economist and Professor of Public Health with an active research program aimed at understanding the role institutional, governance, organizational and political factors on response to the pandemic.

Acknowledgements

We dedicate this volume to all people who have come together in response to the most serious respiratory pandemic in a century. Public health measures and scientific advances can have but limited effects without individuals pulling together for the common good. For all who kept their distance, wore a mask, adapted their work, dealt with hardship, cared for children and family, and stepped forward for a vaccine, we acknowledge your role. For all who took the time to pursue the most reliable information to protect your loved ones and communities, you have our gratitude. For all who lost a loved one, we grieve with you and acknowledge that the best way we can honour the fallen is to create conditions where the worst ravages of this, and future pandemics, are prevented.

We also acknowledge that a true global response to the pandemic remains largely aspirational. While it is true that governments and industry collaborated to advance science and vaccine development as never before, the equitable distribution of benefits accrued did not follow suit. At the time of writing, vaccine roll-out to most of the world's population remains a long way off. We must acknowledge the responsibility to value and protect all lives with equal passion. Indeed, one of our lessons from COVID has been the intricate interconnectivity of our global society — and the rippling impacts of one life, or one case, on us all. Pandemic responses must adapt to become increasingly global, as there is no true end to a pandemic until it is controlled everywhere.

As a group of authors from Canadian Universities, we also recognize that inequitable treatment of people is very much our problem to solve. As we write, the remains of hundreds who died of infectious disease and neglect at residential schools for Indigenous children during the 20th century have come to light. Unfortunately, the same insidious injustices that supported the personification of these children and their peoples as "other," are still entrenched within society today. It is this fearsome virus woven into our global fabric that allows us to accept that low and middle-income countries can somehow afford to wait additional years for vaccine. As we work to put COVID-19 behind us, we must turn and face this older and deadlier affliction spread during the colonial era and that is, tragically, very much alive today. We speak not only of controlling a pathogen, but also to address the conditions, including systemic racism, that enable pandemics to thrive.

Contents

Part 1

Introduction

Chapter 1

A Framework for COVID-19 Response

Ali Okhowat

*School of Population and Public Health, University of British Columbia,
Vancouver, Canada*

*Department of Family Practice, Faculty of Medicine, University of British
Columbia, Vancouver, Canada*

*Division of Global Health, Faculty of Medicine, University of British Columbia,
Vancouver, Canada*

1. Introduction

"We now have a name for the disease: COVID-19. I'll spell it: C-O-V-I-D hyphen one nine — COVID-19. … we're keeping the public informed about what everyone can do to protect their own health and that of others. It's when each and every individual becomes part of the containment strategy that we can succeed." — Dr. Tedros Adhanom Ghebreyesus (February 11, 2020). "WHO Director-General's remarks at the media briefing on 2019-nCoV"

At 02:00 AM on January 23, residents of the then epicentre of the 2019 novel coronavirus in Wuhan, China, were informed of a lockdown that would come into effect at 10:00 AM later that morning. The world had known for weeks of the existence of an outbreak in Wuhan that had started as a cluster of pneumonia cases first reported to the WHO China Country Office on December 31. Yet the scale and scope of the shelter-in-place restrictions of approximately 11 million people was astounding. News organisations broadcast images of desolate streets, taped doorways and health workers in full-body personal protective equipment.

By February 11, 2020 — when the world came to know for the first time the name of the disease caused by the 2019 novel coronavirus — China had reported 42,708 cases and 1,017 deaths and only 393 cases and one death had been recorded across 24 countries (Figure 1). In the day's press conference, WHO's Director-General announced the launch of a research conference of 400 scientists to discuss the plethora of questions that had arisen about COVID-19 and how best to contain it. He stressed, "the main outcome we expect from this meeting is not immediate answers to every question that we have; [rather] the main outcome is a agreed roadmap on what questions we need to ask, and how we will go about answering those questions." The first vaccine could be ready in an unprecedented 18 months, he remarked, and followed with a call for $675 million to support preparedness and response operations in countries.

On February 24, 2021, a little over one year after the term COVID-19 was coined, the WHO released its updated *COVID-19 Strategic Preparedness and Response Plan (SPRP, 2021)*. The figure in its introductory text showing a steady march to over 107 million cases could hardly be imagined a year prior (Figure 2). Lost among the numbers of case counts and graphs of flattening curves, however, were three devastating developments. First, COVID's spread had exposed fractures in the safety nets that were supposed to be in place for those underserved by health systems. From long term care facilities to under-resourced communities to front-line workers, the virus's toll was shown to be disproportionately severe for those who had long been neglected by health and social systems. Second, the chart crystallised the speed at which a novel pathogen could exhibit runaway transmission dynamics. This had occurred despite an unprecedented level of global research and collaboration on COVID-19 related diagnostics, treatments and vaccinations. Lastly, COVID-19's exponential spread overwhelmed even the highest resource health systems in the world and touched every aspect of daily life. The delicate calculus between saving lives and livelihoods sparked debate and division at every

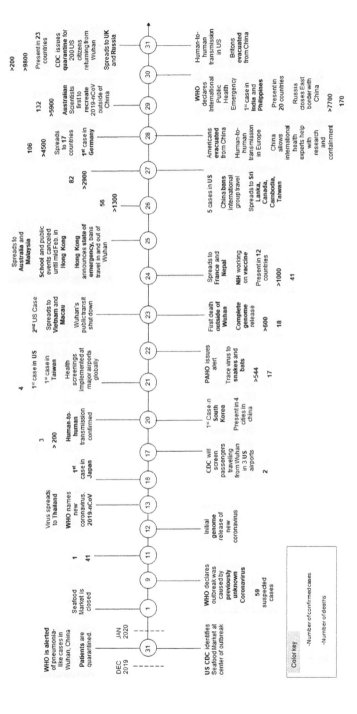

Figure 1: Timeline of COVID-19 cases worldwide (December 31, 2019–January 31, 2020).

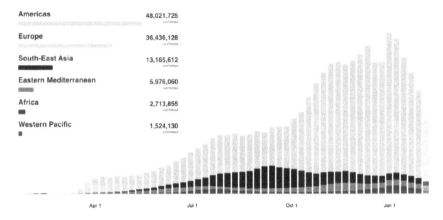

Americas	48,021,725
	confirmed
Europe	36,436,128
	confirmed
South-East Asia	13,165,612
	confirmed
Eastern Mediterranean	5,976,060
	confirmed
Africa	2,713,855
	confirmed
Western Pacific	1,524,130
	confirmed

Apr 1   Jul 1   Oct 1   Jan 1

Figure 2:   Reported weekly COVID-19 cases and deaths to February 13, 2021.

level of government the world over. While these challenges united countries and communities in a common fight, they paradoxically reinforced borders, fragmented freedoms and resulted in transactional diplomacy measured, at time, in doses of vaccines delivered.

2. Disentangling COVID-19's Infodemic

That we are living in a hyper connected world, where a seemingly innocuous cluster of symptoms in one part may have disastrous consequences on the other side, is a truth that cannot be ignored. We need look no further than the travel restrictions that cascaded around the world at the pandemic's onset and that continue to ebb and flow. Restricting travel and quarantines at ports of entry are among humanity's most primitive yet persistent policy tools in combating the outbreak of disease. Yet despite all our scientific advances, we have returned to them. With that return has come waves of information that we are witness to daily regarding the virus' spread, our understanding of its inner workings and the ways in which we're attempting to control its effects.

As a well-informed individual or even a seasoned scientist, managing to keep up-to-date on the depth and breadth of information on what has probably become one of the most studied diseases in history is as overwhelming as it is all-consuming. We know so much about the SARS-CoV-2 virus and the disease state of COVID-19 yet there is also so much more to be known. It is said that where there is a wealth of information yet a dearth of knowledge, rumours and speculation prevail. This has unfortunately been the truth for some aspects of our understanding of COVID-19 and one of the primary motivations for the drafting of this book.

There has been a mass of disinformation, misinformation, and general confusion about the SARS-CoV-2 virus and its clinical manifestation as COVID-19 disease. Few things travel faster than the spread of a highly transmissible contagion, save the stories that may travel ahead of its wake. This is the very definition of an infodemic, which refers to the overabundance and mix of facts, fears, and sometimes falsehoods that influence the public's understanding of a disease. There's no doubt that there can be serious consequences to this.

Dis- and misinformation can lead to a reduced adherence to public health and social measures to contain a disease; threaten people's health and well-being; and reduce the effectiveness of health stakeholders in combating the spread of a disease. This has been such a prominent problem since the first days of the COVID-19 pandemic that in the May 2020 World Health Assembly, Resolution WHA 73.1 was passed on the COVID-19. Response called on Member States to, among other commitments, "provide the population with reliable and comprehensive information on COVID-19 and the measures taken by authorities in response to the pandemic, and to take measures to counter misinformation and disinformation as well as malicious cyber activities."

Nowhere has it been more difficult to discern the difference between fact and fiction, truth and half-truths, and the impact that these have on the health of the public, than when the information is applied to decision-making at the level of plans and policies that affect lives and livelihoods. It was with this goal in mind that the authors of this volume approached their topics. They endeavoured to draft a succinct yet comprehensive summary of the knowledge — based on quality evidence — that we have to date on various aspects of COVID-19.

3. Knowledge is Power ... and Health

With such a range of readers in mind, we have followed three principles in developing this text centered on three pillars of science, solidarity and solutions. Our focus on science has led us through a rigorous, evidence-informed review of the content we have included. Where uncertainties exist, we have attempted to highlight them and where gaps for further research exist or are being actively pursued, we have strived to link to the prominent teams and institutions leading this work. Our search of the primary literature included pre-print archives, such as *Medrxiv*, as well as gray literature including reports by the World Health Organization and affiliated organisations, academic institutions and public health organisations. Our belief in solidarity has meant scoping for information on all sections relevant to a global audience and not limiting it to a specific geography or population subgroup. Our goal is that this text will be read, translated and, ultimately, contributed to by readers all over the world and this can only be done if the content is accurate, timely and informative in a way that furthers our shared struggle to overcome this pandemic. Lastly, our focus on solutions has framed our section on public health control of the virus' spread, clinical management of COVID-19, and vaccination characteristics and strategies.

With these principles in mind, three groups of readers hovered over our shoulders as we drafted these chapters. The first were the scientists, researchers and clinicians who have demanded accurate information and precise wording regarding what we know and the limits of that knowledge. They have served not only as metaphorical critics in our drafts but we have been privileged by the participation of subject matter experts who have provided invaluable contributions to the development of every chapter of this book.

The second group consisted of public health practitioners, policymakers and politicians who imagined threading sections of this text into their policy briefs and Teleprompters. This group sat with furrowed brows as we wrote about nucleic acid amplification tests, vaccine platforms and the efficacy of mask-wearing mandates. As a tome with global ambition, they argued against including content that was too local in scope, applicable to very specific subpopulations or that could not be widely shared. At the same time, they pushed us to mainstream ethical considerations and equity-based factors into all of the chapters, reminding us that until the virus is present anywhere, we are at risk everywhere.

Lastly, we were joined by the lay public who challenged us to render a final version that was informative, yet easy to read. This reader winced, at times, at the jargon that was used, at the statistics that were overshared, and at the depth of some sections. Their constant presence compelled us to write with an eye to the general reader in mind. One of the tradeoffs of writing for such an audience is that while we've rigorously reviewed the content in this book, we have not assigned grades of evidence to specific points, though references have been provided to summary texts that may do so. Where possible, we have referenced open-source material or versions of material that has later been published, in the interests of maximising the accessibility of our readers to the research that underlies this work.

4. Dissecting SARS-CoV-2 by Section and Chapter

In being guided by the WHO's *COVID-19 SPRP (SPRP, 2021)*, this volume's chapters map on to the plan's ten pillars:

1. Coordination, planning, financing, and monitoring.
2. Risk communication, community engagement (RCCE), and infodemic management.
3. Surveillance, epidemiological investigation, contact tracing, and adjustment of public health and social measures.
4. Points of entry, international travel and transport, and mass gatherings.
5. Laboratories and diagnostics.
6. Infection prevention and control, and protection of the health workforce.
7. Case management, clinical operations, and therapeutics.
8. Operational support and logistics, and supply chains.
9. Maintaining essential health services and systems.
10. Vaccination.

The content in this book touches on all of the pillars yet those that are bolded above are covered in most detail. Pillars 1 and 8 are covered in other volumes of this series. This volume may therefore serve to introduce anyone looking for a systematic approach to tackling the spread of COVID-19 at home or abroad with detailed background information on the majority of the WHO preparedness and response pillars.

While no volume can ever hope to review all that is known about COVID-19, this book attempts to provide the reader with an in-depth understanding of the knowledge that we have gleaned to date. It covers up-to-date information (as of May 2021) on the biology of the SARS-CoV-2 virus, its transmission dynamics, diagnostics and the role of laboratories, public health measures in the community, healthcare facility-specific interventions, therapeutics, vaccines and public engagement in combating the infodemic.

This book's 15 content chapters are categorised into seven parts that review details about the basic biology, clinical considerations and public health interventions relevant to COVID-19.

In *Part 2: The Biological Underpinnings of Infection and Transmission*, three chapters explore the biology of the SARS-CoV-2 virus, its pathogenesis and factors influencing its transmission dynamics.

Chapter 2, *SARS-CoV-2: The Virus*, focuses on the biology of the SARS-CoV-2 virus. It reviews the virology and pathophysiology of SARS-CoV-2, clinical features of COVID-19, modes of transmission and the rise of variants and related public health concerns.

In exploring interactions between host and virus, Chapter 3, *Virus Meets Host: SARS-CoV-2 Pathogenesis*, examines the process of viral entry into cells and the roles of innate versus adaptive immunity against SARS-CoV-2. Viral immune evasion, as well as host, viral and environmental factors affecting pathogenicity are also reviewed.

Chapter 4, *Transmission Dynamics of COVID-19*, delves into the factors affecting the spread of SARS-CoV-2, with a focus on explaining the fundamentals of the basic versus effective reproduction number. It goes on to highlight how various public health and social measures may reduce the reproduction number or how overdispersion and super-spreader events may have the opposite effect. It also discusses how characteristics of contacts and venues of transmission affect spread before concluding with a brief discussion of modelling, specifically the susceptible-exposed-infectious-recovered (SEIR) compartmental model.

Part 3: Diagnostics and the Role of Laboratories, contains two chapters that investigate nucleic acid amplification versus protein-based testing methods.

Chapter 5, *The Role of Nucleic Acid Amplification and Sequencing*, focuses on reverse transcriptase polymerase chain reaction (RT-PCR) as the dominant nucleic acid amplification test of choice around the world and discusses its analytic and clinical performance characteristics, the impact of RT-PCR testing on the reproductive rate and the promise and pitfalls of mass testing. The penultimate section looks forward to outbreak investigations and ongoing surveillance using whole genome sequencing and the challenges faced by health systems that have added this to their testing arsenals.

Chapter 6, *Antigen and Antibody Testing*, begins by summarising the two, general protein-based testing methods noted in its title according to their targets, time for sampling, sample site and uses. It proceeds to review in detail antigen versus antibody tests and their respective utilities. While acknowledging the existence of laboratory-based tests for antibodies and their potential shortcomings in terms of turnaround times and resource costs, it concludes with a review of point of care test considerations according to sampling site and quality assurance considerations and test performance characteristics.

Part 4: Public Health Measures in the Community, studies how public health policies and practices have sought to detect, prevent and mitigate the spread of SARS-CoV-2.

Chapter 7, *Contact Tracing, Screening, Self-Isolation and Quarantine*, highlights the non-pharmaceutical interventions that have been deployed in community contexts around the world. It starts with screening principles before turning the reader's attention to the methods and appropriateness of various screening approaches. Contact tracing is tackled next using the WHO definition of a contact to review inclusion criteria and various approaches to contact tracing, including forward, backward and bidirectional tracing and the means of doing so — whether manual or digital. The chapter concludes by touching on timeliness and privacy concern considerations.

Chapter 8, *Restrictions on Travel*, tackles travel restrictions and the need for international coordination before reviewing evidence of importation risk by air versus land ports of entry. Mass gathering restrictions are also addressed with a focus on the importance of these restrictions worldwide and how they have been implemented in Canada.

Chapter 9, *Non-Medical Masking, Hygiene and Social Distancing*, begins by assessing the evidence on the function and effectiveness non-medical masks. It goes on to address the role of hygiene and social distancing measures — the latter in high versus low occupancy settings — in decreasing COVID-19 transmission.

The two chapters of *Part 5: Interventions in Healthcare*, examine COVID-19 control measures in hospitals versus long-term care facilities.

Chapter 10, *Hospital Infection Control*, situates the discussion on infection prevention within the framework of a hierarchy of controls and then systematically tackles each one. Elimination and substitution reviews screening, isolation and non-essential visitor policies and procedures before moving on to engineering and environmental controls. This latter section discusses physical separation and spatial barriers, ventilation, routine cleaning and disinfection, and waste management measures. A discussion of administrative controls follows, staffing and personnel surge considerations, as well as the protection — via training, vaccination and communication — of health human resources. Protocols of hospital sub-departments, such as surgery, obstetrics and critical care are reviewed in this section. This section would not be complete without an exploration of personal protective equipment requirements.

Chapter 11, *Long-Term Care Facilities*, studies why transmission dynamics and deaths have been disproportionately severe in long-term care facilities. It begins by recounting population-based risk factors inherent in long-term care residences before reviewing strategies, including vaccination, aimed at reducing transmission as well as a four-part framework to address outcome disparities. It concludes with a brief discussion about priorities for pandemic preparedness, including adequate resourcing of essential health supplies as well as standardising data collection requirements and comparisons of US Centres for Disease Control, WHO and the Public Health Agency of Canada guidelines.

Part 6: Therapeutics, runs headlong into the fascinating world of therapeutics by assessing the evidence of different types of treatments for COVID-19.

Specifically, Chapter 12, *Therapeutics for COVID-19*, is structured according to the three stages of COVID-19 manifestation that are outlined in the introductory section: early infection, pulmonary phase, and hyper inflammation phase. It then goes on to discuss pre- versus post-exposure prophylaxis considerations, including the role of polyclonal antibodies. The next section examines the treatment of non-severe COVID-19 patients with a synthesis of evidence on the efficacy of colchicine, proxulatamide, and convalescent plasma. Two viral-based treatment options for the pulmonary phase are thereafter reviewed, specifically remdesivir and human recombinant soluble ACE-2. Lastly, host-based treatment options for the pulmonary and inflammatory phases are examined, including dexamethasone and other corticosteroids, interleukin-6 pathway inhibitors, Janus kinase inhibitors, and other drugs interfering with interleukin and interferon-related pathways. Finally, other therapies such as antibacterial, antithrombotic and supportive care, are highlighted, including extracorporeal membrane oxygenation.

The next section provides an overview of one of the most critical topics in our fight against the spread of COVID-19: vaccination. *Part 7: Vaccines*, reviews vaccine design, allocation and safety measures.

Chapter 13, *Overview of Vaccine Designs and Performance*, delves into the four main types of vaccines platforms: whole, inactivated virus vaccines; protein subunit vaccines; non-replicating viral vector vaccines; and Ribonucleic Acid-based vaccines. Current vaccines are traced to their respective platform sections and their manufacturing and relative performance characteristics are reviewed. The section concludes with a summary table of what we know about each vaccine with respect to its dosing frequency, storage temperatures, and efficacy in phase 3 trial results, among other data.

Chapter 14, *Vaccine Allocation and Prioritisation*, reviews the global allocation of COVID-19 vaccines through bilateral agreements and the multi-institution led global COVAX facility. Various vaccine allocation frameworks are next explored with a focus on the *WHO Framework for Allocation and Prioritisation of COVID-19 Vaccination*. Strategies for informing priority decisions are thereafter explored, with the case of the Canadian province of British Columbia's vaccine rollout reviewed as an example. Comments on other considerations that may influence the aforementioned allocation schemes are then evaluated, including logistical challenges such as cold-chain, storage or last-mile delivery considerations, the emergence of variants of concern, and vaccine coverage versus hesitancy concerns. The chapter concludes with a synthesis of lessons from Israel's vaccine rollout.

Chapter 15, *COVID-19 Vaccine Safety*, consists of three parts. The first highlights key considerations of vaccine safety from pre-clinical and clinical (Phase 1 through Phase 3) trials and licensure. The second summarises the most up-to-date information on vaccine safety as of mid-April 2021. A helpful table summarising safety assessments of COVID-19 vaccines categorised as one of four vaccine types is provided, as well as a summary of the objectives and reportable versus unreportable events related to Phase 4 post-market surveillance data. Lastly, the third reviews local, regional and global strategies that have been instituted to monitor vaccine safety. Vaccine surveillance safety systems, including passive and active varieties, are touched on, with a case study highlighting post-market safety surveillance of the Oxford/AstraZeneca vaccine. Vaccine safety considerations for special population, including contraindications, as well as vaccine types and adjuvants are also discussed. The chapter concludes with a discussion of the challenges inherent in detecting safety signals in such a short period of time for vaccines that have been developed with unprecedented speed and, in some cases, using relatively novel technologies.

Part 8: Public Engagement and Combating the Infodemic, details how information related to COVID-19 has travelled from various sources to the public and specific stakeholders involved in the response to COVID-19.

Chapter 16, *Public Engagement*, describes how various media have been used to disseminate information related to COVID-19 — though not always rooted in evidence or good faith. To this end, it also reviews examples of how mis- and disinformation have been attempted to be countered through special partnerships with traditional and social media outlets. All media have strived yet struggled to balance open conversations about COVID-19 with the filtering out of potentially harmful content. As the penultimate chapter, it provides a thought-provoking segway into structural factors that frame risk and inequity in society.

The volume concludes with Chapter 17, *Preventing the Next Pandemic*, which provides a look back on how the world has irrevocably changed and which initiatives, institutions and ideas will need to prevail to help us prevent the next pandemic. This chapter rounds out the book by critically looking at the role of institutions, governance and governments whose actions and policies have become ever important as harbingers to both injustice and equity in different contexts around the world. This section reviews how various jurisdictions have responded to the spread of COVID-19 through public health campaigns, policies, and the enforcement of soft and hard law. Embedded in this discussion is a consideration of cultural factors that influence the acceptability of these interventions and willingness of the population to engage in or be bound by conditions and restrictions related to preventing or mitigating the spread of COVID-19.

5. An Origin Story of Remote Beginnings

This book is the result of an immense effort by the editors and a team of authors from the University of British Columbia's School of Population and Public Health SPPH 520 course, Control of Communicable Diseases, led by Dr. David Patrick and assisted by Ariana Saatchi. Students in the class ranged in attendance from three continents and drafted these chapters with subject matter experts as the pandemic unfolded and, in some places, returned with a vengeance in subsequent waves that battered their communities and countries. Almost all of the original research, consultations and review of the work were undertaken through the distributed teams and remote work that have become a mainstay of the pandemic.

6. Of Scope and Boundaries

As ambitious as this project has been in providing an overview of many of the more salient points from research and practice relevant to COVID-19, it is focused on providing evidence-informed and practical information. This volume does not provide an exhaustive evaluation of the cornucopia of primary and secondary literature that has emerged on COVID-19. It also does not endeavour to be used as a point of care reference — though many chapters lend themselves to a cursory review of the topics they cover. Lastly, it should not be construed as forwarding a definitive viewpoint on many of the topics addressed. Our knowledge of COVID-19 is continuously emerging and some of the points mentioned in this textbook may very well be challenged in the coming months and years. It is with this in mind that the editors endeavour to treat this text as a living volume that will be frequently updated.

7. A Call to Action

The target audience for this volume includes both lay reader and the policy wonk, the informed citizen and the popular press, students of science and sociology through critics and sceptics of them both. Our intent in writing this volume was to make accessible to all of the above groups in the most accessible manner a structured approach to understanding COVID-19. Yet we would be remiss to admit that if there are ideas that spur you to action, compel you to become involved, to create, to advocate or simply to nudge a correction online, we will feel fulfilled in having not simply achieved our purpose but added to yours. As you explore the contents of these pages, consider how what you learn aligns with what was done or could have been done differently in the early days of the pandemic. Think about which of the pillars of the WHO's COVID-19 SPRP need to be most strengthened in your local region, country or globally for there to be a true resolution to this pandemic. And reflect on how the world has and perhaps should change to prevent or mitigate the spread of the next novel pathogen. The cost of inaction is too high and the actions of every person matter in combating COVID-19. As Dr. Tedros said in his opening speech on February 11, 2020, "It's when each and every individual becomes part of the containment strategy that we can succeed."

References

1. El Zowalaty ME, Järhult JD. From SARS to COVID-19: A previously unknown SARS- related coronavirus (SARS-CoV-2) of pandemic potential infecting humans — Call for a One Health approach. One Health. 2020 Feb 24;9:100124.
2. *COVID-19 Strategic Preparedness and Response Plan.* Geneva: World Health Organization; 2021, p. 4.

Part 2

The Biological Underpinnings
of Infection and Transmission

Chapter 2

SARS-CoV-2: The Virus

Kishore Hari[*] and Mel Krajden[†,‡]

[*]*School of Population and Public Health, University of British Columbia, Vancouver, Canada*

[†]*Department of Pathology and Laboratory Medicine, Faculty of Medicine, University of British Columbia, Vancouver, Canada*

[‡]*Public Health Microbiology and Reference Laboratory, BC Centre for Disease Control, Vancouver, Canada*

Key Message

- A thorough understanding of the biological mechanisms responsible for SARS-CoV-2 transmission and disease is essential in order for public health professionals and clinicians to adequately implement intervention and control measures.
- Entry of SARS-CoV-2 occurs predominantly through the host ACE2 receptor, which binds the S1 subunit of the SARS-CoV-2 spike protein domain contained within the viral envelope.
- Transmission of SARS-CoV-2 occurs primarily through direct or indirect contact with infected respiratory droplets and aerosols. Other possible modes of transmission include fecal–oral transmission, and

transplacental transmission, although more evidence is needed to confirm these findings.

- Common COVID-19 symptoms include fever, shortness of breath, myalgia, and sore throat. More severe symptoms requiring potential ICU admission and direct intervention include respiratory failure and pneumonia.
- Several factors, such as the presence of multiple comorbidities and age, have been shown to be correlated with increased COVID-19 severity and worsened prognosis. Additionally, evidence demonstrates that males exhibit higher rates of hospitalisation and mortality relative to females, suggesting biological sex may play a role in COVID-19 prognosis.
- While SARS-CoV-2 exhibits lower rates of mutation compared to seasonal influenza, the rise of variants (D614G, B.1.1.7, etc.) present significant concerns related to future control efforts as increases in transmissibility impacts the basic reproductive number (R_0).

1. Introduction

The ongoing COVID-19 pandemic has dramatically altered the daily lives of millions of people worldwide. While many features of SARS-CoV-2 remain unknown, an understanding of the biological mechanisms responsible for SARS-CoV-2 transmission and disease is fundamental to advance the field of public health during this unprecedented respiratory pandemic. Furthermore, while ongoing intervention measures such as the use of masks, social distancing, and vaccination have helped mitigate the effects of COVID-19, the enhancement of knowledge with respect to the biology of SARS-CoV-2 is essential for planning and implementation of future control measures. Thus, this chapter will address the following aspects of SARS-CoV-2:

- Virology and morphology of the virus.
- Clinical features, physiological implications, and prognosis.
- Modes of transmission.
- The rise of variants and related public health concerns.

2. Virology

2.1 *Basic structure and morphology*

The SARS-CoV-2 virus is a positive-sense, single-stranded RNA virus with Spike (S), Envelope (E), and Membrane (M) glycoproteins contained within its viral envelope.[1-3] Based on its genetic structure, it can be classified as a beta-coronavirus (betaCoVs).[1] Similar to other betaCoVs, SARS-CoV-2 is associated with epidemic outbreaks that give rise to respiratory and non-respiratory related symptoms which may vary greatly in terms of clinical severity,[1] and also have the ability to cross the animal-human transmission barrier to establish itself as a human pathogen.[3] In terms of morphology, the virus is spherical with a diameter of 60–140 nm and a genomic size of 29.9 kilobases (kb).[1,3,4] Furthermore, genomic analysis has demonstrated that the SARS-CoV-2 virus is similar to other coronaviruses such as SARS-CoV-1 (79.9%), bat coronavirus (RaTG13) (92.4%–96.2%), and MERS-CoV (50%).[1-4] A summary comparing different subtypes and genera of common coronaviruses can be found in Table 1.

SARS-CoV-2, like other human coronaviruses (hCoVs), contains a genetic structure featuring a 5'-methylated cap and 3'-polyadenylated tail.[3] Structural proteins, including the spike protein, envelope protein, membrane protein, and nucleocapsid protein are encoded by the 3'-terminal region,[3] while non-structural proteins essential for viral replication are encoded by the 5'-terminal region.[3] Given the high mutation rate typical for RNA viruses and the evolution of various strains of SARS-CoV-2 since the beginning of the pandemic,[5,6] public health considerations regarding the implications of new variants on aspects such as vaccine efficacy and transmission dynamics should remain a top priority. This topic will be discussed in more detail later in the chapter.

Similar to other coronaviruses, SARS-CoV-2 may be inactivated by ultraviolet (UV) radiation and heating,[1] at 56°C and 70°C for 30 minutes and 5 minutes of UV exposure, respectively.[4] The survivability of SARS-CoV-2 is highly variable depending on surface type and texture; for example, the stability of the virus on smooth surfaces, such as plastic and stainless steel, is much longer than its stability on less robust surfaces

Table 1:   Comparison of SARS-CoV-2 with other coronaviruses.

	Genera[3]	Illness[3]	Genomic similarity[3]
SARS-CoV-2	• Beta-coronavirus	• Highly pathogenic and lethal • Infects lower respiratory tract • May cause: Acute Lung Injury (ALI), Acute Respiratory Distress syndrome (ARDS), septic shock, and multi-organ failure	N/A (reference strain)
SARS-CoV-1	• Beta-coronavirus	• Highly pathogenic and lethal • Infects lower respiratory tract • May cause: Acute Lung Injury (ALI), Acute Respiratory Distress Syndrome (ARDS), septic shock, and multi-organ failure	• Shares 80% genomic similarity with SARS-CoV-2
MERS-CoV	• Beta-coronavirus	• Infects lower respiratory tract • May cause: Acute Lung Injury (ALI), Acute Respiratory Distress Syndrome (ARDS), septic shock, and multi-organ failure	• Shares 50% genomic similarity with SARS-CoV-2
SARS-CoV hCoV-HKU1	• Beta-coronavirus	• Mainly asymptomatic, mild respiratory, or gastrointestinal infections	N/A
hCoV-OC43	• Beta-coronavirus	• Mainly asymptomatic, mild respiratory, or gastrointestinal infections	N/A
hCoV-NL63	• Alpha-coronavirus	• Mainly asymptomatic, mild respiratory, or gastrointestinal infections	N/A
hCoV-229E	• Alpha-coronavirus	• Mainly asymptomatic, mild respiratory, or gastrointestinal infections	N/A

such as paper (2–4 days and 3 hours, respectively).[4] Moreover, with respect to sanitation and hygiene, SARS-CoV-2, as with several other viruses, can be inactivated by disinfectants such as ethanol and chlorine.[1] However, despite this rather sensitive susceptibility profile, SARS-CoV-2 can remain stable with minimal impact to its infectivity for up to 24 hours at room temperature,[4] a feature which may raise concerns related to adequate sanitation and its impact on community transmission.

2.2 *Mechanism of entry*

SARS-CoV-2 utilises angiotensin-converting enzyme-2 (ACE2) as the host target cell receptor for viral entry in human hosts.[2,4] The S1 subunit of the spike protein contained within the viral envelope acts as the receptor binding domain (RBD) for the ACE2 receptor.[2] Following receptor attachment, the S2 subunit facilitates fusion of the virus and host membranes, resulting in the viral RNA being injected into the host cell cytoplasm.[3] Furthermore, spike protein priming via proteases such as cathepsin B/L and TMPRSS2 serve as an essential component to facilitate viral entry of SARS-CoV-2 into host cells,[3,4] with cathepsin B/L being the therapeutic focus of many pharmacological-based interventions to potentially prevent viral entry.[4] In addition to the ACE2-mediated mechanism of entry, a strong body of evidence has suggested that an alternative route through CD147-SP may serve as a pathway to host cell invasion.[3,7]

Compared to other coronaviruses and seasonal influenza (Table 2), SARS-CoV-2 has a higher basic reproductive number (R_0),[8–10] and therefore has more potential for higher rates of transmission and consequently increases the risk of outbreaks.[4,8] This increased risk of transmission

Table 2: Comparison of estimated R_0 values of beta-coronaviruses and seasonal influenza.

	Basic reproductive number (R_0)
SARS-CoV-2	~2.5 (range 1.8–3.6)[10]
SARS-CoV-1	~2.0–3.0[10]
MERS-CoV	~0.9[10]
Seasonal influenza	~1.28 (IQR:1.19–1.37)[8,9]

poses challenges regarding the herd immunity threshold, which would require an estimated 60% of the population to become immune to halt the ongoing epidemic.[8] Furthermore, various structural components of SARS-CoV-2 may account for this difference in transmissibility; for example, SARS-CoV-2 appears to have increased binding affinity for ACE2,[3] particularly in the upper respiratory tract and conjunctival membranes, increasing the efficiency of infection in these areas.[4] This is a topic that will be discussed in more detail later in the chapter.

3. Clinical Features of Disease, Physiological Implications, and Prognosis

3.1 *Common symptoms and complications*

SARS-CoV-2 infections produce a spectrum of symptoms including fever, chills, cough, shortness of breath, fatigue, muscle/body aches, sore throat, and diarrhea.[3,11] More severe complications include viral pneumonia, respiratory failure, hypoxia, lung damage, sepsis, and potential cardiac injury.[1,2,12] Furthermore, in terms of chest radiology, ultrasound features of COVID-19 patients typically include bilaterally thickened and abnormal pleural lines,[3,13] but low rates of pleural effusion (PE).[3,13–15] Interestingly, however, the presence of PE in COVID-19 patients has recently been hypothesised to be a predictor of disease progression to critical stages,[15] although more evidence is needed to confirm these findings.

Concerns related specifically to SARS-CoV-2 induced pneumonia have become prominent since the beginning of the pandemic. Thus, while several aspects of the pneumonia-inducing cascade remain unknown, studies suggest that an over-amplified host immune response is one of the primary reasons that could account for the severity of illness associated with respiratory complications and subsequent lung damage.[1] This will be elucidated further in the next section of this chapter detailing the role of the host immune response with regard to SARS-CoV-2 induced illness.

3.2 *Physiological implications*

The clinical manifestations of COVID-19 can vary greatly, with symptoms ranging from mild/moderate to severe/critical.[11,12] Furthermore, the severity of symptoms influences subsequent treatment and management of those with COVID-19; for example, patients experiencing severe respiratory failure and pneumonia often require mechanical ventilation and supplemental oxygen, along with admission to the ICU,[1,12] while milder cases may only require isolation and close monitoring. Non-respiratory related complications may also lead to severe health outcomes requiring more direct intervention; for example, COVID-19 induced kidney damage and acute kidney injury may necessitate ICU admission and renal replacement therapy.[1] Hospitalised cases have also shown clinical improvement in response to treatment with the antiviral Remdesivir,[16–18] which will be discussed in a later chapter.

3.3 *Prognosis*

On average, the clinical incubation period for SARS-CoV-2 is 1–14 days.[12,19] Furthermore, while the overall prognosis for the general population remains in good standing, complications related to COVID-19 have proven to be more devastating with increasing age, [19–22] with people over the age of 70 demonstrating the highest rates of critical illness.[10] Thus, while the infection rate of all age demographics is relatively uniform,[23] both hospitalisation and mortality rates increase substantially with age.[23] [25] In addition to age, however, other factors, such as cardiovascular disease, the presence of myocardial injury, obesity, diabetes, chronic heart disease, chronic obstructive pulmonary disease (COPD), hypertension, frailty, and pre-existing respiratory disease seem to negatively impact prognosis and are correlated with ICU admission and mortality.[1,2,19,20,22,24–26]

Interestingly, studies have shown that biological sex may be a prognostic factor correlated with severity of illness and mortality. Thus, there appears to be a significant association with males being at risk for higher rates of hospitalisation, severe illness, and mortality.[20,21,24–27] One possible explanation for these findings is the tendency for males to have more comorbidities than their female counterparts.[28] Additionally, evidence suggests that the immune system response between males and females differs with respect to T-lymphocyte count and responsiveness,[21,26,28] as well as males having an increased neutrophil-to-lymphocyte ratio (NLR).[21,28] This will be addressed further in sections discussing the host immune response.

The impact of ACE2 with regard to prognosis has also been widely discussed. In particular, studies have highlighted the protective role of ACE2 with respect to lung inflammation and injury.[29–32] Thus, a diminished presence of ACE2 following infection may exacerbate the harmful inflammatory effects of SARS-CoV-2, as ACE2-mediated protection via the MAS receptor axis may become down-regulated, leading to subsequent lung injury.[29–32] Potential sex differences in ACE2 expression would also support the aforementioned findings related to increased mortality and severity of illness among males.[27] Furthermore, it should also be noted that while SARS-CoV-2 infection occurs predominantly in tissues exhibiting high ACE2 expression,[33] Zoufaly *et al.* found that the presence of human recombinant soluble ACE2 (hrsACE2) could potentially benefit patients with COVID-19 by neutralising SARS-CoV-2, reducing injury to vital organs (i.e. the kidneys, heart, and lungs), and significantly reduce the viral load of SARS-CoV-2.[34] As such, it appears that while transmembrane ACE2 presence is positively correlated with the probability of infection, the effects of soluble ACE2 treatment may protect those infected with SARS-CoV-2 and may influence prognosis.

4. Modes of Transmission

4.1 *Target host receptors*

As with other infectious diseases, the mode of transmission for SARS-CoV-2 is largely dependent on the location and density of target host receptors. As mentioned previously, the spike binding domain of SARS-CoV-2 binds to host ACE2 receptors, which is the first step in the pathogenic cascade.[1] ACE2 receptors are found predominantly within the respiratory tract.[2] However, ACE2 receptors have also been isolated within the conjunctival membrane and gastrointestinal tract, raising concerns related to the possibility of infections in these areas as well.[2]

4.2 *Transmission routes*

SARS-CoV-2 transmission occurs primarily via direct or indirect contact with infected respiratory droplets and aerosols,[2,3,35] which are most often produced by coughing and sneezing.[1] Studies have shown that most transmission occurs during face-to-face contact (up to 2 meters apart) between an infectious and susceptible individual.[1-3] Other activities, such as sleeping in the same room as an infected individual, sharing food, and remaining in enclosed settings increases the risk of transmission significantly.[1,2] Furthermore, while close-range transmission appears to be the most common scenario for infection, some studies suggest that transmission in indoor environments with poor or underdeveloped ventilation is driven by aerosol transmission.[1,2] This has implications for control measures in closed environments.

With regard to other potential routes of transmission, it is important to note that isolation of SARS-CoV-2 RNA from stool samples has been reported.[2] However, while there have been no reported cases linked to fecal–oral transmission of COVID-19 to date,[2] these findings should re-emphasise the importance of adequate sanitation and hygiene measures at the individual, institutional, and community levels. Moreover, an emerging (albeit scarce) body of evidence has demonstrated the potential for transplacental transmission of SARS-CoV-2, raising concerns related to maternal-fetal transmission,[3,35] although the likelihood of this is quite rare.[3]

5. The Rise of Variants and Related Public Health Concerns

5.1 *Expected rates of mutation*

As mentioned previously, SARS-CoV-2 is an RNA virus and is therefore expected to exhibit high rates of mutation,[5] presenting significant concerns for viral evolution and public health safety.[36] Interestingly, early research has shown that when compared to seasonal influenza, SARS-CoV-2 demonstrates lower rates of mutation due to its intrinsic proofreading mechanism.[37] These findings are supported by recent evidence suggesting the slow accumulation of mutations of the SARS-CoV-2 proteome.[38] However, as transmission persists for longer periods of time, the potential for viral evolution and adaptation to succeed in host environments is an aspect of COVID-19 that must not be ignored.[39]

Thus, while more research is needed in order to understand the mutational dynamics of SARS-CoV-2, investigation of phenotypical differences of current variants is necessary to inform future public health measures and vaccine planning.

5.2 *Variants of interest*

Since the beginning of the COVID-19 pandemic, various mutations of interest have been recorded and analyzed across the globe. Fortunately, most of the variants observed have been shown not to alter pathogenesis.[40] Despite these findings, specific variants of SARS-CoV-2 have raised significant public health concerns with respect to transmissibility, infectivity, and illness severity.

The D614G variant, which encompasses an Aspartate-614 to Glycine mutation in the spike protein domain,[41] appears to enhance the viral infectivity of SARS-CoV-2.[40] For example, studies suggest that the D614G variant demonstrates higher rates of transmissibility,[41] as well as increased infectiousness relative to the wildtype strain.[40] However, recent data suggests that while more transmissible, the mortality and severity of illness of the D614G variant does not significantly deviate from the wildtype strain.[42,43] These findings offer a somewhat optimistic perspective with regard to the virulence of one of the most common strains of SARS-CoV-2.

Other prominent strains include the UK variant (B.1.1.7) and the South African variant (B.1.351).[44,45] The B.1.1.7 variant exhibits both increased transmissibility and mortality,[44] while the B.1.351 variant seems to demonstrate increased transmissibility alone.[45] This information highlights the increased need for research into the transmission dynamics of known variants of interest, as well as the potential implications regarding public health intervention.

5.3 *Vaccine effectiveness*

Despite the concerns related to newly established variants, some studies have shown promise regarding the sustained benefit of vaccines. For example, Weissman *et al.* demonstrated that the D614G variant was susceptible to monoclonal antibody-mediated neutralisation in individuals infected with either the D614 or G614 variant.[46] Furthermore, Emary *et al.* showed that the ChAdOx1 nCoV-19 vaccine was effective for the neutralisation of the B.1.1.7 variant, although it was less efficacious when compared to the non-B.1.1.7 variant (70.4% versus 81.5%, respectively).[47] However, while these findings offer some optimism, it should also be noted that the ChAdOx1 nCoV-19 was not found to provide adequate protection against the B.1.351 variant,[48] demonstrating potential obstacles as new variant strains evolve over the course of transmission.

5.4 *Public health concerns and implications for R_0*

The aforementioned variants undoubtedly pose concerns related to the heightened risk for transmission events within the general population. More specifically, the increased transmissibility of the B.1.1.7, D614G, and B.1.351 variants will significantly impact the R_0 of SARS-CoV-2 in the absence of appropriate and effective public health measures. The control of both current and future SARS-CoV-2 variants is therefore contingent on our biological understanding of vaccine efficacy and drug responsiveness, as well as our efforts pertaining to the monitoring and surveillance of both active cases and potential contacts. With an already remarkable R_0 value of ~2.5,[10] it is essential for public health professionals to understand the safety risks associated with the rise of variants with increased transmissibility. Thus, current control measures should continue to adapt in order to adequately address public health guidelines and ultimately curb transmission to bring the R_0 below 1.0 and end epidemic transmission.

6. Conclusion

While the information highlighted provides a comprehensive description of the biological properties and implications of the SARS-CoV-2 virus and its related variants, further research involving the study of host–virus interactions should be conducted to facilitate a higher-level understanding of how the virus, once internalised, contributes to the disruption of normal physiological mechanisms and how it elicits severe illness. Once eluci-dated, these findings will ultimately help policy makers, public health professionals, and clinicians adequately control the spread of COVID-19 and future respiratory outbreaks related to the *Coronaviridae* family through appropriate intervention strategies.

References

1. Cascella M, Rajnik M, Cuomo A, Dulebohn SC, Di Napoli R. Features, evaluation, and treatment of coronavirus (COVID-19). In: *StatPearls* [Internet]. Treasure Island (FL): StatPearls Publishing; 2021 [cited 2021 Apr 6]. Available from: http://www.ncbi.nlm.nih.gov/books/NBK554776/.

2. Cevik M, Kuppalli K, Kindrachuk J, Peiris M. Virology, transmission, and pathogenesis of SARS-CoV-2. *BMJ*. 2020;371:m3862.

3. Zhu Z, Lian X, Su X, Wu W, Marraro GA, Zeng Y. From SARS and MERS to COVID-19: A brief summary and comparison of severe acute respiratory infections caused by three highly pathogenic human coronaviruses. *Respiratory Research*. 2020;21(1):224.

4. Neerukonda SN, Katneni U. A review on SARS-CoV-2 virology, pathophysi-ology, animal models, and anti-viral interventions. *Pathogens* [Internet]. 2020 May 29 [cited 2021 Apr 6];9(6). Available from: https://www.ncbi.nlm.nih.gov/pmc/articles/PMC7350325/.

5. Pachetti M, Marini B, Benedetti F, Giudici F, Mauro E, Storici P, *et al.* Emerging SARS-CoV-2 mutation hot spots include a novel RNA-dependent-RNA polymerase variant. *Journal of Translational Medicine*. 2020;18(1):179.

6. Garvin MR, T. Prates E, Pavicic M, Jones P, Amos BK, Geiger A, *et al.* Potentially adaptive SARS-CoV-2 mutations discovered with novel spatio-temporal and explainable AI models. *Genome Biology*. 2020;21(1):304.

7. Ulrich H, Pillat MM. CD147 as a target for COVID-19 treatment: Suggested effects of azithromycin and stem cell engagement. *Stem Cell Reviews and Reports*. 2020;1–7.

8. Cevik M, Bamford CGG, Ho A. COVID-19 pandemic — a focused review for clinicians. *Clinical Microbiology and Infection*. 2020;26(7):842–847.

9. Biggerstaff M, Cauchemez S, Reed C, Gambhir M, Finelli L. Estimates of the reproduction number for seasonal, pandemic, and zoonotic influenza: A systematic review of the literature. *BMC Infectious Diseases*. 2014; 14(1):480.

10. Petersen E, Koopmans M, Go U, Hamer DH, Petrosillo N, Castelli F, *et al.* Comparing SARS-CoV-2 with SARS-CoV and influenza pandemics. *The Lancet Infectious Diseases.* 2020;20(9):e238–244.

11. CDC. Coronavirus disease 2019 (COVID-19) — symptoms [Internet]. *Centers for Disease Control and Prevention,* 2021 [cited 2021 Mar 11]. Available from: https://www.cdc.gov/coronavirus/2019-ncov/symptoms-testing/symptoms.html.

12. CDC. Healthcare workers [Internet]. Centers for Disease Control and Prevention, 2020 [cited 2021 Apr 6]. Available from: https://www.cdc.gov/coronavirus/2019-ncov/hcp/clinical-guidance-management-patients.html.

13. Tan G, Lian X, Zhu Z, Wang Z, Huang F, Zhang Y *et al.* Use of lung ultrasound to differentiate coronavirus disease 2019 (COVID-19) pneumonia from community-acquired pneumonia. *Ultrasound in Medicine and Biology.* 2020;46(10):2651–2658.

14. Malik J, Javed N, Naeem H, Sattar RA, Ikram U. Covid-19 associated pneumonia and pleural effusion masquerading as heart failure in rheumatic heart disease. *European Journal of Case Reports in Internal Medicine* [Internet]. 2020 Jul 10 [cited 2021 Apr 6];7(8). Available from: https://www.ncbi.nlm.nih.gov/pmc/articles/PMC7417058/.

15. Zhan N, Guo Y, Tian S, Huang B, Tian X, Zou J *et al.* Clinical characteristics of COVID-19 complicated with pleural effusion. *BMC Infectious Diseases.* 2021;21(1):176.

16. CDC. Healthcare workers [Internet]. Centers for Disease Control and Prevention, 2020 [cited 2021 Apr 6]. Available from: https://www.cdc.gov/coronavirus/2019-ncov/hcp/therapeutic-options.html.

17. Grein J, Ohmagari N, Shin D, Diaz G, Asperges E, Castagna A *et al.* Compassionate use of remdesivir for patients with severe covid-19. *New England Journal of Medicine.* 2020;382(24):2327–2336.

18. Beigel JH, Tomashek KM, Dodd LE, Mehta AK, Zingman BS, Kalil AC *et al.* Remdesivir for the treatment of covid-19 — final report. *New England Journal of Medicine.* 2020;383(19):1813–1826.

19. Li X, Li T, Wang H. Treatment and prognosis of COVID-19: Current scenario and prospects (Review). *Exp Ther Med* [Internet]. 2021 Jan [cited 2021 Apr 6];21(1). Available from: https://www.ncbi.nlm.nih.gov/pmc/articles/PMC7678645/.

20. Ciceri F, Castagna A, Rovere-Querini P, De Cobelli F, Ruggeri A, Galli L *et al.* Early predictors of clinical outcomes of COVID-19 outbreak in Milan, Italy. *Clinical Immunology.* 2020;217:108509.

21. Sun Z-H. Clinical outcomes of COVID-19 in elderly male patients. *Journal of Geriatric Cardiology*. 2020;17(5):243–245.

22. Aoun M, Khalil R, Mahfoud W, Fatfat H, Bou Khalil L, Alameddine R *et al*. Age and multimorbidities as poor prognostic factors for COVID-19 in hemo-dialysis: a Lebanese national study. *BMC Nephrology*. 2021;22(1):73.

23. CDC. Cases, data, and surveillance [Internet]. Centers for Disease Control and Prevention, 2020 [cited 2021 Apr 6]. Available from: https://www.cdc.gov/coronavirus/2019-ncov/covid-data/investigations-discovery/hospitalization-death-by-age.html.

24. Hägg S, Jylhävä J, Wang Y, Xu H, Metzner C, Annetorp M *et al*. Age, frailty, and comorbidity as prognostic factors for short-term outcomes in patients with coronavirus disease 2019 in geriatric care. *Journal of the American Medical Directors Association*. 2020;21(11):1555–1559.e2.

25. Cunningham JW, Vaduganathan M, Claggett BL, Jering KS, Bhatt AS, Rosenthal N *et al*. Clinical outcomes in young us adults hospitalized with Covid-19. *JAMA Internal Medicine*. 2021;181(3):379.

26. Ludwig M, Jacob J, Basedow F, Andersohn F, Walker J. Clinical outcomes and characteristics of patients hospitalized for Influenza or COVID-19 in Germany. *International Journal of Infectious Diseases*. 2021;103:316–322.

27. Majdic G. Could sex/gender differences in ace2 expression in the lungs con-tribute to the large gender disparity in the morbidity and mortality of patients infected with the SARS-CoV-2 virus? *Frontiers in Cellular and Infection Microbiology* [Internet]. 2020 Jun 9 [cited 2021 Apr 6];10. Available from: https://www.ncbi.nlm.nih.gov/pmc/articles/PMC7295901/.

28. Meng Y, Wu P, Lu W, Liu K, Ma K, Huang L *et al*. Sex-specific clinical characteristics and prognosis of coronavirus disease-19 infection in Wuhan, China: A retrospective study of 168 severe patients. *PLoS Pathogens* [Internet]. 2020 Apr 28 [cited 2021 Apr 6];16(4). Available from: https://www.ncbi.nlm.nih.gov/pmc/articles/PMC7209966/.

29. Verdecchia P, Cavallini C, Spanevello A, Angeli F. The pivotal link between ACE2 deficiency and SARS-CoV-2 infection. *European Journal of Internal Medicine*. 2020;76:14–20.

30. Chaudhry F, Lavandero S, Xie X, Sabharwal B, Zheng Y-Y, Correa A *et al*. Manipulation of ACE2 expression in COVID-19. *Open Heart*. 2020; 7(2):e001424.

31. Samavati L, Uhal BD. Ace2, much more than just a receptor for SARS-CoV-2. Front *Cell Infect Microbiol* [Internet]. 2020 [cited 2021 Apr 6];10. Available from: https://www.frontiersin.org/articles/10.3389/fcimb.2020.00317/full.

32. Viveiros A, Rasmuson J, Vu J, Mulvagh SL, Yip CYY, Norris CM *et al.* Sex differences in COVID-19: Candidate pathways, genetics of ACE2, and sex hormones. *American Journal of Physiology-Heart and Circulatory Physiology.* 2020;320(1):H296–304.
33. Ni W, Yang X, Yang D, Bao J, Li R, Xiao Y *et al.* Role of angiotensin-converting enzyme 2 (Ace2) in COVID-19. *Critical Care.* 2020;24(1):422.
34. Zoufaly A, Poglitsch M, Aberle JH, Hoepler W, Seitz T, Traugott M *et al.* Human recombinant soluble ACE2 in severe COVID-19. *The Lancet Respiratory Medicine.* 2020;8(11):1154–1158.
35. Vivanti AJ, Vauloup-Fellous C, Prevot S, Zupan V, Suffee C, Do Cao J *et al.* Transplacental transmission of SARS-CoV-2 infection. *Nature Communications.* 2020;11(1):3572.
36. Wu S, Tian C, Liu P, Guo D, Zheng W, Huang X *et al.* Effects of SARS-CoV-2 mutations on protein structures and intraviral protein–protein interactions. *Journal of Medical Virology.* 2021;93(4):2132–2140.
37. Manzanares-Meza LD, Medina-Contreras O. SARS-CoV-2 and Influenza: A comparative overview and treatment implications. *BMHIM.* 2020;77(5):4621.
38. Vilar S, Isom DG. One year of SARS-CoV-2: How much has the virus changed? *Biology.* 2021;10(2):91.
39. Luo R, Delaunay-Moisan A, Timmis K, Danchin A. SARS-CoV-2 biology and variants: Anticipation of viral evolution and what needs to be done. *Environmental Microbiology.* 2021;1462–2920.15487.
40. Chen J, Wang R, Wang M, Wei G-W. Mutations strengthened SARS-CoV-2 infectivity. *Journal of Molecular Biology.* 2020;432(19):5212–5226.
41. Hou YJ, Chiba S, Halfmann P, Ehre C, Kuroda M, Dinnon KH, *et al.* SARS-CoV-2 D614G variant exhibits efficient replication ex vivo and transmission in vivo. *Science.* 2020;370(6523):1464–1468.
42. Volz E, Hill V, McCrone JT, Price A, Jorgensen D, O'Toole Á *et al.* Evaluating the effects of SARS-CoV-2 spike mutation D614g on transmissibility and pathogenicity. *Cell.* 2021;184(1):64–75.e11.
43. Groves DC, Rowland-Jones SL, Angyal A. The D614G mutations in the SARS-CoV-2 spike protein: Implications for viral infectivity, disease severity and vaccine design. *Biochemical and Biophysical Research Communications.* 2021;538:104–107.
44. Challen R, Brooks-Pollock E, Read JM, Dyson L, Tsaneva-Atanasova K, Danon L. Risk of mortality in patients infected with SARS-CoV-2 variant of concern 202012/1: Matched cohort study. *BMJ.* 2021;372:n579.

45. Tang JW, Toovey OTR, Harvey KN, Hui DDS. Introduction of the South African SARS-CoV-2 variant 501y.V2 into the UK. *Journal of Infection.* 2021;82(4):e8–10.

46. Weissman D, Alameh M-G, de Silva T, Collini P, Hornsby H, Brown R *et al.* D614g spike mutation increases SARS-CoV-2 susceptibility to neutralization. *Cell Host & Microbe.* 2021;29(1):23–31.e4.

47. Emary KRW, Golubchik T, Aley PK, Ariani CV, Angus B, Bibi S *et al.* Efficacy of ChAdOx1 nCoV-19 (Azd1222) vaccine against SARS-CoV-2 variant of concern 202012/01 (B.1.1.7): An exploratory analysis of a randomised controlled trial. *The Lancet* [Internet]. 2021 Mar 30 [cited 2021 Apr 6];0(0). Available from: https://www.thelancet.com/journals/lancet/article/PIIS0140-6736(21)00628-0/abstract.

48. Madhi SA, Baillie V, Cutland CL, Voysey M, Koen AL, Fairlie L *et al.* Efficacy of the ChAdOx1 nCoV-19 Covid-19 Vaccine against the B.1.351 Variant. *New England Journal of Medicine.* 2021;0(0):null.

Chapter 3

Virus Meets Host: SARS-CoV-2 Pathogenesis

Cameron Geddes[*] and James A. Russell [†,‡]

*Faculty of Medicine, University of British Columbia,
Vancouver, Canada*

†*Centre for Heart Lung Innovation, St. Paul's Hospital,
Vancouver, Canada*

‡ *Adults Critical Care Medicine, Vancouver General Hospital,
Vancouver, Canada*

Key Message

- The SARS-CoV-2 virus has adapted to proficiently infect and cause disease in its hosts, leading to the events of the COVID-19 pandemic. SARS-CoV-2 infection impacts multiple organ systems which approaches to control and treatment must consider to appropriately manage COVID-19 cases.
- The use of the ACE2 receptor as part of the virus' cell entry strategy has negative consequences for the host renin angiotensin system. The dysregulation of this system may explain some aspects of disease in COVID-19 and may be a therapeutic target.
- The host's immune system plays an important role in reducing harm caused by the infection and facilitating viral clearance. However, the

innate inflammatory host response can increase the severity of disease in some COVID-19 cases and should be therapeutically controlled.

- SARS-CoV-2 is able to decrease the effectiveness of the host's innate and adaptive immune responses using specific methods. Some therapies have been proposed to mitigate these strategies and aid the immune system.
- Different variations of host, agent, and environmental factors have been shown to affect the infectivity and virulence of COVID-19.

1. Introduction

Pathogenesis of infection describes the complex interplay between the infectious agent and host response, particularly the immune system of which we focus on herein.[1] In this chapter, we discuss the mechanisms used by SARS-CoV-2 to infect its hosts, strategies used by the host immune system to defend itself from the virus, and how the conflicting efforts of these two parties leads to disease, progression, and death or recovery. We will also discuss how differing variations of the virus, host, and environment affect infection progression and disease both positively and negatively. The SARS-CoV-2 virus binds to and down-regulates the ubiquitous receptor angiotensin converting enzyme 2 (ACE 2) which has profound effects on the renin angiotensin system (RAS) of the host; accordingly, we discuss aspects of this interaction and related therapeutic strategies.

2. Viral Entry into Cells and the Renin Angiotensin System

2.1 *Viral entry via ACE2 receptor*

A key component of the viral life cycle is the method used by the virus to gain entry into host cells to propagate. Various strategies are utilised by viruses to accomplish this; in the case of SARS-CoV-2, the virus uses endocytosis which is the same mechanism by which the host cell takes in ordinary resources. SARS-CoV-2 primarily attaches to ACE2 on the cell membrane.[2] This receptor is prolifically prevalent in the epithelia of the lung and intestine.[3] but is also found in conjunctival membrane,[4] blood vessels, and many other organs at lower levels.[3] The binding between the virus and the host's ACE2 receptor is mediated by the virus' spike glyco-protein.[5] Once these two elements bind, the virus is able to fuse its membrane to the membrane of the host cell to enter the host cell.

In addition to its membrane-bound form, ACE2 also exists in a soluble form (sACE2) by releasing from the membrane into the circulation as plasma ACE2.[6] Plasma ACE2 has a dual role in SARS-CoV-2 infection. Under normal physiological concentrations of plasma ACE2, the soluble receptor appears to continue to mediate SARS-CoV-2 entry into the cell via receptor-mediated endocytosis.[6] On the other hand, infused soluble (human recombinant) ACE2 has been shown to be a potential therapy for COVID-19.[7,8]

2.2 *Effects on the renin angiotensin system*

ACE2 is a central player of the RAS, which plays a key role in regulating blood pressure.[9] ACE2 is a counter-regulatory component of RAS. Angiotensin II is a potent vasoconstrictor which raises blood pressure and is converted to angiotensin I-7 (a vasodilator) by ACE2.

However, in COVID-19 patients, SARS-CoV-2 down regulates ACE2, leading to elevated angiotensin II levels which causes vasoconstriction, increased permeability, and hyperinflammation potentially leading to organ damage.[10] In particular, angiotensin II has been shown to accumulate in lung tissue when ACE2 is inhibited in influenza models, which is a potential explanation for the prevalence of lung injury in COVID-19.[11] The critical illness complications of COVID-19 — septic shock, acute respiratory distress syndrome, and acute kidney injury — may be caused in part by dysregulation of the host RAS response.[12–14]

Figure 1 shows membrane-bound tissue and circulating peptides of the RAS compose an intersecting network of regulatory and counterregulatory peptides. ACE2 is a key counterregulatory enzyme that degrades angiotensin II to angiotensin I, thereby attenuating its effects on vasoconstriction, sodium retention, and fibrosis. ACE2 is down-regulated by SARS-CoV-2 in COVID-19.

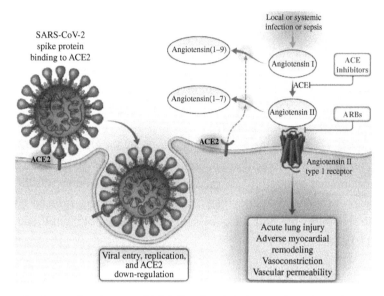

Figure 1: Interactions between SARS-CoV-2 and the host renin angiotensin system.[15]

The underlying mechanisms leading to organ injury after SARS-CoV-2 infection include increased angiotensin II[16] that can cause microvascular damage, increased vascular permeability, secondary production of inflammatory cytokines, accelerated apoptosis, and fibrosis. Local activation of the renin–angiotensin–aldosterone system may mediate lung and cardiac injury responses to SARS-CoV-2 by increasing lung and coronary microvascular thrombosis and coagulation (increased D-dimers), which is associated with increased COVID-19 mortality.[17,18] Angiotensin II binds the angiotensin II receptor 1 (AGTR1) which increases expression of tissue factor and plasminogen activator inhibitor-1.[19]

For these reasons, angiotensin receptor blockers and ACE inhibitors have been proposed as potential therapeutic interventions, although the evidence of efficacy is mixed at present.[12–14] Only one study has adjusted for underlying co-morbidities that addresses indication bias, and that study showed an association of ARBs and ACE inhibitors with decreased mortality of COVID-19.[20] Many groups are investigating the association of use of angiotensin receptor blockers and ACE inhibitors in cohort studies and in randomised controlled trials.

3. Immune System Responses and Viral Evasion

The immune system consists of a variety of constituents that protect the host from infectious agents. Comprised of two main components, namely innate and adaptive immunity, that differ importantly in specificity and timing of response (Figure 2).

3.1 *Innate immune system*

The innate immune system is the body's first line of defense against pathogens, and is not specific to any pathogen. This includes a broad scope of organ systems anatomically and functionally; skin, leukocytes such as neutrophils and macrophages, and proteins like complement and interferon. The cells of the innate system recognise common features broadly found among pathogens, and are quickly activated as soon as a pathogen enters the body. A related critical role of these cells is to "alert" the cells of the adaptive system by "presenting" them with a molecular structure, called an antigen, from the pathogen itself.[22] These cells are aptly named antigen presenting cells, and are a crucial link between the innate and adaptive systems.

In the body, SARS-CoV-2 is first recognised by toll-like receptors (TLRs). TLRs recognise molecular structures that are common to pathogens, called pathogen-associated molecular patterns (PAMPs), and use this information to activate the immune system by triggering the release of cytokines, which serve as intercellular messengers that promote the inflammatory response and recruit other immune cells to the

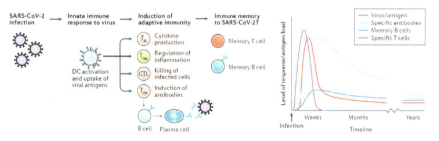

Figure 2:   Overview of cell responses to SARS-CoV-2 and predicted time courses.[21]

site of infection.[23] The complement system, a large number of proteins that "complement" the immune response, also plays a prominent role in SARS-CoV-2 infections.[23] There is also significant evidence that monocytes, macrophages, neutrophils, and interferons contribute to the innate response as well.[23]

3.1.1 *Innate immune response*

During initial stage of infection — the viral response phase — (Figure 3)[24] macrophages and monocytes infiltrate the infected tissue in defense, associated with mild symptoms such as fever, cough, fatigue, sore throat, and headache.[25] At this stage, the innate system is "buying time" for the adaptive immune system to initiate because the adaptive system is required to fully eliminate the virus and prevent disease progression.[26] The majority of COVID-19 patients do not progress beyond this early stage because of successful viral removal and have a very optimistic prognosis and recovery. Treatment at this stage is generally targeted towards managing the symptoms of inflammation rather than directly combating the virus.[24] Anti-viral drug strategies have unfortunately had mixed results at the time of writing.

The more severe stages of infection (Figure 3)[24] involve significant increases in viral load and localised inflammation in the lung; this can be followed by a more diffuse "hyper" immune response that can damage host organs leading to vital organ dysfunction. This often occurs when the

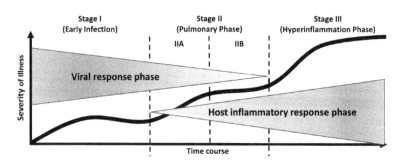

Figure 3: Classification of COVID-19 disease states incorporating virus and host dynamics.[24]

host is unable to mount an effective innate immune response, leading inflammation to increase to critical levels via macrophage and granulocyte activity.[26]

Those who progress to more severe (host inflammatory) stages of COVID-19 usually need to be hospitalised to receive supportive measures such as oxygen anti-viral therapies.[24] Patients at these stages develop respiratory failure, shock, and/or multiorgan failure.[25]

The central role of the immune system in severe disease — i.e. a hyperinflammatory response — has been highlighted by finding that a potent anti-inflammatory agent (dexamethasone, a corticosteroid) significantly decreases the mortality of COVID-19 and has become standard of care for hospitalised patients who require oxygen to decrease risk of ICU admission and death.[27,28]

3.1.2 *Viral evasion of the innate system*

Despite the body's plethora of defenses, SARS-CoV-2 also has some schemes of its own to avoid being eliminated from the host. One method used to preserve itself is to inhibit interferon production, because interferon is one of the body's most potent antiviral machinery, by translating proteins once inside the host cell that down-regulate its production.[29] This allows the virus to replicate and infect neighbouring cells without the standard "neighborhood alert" that interferons normally provide in host tissue. Interferon (inhaled or systemic) is being evaluated as a therapy for COVID-19.

3.2 *Adaptive immune system*

In comparison to the innate response, the adaptive response is much slower, but is highly specific to the pathogen involved due to its prior exposure to and consequent knowledge of the pathogen and its antigens. The longer length of time for this adaptive immune response to occur is attributable to the manufacturing process of lymphocytes that are specific to the pathogen involved. B-lymphocytes secrete antibodies that are complementary and therefore bind to the pathogen's antigens (similar to a lock and key), latching onto and inactivating the pathogen. This is called "humoral immunity", and is the mechanism that vaccines mimic. Alternatively, "cellular immunity" of the adaptive system involves T-lymphocyte cells, which target cells bearing the presented antigen and destroys them directly.

3.2.1 *Adaptive response*

The adaptive response follows and is closely coordinated by the innate immune response. Once they have been presented with viral antigen, B-cells contribute early to SARS-CoV-2 infection; first against the nucleocapsid protein, then the spike protein.[30] B-cells produce different types of antibodies in response to the virus, including IgM, which is quickly produced and provides short-term protection, IgA, which provides protection in mucosa, and IgG, which is the most prevalent antibody found in the blood and prevents re-infection in the long-term. IgM and IgA antibodies have been detected within five days after initial symptom onset in COVID-19, while IgG has been detected after 14 days.[31,32].

T-cell-mediated immunity is also crucial to viral clearance of SARS-CoV-2. Lower T-cell counts are associated with higher mortality in COVID-19 patients.[33] Both major types of T cells (CD^{4+} and CD^{8+}) have been observed in convalescent COVID-19 patients, and these cells were reactive to a variety of viral features of SARS-CoV-2.[21] As mentioned above, a strong T-cell response is perhaps more important than the presence of antibodies; therefore recruiting an effective T-cell response during the clinical course of COVID-19 is an important consideration for vaccine design.[34]

3.2.2 *Viral evasion of the adaptive system*

SARS-CoV-2 is also able to negatively affect the adaptive immune system. Infection has been shown to functionally exhaust T cells as the disease progresses and hyperinflammation occurs,[35] which can be attributed to the increase in cytokine levels during the COVID-19 clinical course which increases inhibitory factors on T cells. To counteract this process, cytokines have been proposed as potential therapeutic targets to increase T cell capacity.[34]

4. Factors Affecting Pathogenesis

4.1 *The host*

4.1.1 *Age*

One of the most crucial factors affecting the development and severity of COVID-19 is the age of the patient. Severity of disease follows an age gradient, with younger individuals unlikely to develop severe symptoms and older individuals having the most risk of severe disease. Several aspects of SARS-CoV-2 infection have been speculated to contribute to this phenomenon. First, older individuals are more likely to have comorbid conditions that in themselves increase the risk of severe disease and also may be associated with the use of ACE inhibitors and AT1R blockers, both of which up-regulate the expression of ACE2, which as mentioned is the primary receptor for SARS-CoV-2 entry into host cells.[36] Nonetheless, mSARS-CoV-2 could also be more harmful to older individuals due to a process called antibody-dependent enhancement (ADE).

In ADE, viruses are better able to infect host cells due to the binding of a non-neutralising antibody (usually from an antigen from a related pathogen) that allows it to be more easily taken up into host cell membranes due to the presence of host cell antigen. Since older individuals on average have been exposed to more coronaviruses (such as the viruses responsible for the "common cold"), it remains a possibility that the older population is more susceptible to ADE and consequently more susceptible to COVID-19.[36] A decreased capacity for T-cells may also play a role in increased virulence in this population.[37]

4.1.2 *Sex*

There is also significant evidence that males have a higher risk of hospitalisation and mortality compared to females.[38] 45% of COVID-19 Canadian cases are male, but males have higher hospital (56%), ICU admission (65%) and mortality rates than females ($p < 0.0001$).[39] This may be explained by intrinsic advantages of the female immune system compared to males'. Females produce more interferon upon sensing viral RNA,[40] have a greater count and level of activity in T-cells,[41,42] and increased antibody production from B-cells.[41] As discussed above, these elements are key to neutralising SARS-CoV-2.

In addition, ACE2 is encoded on the X-chromosome and expressed differently in males compared to females, which could explain increased male risk for severe COVID-19. Plasma ACE2 is increased in men with kidney disease[43] and diabetes,[44] and is lower with increased age in men.[45]

4.1.3 *Species*

As an interesting aside, there is strong molecular evidence that SARS-CoV-2 can affect many animal species. Bats are the main reservoir for many coronaviruses and it has been suggested they may be a potential origin of SARS-CoV-2, with pangolins being an intermediate host. Studies have shown that SARS-CoV-2 is about 96.2% similar to bat-CoV and more so similar to pangolin-CoV.[46] In addition, the receptor-binding domain of the pangolin-CoV has strong binding ability to the human ACE2 receptor. Cats, dogs, and mink have also been shown to be susceptible to the virus and may act as additional reservoirs.

4.2 *The virus — SARS-COV-2 mutants*

As a result of random chance and natural selection, the SARS-CoV-2 virus has mutated in certain populations, thus creating variants with potentially differing levels of pathogenicity and/or infectivity.[47] Many of these variants are defined by mutations in the virus' spike protein near the ACE2 binding interface, however their effect on binding to ACE2 is unknown.[48] SARS-CoV-2 mutants are emerging and spreading globally, severely altering the prevalence and in some cases the severity of COVID-19. It is also uncertain as yet how SARS-COV-2 mutants will ultimately alter vaccine efficacy globally.

4.3 *The environment*

Several environmental conditions affect the SARS-CoV-2 virus in humans, the most-studied of which being temperature. As environmental temperature increases, COVID-19 prevalence decreases.[49] This trend is also observed in other coronaviruses, such as those causing the common cold. In higher temperatures, viral proteins and nucleic acids are more likely to denature,[50] making the virus less capable of host cell entry, replication of its DNA, and defense from the host immune system.

Humidity also seems to affect the virus' pathogenicity. This may be attributable to simple mechanics: increased humidity decreases the speed of a projectile viral droplet from an infected individual, decreasing its reach to potential new hosts.[51] In addition, given that SARS-CoV-2 has a lipid envelope, hydrophobic effects may lead the virus to travel more efficiently in less-humid environments.[52]

References

1. Pathogenesis: Of host and pathogen. *Nature Immunology*. 2006;7(3):217.
2. Zamorano Cuervo N, Grandvaux N. ACE2: Evidence of role as entry receptor for SARS-CoV-2 and implications in comorbidities. *eLife* 2020;9.
3. Hamming [V, Timens W, Bulthuis M, Lely AT, Navis GJ, van Goor H. Tissue distribution of ACE2 protein, the functional receptor for SARS Coronavirus. A first step in understanding SARS pathogenesis. *Journal of Pathology*. 2004;203(2):631–637.
4. Leonardi A, Rosani U, Brun P. Ocular surface expression of SARS-CoV-2 receptors. *Ocular Immunology Inflammation*. 2020;28(5):735–738.
5. Yang J, Petitjean SJL, Koehler M, Zhang Q, Dumitru AC, Chen W *et al.* Molecular interaction and inhibition of SARS-CoV-2 binding to the ACE2 receptor. *Nature Communications*. 2020;11(1):4541.
6. Yeung ML, Teng JLL, Jia L, Zhang C, Huang C, Cai J *et al.* Soluble ACE2-mediated cell entry of SARS-CoV-2 via interaction with proteins related to the renin-angiotensin system. *Cell*. 2021.
7. Zoufaly A, Poglitsch M, Aberle JH, Hoepler W, Seitz T, Traugott M *et al.* Human recombinant soluble ACE2 in severe COVID-19. *The Lancet Respiratory Medicine*. 2020;8(11):1154–1158.
8. Krishnamurthy S, Lockey RF, Kolliputi N. Soluble ACE2 as a potential therapy for COVID-19. *American Journal of Physiology: Cell Physiology* 2021;320(3):C279–C281.
9. DeMello WC, Frohlich ED, SpringerLink ebooks — Medicine. *Renin Angiotensin System and Cardiovascular Disease*. 1. Aufl. ed. New York, NY: Humana Press, 2014.

10. Henry BM, Vikse J, Benoit S, Favaloro EJ, Lippi G. Hyperinflammation and derangement of renin-angiotensin-aldosterone system in COVID-19: A novel hypothesis for clinically suspected hypercoagulopathy and microvascular immunothrombosis. *Clinica Chimica Acta*. 2020;507:167–173.
11. Yang P, Gu H, Zhao Z, Wang W, Cao B, Lai C *et al*. Angiotensin-converting enzyme 2 (ACE2) mediates influenza H7N9 virus-induced acute lung injury. *Scientific Reports*. 2014;4(1):7027.
12. Pirola CJ, Sookoian S. Estimation of Renin-Angiotensin-Aldosterone-System (RAAS)-Inhibitor effect on COVID-19 outcome: A meta-analysis. *Journal of Infection*. 2020;81(2):276–281.
13. Hasan SS, Kow CS, Hadi MA, Zaidi STR, Merchant HA. Mortality and disease severity among COVID-19 patients receiving renin-angiotensin system inhibitors: A systematic review and meta-analysis. *American Journal of Cardiovascular Drugs*. 2020;20(6):571–590.
14. Liu X, Long C, Xiong Q, Chen C, Ma J, Su Y *et al*. Association of angiotensin converting enzyme inhibitors and angiotensin II receptor blockers with risk of COVID-19, inflammation level, severity, and death in patients with COVID-19: A rapid systematic review and meta-analysis. *Clinical Cardiology*. (Mahwah, N.J.) 2020.
15. Vaduganathan M, Vardeny O, Michel T, McMurray JJV, Pfeffer MA, Solomon SD. Renin–angiotensin–aldosterone system inhibitors in patients with Covid-19. *New England Journal of Medicine*. 2020;382(17):1653–1659.
16. Henry BM, Vikse J, Benoit S, Favaloro EJ, Lippi G. Hyperinflammation and derangement of renin–angiotensin–aldosterone system in COVID-19: A novel hypothesis for clinically suspected hypercoagulopathy and microvascular immunothrombosis. *Clinica Chimica Acta*. 2020;507:167–173.
17. Zhou F, Yu T, Du R, Fan G, Liu Y, Liu Z, *et al*. Clinical course and risk factors for mortality of adult inpatients with COVID-19 in Wuhan, China: A retrospective cohort study. *The Lancet* (British edition) 2020;395(10229):1054–1062.
18. Yin S, Huang M, Li D, Tang N. Difference of coagulation features between severe pneumonia induced by SARS-CoV2 and non-SARS-CoV2. *Journal of Thrombosis and Thrombolysis*. 2020.
19. D'Elia JA, Bayliss G, Gleason RE, Weinrauch LA. Cardiovascular-renal complications and the possible role of plasminogen activator inhibitor: A review. *Clinical Kidney Journal*. 2016;9(5):705–712.
20. Lee T, Cau A, Cheng MP, Levin A, Lee TC, Vinh DC, *et al*. Angiotensin receptor blockers and angiotensin converting enzyme inhibitors in Covid-19 — meta-analysis/meta-regression adjusted for confounding factors. *CJC Open*. (Online) 2021.

21. Cox RJ, Brokstad KA. Not just antibodies: B cells and T cells mediate immunity to COVID-19. *Nature Reviews Immunology.* 2020;20(10): 581–582.
22. Calis J, van Woensel J, Lemson J, De Blasi RA, Moreira J, Angus DC *et al.* Severe Sepsis and Septic Shock. *New England Journal of Medicine.* 2013;369(21):2062–2063.
23. Birra D, Benucci M, Landolfi L, Merchionda A, Loi G, Amato P *et al.* COVID 19: A clue from innate immunity. *Immunologic Research.* 2020;68(3): 161–168.
24. Siddiqi HK, Mehra MR. COVID-19 illness in native and immunosuppressed states: A clinical–therapeutic staging proposal. *The Journal of Heart and Lung Transplantation.* 2020;39(5):405–407.
25. Romagnoli S, Peris A, De Gaudio AR, Geppetti P. SARS-CoV-2 and COVID-19: From the Bench to the Bedside. *Physiological Reviews.* 2020;100(4):1455–1466.
26. Shi Y, Wang Y, Shao C, Huang J, Gan J, Huang X *et al.* COVID-19 infection: The perspectives on immune responses. *Cell Death and Differentiation.* 2020;27(5):1451–1454.
27. Horby P, Lim WS, Emberson JR, Mafham M, Bell JL, Linsell L *et al.* Dexamethasone in hospitalized patients with COVID-19. *New England Journal of Medicine.* 2020 2021;384(8):693–704.
28. WHO COVID-19 Clinical care bundle. World Health Organization 2021 April 23.
29. Shah VK, Firmal P, Alam A, Ganguly D, Chattopadhyay S. Overview of immune response during SARS-CoV-2 infection: Lessons from the past. *Frontiers in Immunology.* 2020;11:1949.
30. Tan Y, Goh P, Fielding BC, Shen S, Chou C, Fu J *et al.* Profiles of antibody responses against severe acute respiratory syndrome coronavirus recombinant proteins and their potential use as diagnostic markers. *Clinical and Diagnostic Laboratory Immunology.* 2004;11(2):362–371.
31. Guo L, Ren L, Yang S, Xiao M, Chang D, Yang F *et al.* Profiling early humoral response to diagnose novel coronavirus disease (COVID-19). *Clinical Infectious Diseases.* 2020;71(15):778–785.
32. Viral kinetics and antibody responses in patients with COVID-19. *Obesity, Fitness & Wellness Week.* 2020:695.
33. Luo M, Liu J, Jiang W, Yue S, Liu H, Wei S. IL-6 and CD^{8+} T cell counts combined are an early predictor of in-hospital mortality of patients with COVID-19. *JCI Insight.* 2020;5(13).
34. de Candia P, Prattichizzo F, Garavelli S, Matarese G. T Cells: Warriors of SARS-CoV-2 infection. *Trends in Immunology.* 2021;42(1):18–30.

35. Diao B, Wang C, Tan Y, Chen X, Liu Y, Ning L *et al.* Reduction and functional exhaustion of T cells in patients with coronavirus disease 2019 (COVID-19). *Frontiers in Immunology.* 2020;11:827.
36. Peron JPS, Nakaya H. Susceptibility of the elderly to SARS-CoV-2 infection: ACE-2 overexpression, shedding, and antibody-dependent enhancement (ADE). *Clinics* (São Paulo, Brazil) 2020;75:e1912.
37. Liu K, Chen Y, Lin R, Han K. Clinical features of COVID-19 in elderly patients: A comparison with young and middle-aged patients. *Journal of Infection.* 2020;80(6):e14–e18.
38. Peckham H, de Gruijter NM, Raine C, Radziszewska A, Ciurtin C, Wedderburn LR, *et al.* Male sex identified by global COVID-19 meta-analysis as a risk factor for death and ITU admission. *Nature Communications.* 2020;11(1):6317.
39. COVID-19 daily epidemiology update. Government of Canada 2021 April 23.
40. Berghöfer B, Frommer T, Haley G, Fink L, Bein G, Hackstein H. TLR7 ligands induce higher IFN-alpha production in females. *The Journal of Immunology.* (1950) 2006;177(4):2088–2096.
41. Abdullah M, Chai P, Chong M, Tohit ERM, Ramasamy R, Pei CP, *et al.* Gender effect on *in vitro* lymphocyte subset levels of healthy individuals. *Cellular Immunology.* 2012;272(2):214–219.
42. Hewagama A, Patel D, Yarlagadda S, Strickland FM, Richardson BC. Stronger inflammatory cytotoxic T-cell response in women identified by microarray analysis. *Genes and Immunity.* 2009;10(5):509–516.
43. Anguiano L, Riera M, Pascual J, Soler MJ. Circulating ACE2 in cardiovascular and kidney diseases. *Current Medicinal Chemistry.* 2017;24(30):3231.
44. Soro-Paavonen A, Gordin D, Forsblom C, Rosengard-Barlund M, Waden J, Thorn L, *et al.* Circulating ACE2 activity is increased in patients with type 1 diabetes and vascular complications. *Journal of Hypertension.* 2012;30(2):375–383.
45. Fernández-Atucha A, Izagirre A, Fraile-Bermúdez AB, Kortajarena M, Larrinaga G, Martinez-Lage P, *et al.* Sex differences in the aging pattern of renin-angiotensin system serum peptidases. *Biology of Sex Differences.* 2017;8(1):5.
46. Mahdy MAA, Younis W, Ewaida Z. An overview of SARS-CoV-2 and animal infection. *Frontiers in Veterinary Science.* 2020;7:596391.
47. Lauring AS, Hodcroft EB. Genetic variants of SARS-CoV-2 — what do they mean? *JAMA: The Journal of the American Medical Association.* 2021;325(6):529–531.

48. Hu B, Guo H, Zhou P, Shi Z. Characteristics of SARS-CoV-2 and COVID-19. *Nature Reviews Microbiology*. 2021;19(3):141–154.
49. Eslami H, Jalili M. The role of environmental factors to transmission of SARS-CoV-2 (COVID-19). *AMB Express*. 2020;10(1):92–8.
50. Zhan J, Liu QS, Sun Z, Zhou Q, Hu L, Qu G, *et al*. Environmental impacts on the transmission and evolution of COVID-19 combing the knowledge of pathogenic respiratory coronaviruses. *Environmental Pollution*. (1987) 2020;267:115621.
51. Nicas M, Nazaroff WW, Hubbard A. Toward understanding the risk of secondary airborne infection: Emission of respirable pathogens. *Journal of Occupational and Environmental Hygiene*. 2005;2(3):143–154.
52. Tang JW. The effect of environmental parameters on the survival of airborne infectious agents. *Journal of the Royal Society Interface*. 2009;6(Suppl 6): S737–S746.

Chapter 4

Transmission Dynamics of COVID-19

Samantha Bardwell* and Daniel Coombs[†,‡]

*School of Population and Public Health, University of British Columbia, Vancouver, Canada

†Department of Mathematics, University of British Columbia, Vancouver, Canada

‡Institute of Applied Mathematics, University of British Columbia, Vancouver, Canada

Key Message

- The dynamics of COVID-19 depend on a number of factors, including the reproduction number; the overdispersion parameter; contacts, networks, and venues of transmission; and other epidemiological characteristics.
- Estimates for the basic reproduction number of COVID-19 fall between 2.2 and 3.9, indicating high initial exponential growth, and a herd immunity threshold (HIT) of 50–75%. Intervention strategies can be targeted to reduce the effective reproduction number.
- COVID-19 has high heterogeneity of transmission, referred to as overdispersion; 80% of secondary transmission is thought to be caused by 10–20% of infected individuals. This overdispersion often leads to superspreading events, however, if intervention methods are

targeted to prevent super-spreading, transmission of COVID-19 is lower than predicted.

- Transmission is higher among adults than children, and susceptibility is the highest among older adults. Households are the most common setting for secondary transmission to occur. Clustering of cases has been reported at several venue types, including elderly care centres, religious gatherings, and meat processing plants.
- Understanding transmission dynamics provides insight into the spread of COVID-19 through the population and can be applied in tools such as mathematical modelling. Modelling is useful for estimating parameters; making predictions on growth; and evaluating intervention methods, vaccination strategies, and variants of concern.

1. Introduction

Like most infectious diseases, the dynamics of COVID-19 are complex and depend on a number of factors. Classification of the reproduction number and the overdispersion parameter are essential for understanding the basic transmission of COVID-19. Additionally, since COVID-19 is spread from person to person, contacts and networks, including venues of transmission, are influential to the dynamics. Other epidemiologic characteristics of COVID-19 also play a role in the details of transmission. Understanding transmission dynamics provides insight into the spread of COVID-19 through the population and can be applied in tools such as mathematical modelling to make predictions on growth and help inform intervention strategies.

2. Exponential Growth and the Reproduction Number

COVID-19 has been predicted to grow exponentially, governed by the reproduction number, R. The reproduction number for a disease is the number of secondary cases attributed to one single case. In a general sense, it is an indication of the transmissibility of the virus. With higher R values, each infected person will transmit the disease to more contacts. Because R represents the slope of exponential growth of infection, with

$R > 1$ the epidemic will continue, and with $R < 1$ the epidemic should die off.[1] Hence, it is very important to keep the reproductive number below one. Variations of the reproduction number often referred to are the basic and the effective reproduction numbers.

2.1 *The basic reproduction number*

The basic reproduction number is the mean number of secondary cases attributed to a single case in a fully susceptible population. The basic reproduction number is commonly denoted as R_0 (R-naught). R_0 is important in disease dynamics because it dictates the initial exponential growth of the infection. The value of R_0 for COVID-19 has been calculated globally using models and data analysis and is estimated to be in the range of 2.2–3.9.[2–9] The interpretation of this value is that any one individual infected with COVID-19 in a fully susceptible population will infect another 2.2–3.9 individuals on average. However, when looking at countries individually, the reported basic reproductive number varies hugely; other key factors that vary R_0 include culture and the stage of the epidemic.[1]

Herd immunity is the indirect protection from infectious disease that occurs when a sufficient percentage of the population has immunity; once this has been achieved, the population is described as having reached the HIT. Herd immunity depends on the basic reproduction number of a disease; the higher the value of R_0, the higher the HIT. Based on the estimated of R_0, the HIT for COVID-19 has been predicted to be between 50% and 75%.[1–9] Theoretically, if 50–75% of the population were to gain immunity, whether through immunisation against or contraction of COVID-19, that would be sufficient to indirectly protect those in the population who were still susceptible.

Although the exact value of R_0 is not precisely agreed on, the estimated range is much higher than one. Exponential growth of COVID-19 was therefore especially problematic at the epidemic onset with a fully susceptible population and no risk mitigation in place. Many examples of rapid exponential growth can be seen across the globe. In the early stages of the Wuhan outbreak, the epidemic doubled every 7.4 days.[2] In Europe,

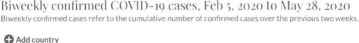

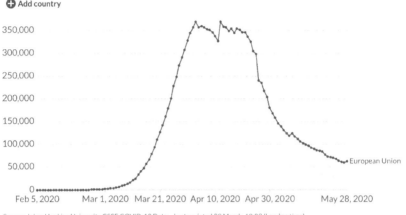

Source: Johns Hopkins University CSSE COVID-19 Data – Last updated 28 March, 10:03 (London time)
OurWorldInData.org/coronavirus • CC BY

Figure 1:   Biweekly confirmed COVID-19 cases in the European Union.[11]

the first case of COVID-19 was reported on January 24, 2020, and within 45 days, all 27 countries of the European Union had been reached.[10] The rapid exponential growth experienced by the European Union is illustrated in Figure 1.

2.2 *The effective reproduction number*

While R_0 provides valuable information on infection growth, this is only in the absence of immunity and mitigation strategies. The dynamics of an epidemic are heavily influenced by a number of factors, including, but not limited to the proportion of the population with immunity; policy implementation to target infection risk; individual behaviour; and disease variants.[12] As the epidemic progresses, the effective reproductive number, R_t, is a much more useful metric. This value accounts for immunity and mitigation strategies when providing the expected number of secondary cases attributed to an infected person at any given time in the epidemic; it does not require a fully susceptible population and can accurately reflect the current precautions in place. For example, in Germany the estimated R_t at the start of the outbreak in March 2020 was approximately 4. In May 2020, after lockdown had been in place for several months, the estimated R_t value was approximately 1.[12] With lockdown measures in place, Germany was more successful in controlling the transmission of COVID-19. This response exemplifies the variance of R_t as factors change throughout time.

In late 2020, the discovery of variants of COVID-19 began. These variants of concern (VOC) pose new problems as some have increased transmission advantages. The B.1.1.7 variant (or the "UK VOC") has particularly high transmission, with an estimated basic reproduction number about 1.5 times that of the original strain.[13–15] As the prevalence of highly transmissible variants of COVID-19 increases, R_t also increases. In Canada, the "third wave" of COVID-19 was driven by the introduction of VOC. As of April 2021, VOC make up more than half of new reported cases in some areas of Canada, contributing to the steady increase of R_t above 1.[16]

By examining current and predicted R values, interventions can be appropriately targeted. Across the world, populations have seen a change in the reproduction number of COVID-19 as behaviours and susceptibility change. The values of R_t in Canada have been calculated over the past year and demonstrate changes in mitigation strategies and behaviours in the country (refer to Table 1).[17] Throughout the month of March 2020, provinces across Canada began declaring states of emergency and implementing lockdowns, which resulted in the large drop in R_t from March to April (refer to Figure 2).[17] After the relaxation of restrictions in the summer months, a slow rise in R_t was observed (refer to Figure 2).[18]

2.3 *Strategies to reduce the reproduction number*

With interventions that are effective in reducing the value of R, there will be a time delay between the implementation of the intervention and the change to infection growth. The number of cases will continue at the same rate for a period of time due to the infections contracted before restrictions were implemented.[20,21] For example, many countries have urged citizens to avoid essential travel, thereby reducing passenger air travel, use of public transit, driving, and walking. A strong correlation between reduction in

Table 1:   Effective reproduction numbers in Canada from March 2020 to February 2021.[17]

Month	Effective reproduction number (R_t)
March 2020	2.52
April 2020	1.16
May 2020	0.91
June 2020	0.81
July 2020	1.17
August 2020	1.04
September 2020	1.21
October 2020	1.22
November 2020	1.06
December 2020	1.03
January 2021	0.89
February 2021	0.95

Canada

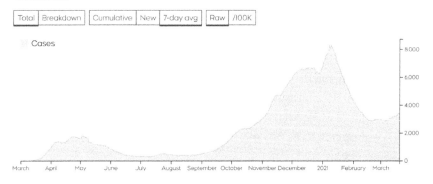

Figure 2:   Seven-day average of new COVID-19 cases in Canada from March 2020 to March 2021.[19]

day-to-day outings and the effective reproduction number has been observed, with a time delay of about two to three weeks between implementation and noticeable impact.[1]

The type and circumstances of a chosen intervention have an obvious relationship with the change in the effective reproduction number.

Restrictions and measurements that are strict result in a greater reduction of R than those considered to be mild. The later that measurements are put into place, the stricter they need to be to contain the spread of COVID-19. If measurements are delayed, the infectious population will continue to grow and will become harder to contain. School closures, partial work-place closures, and curfews are all considered mild restrictions.[20] These mild restrictions will lower R_t, however if the value is above one, the efforts will likely not be strict enough to bring the value below one. Mild restrictions contribute to slowing the epidemic, but they are not enough to control it.[20,21]

2.4 *Unexpected exponential growth*

Examples of failure to recognise exponential growth and implement timely restrictions were frequent at the onset of COVID-19. Outside of Asia, early in the pandemic Italy was the country with the largest out-break. The rapid spread across Italy demonstrates that no mitigation strat-egy can prevent the saturation of hospitals if adopted too late, emphasising the importance of containing COVID-19 as early as possible. The first COVID-19 and intensive care unit (ICU) patient in Lombardy, Italy was reported on February 24, 2020. By March 6, 2020 the number of COVID-19 ICU patients exceeded 100, with a slowing of exponential growth as the number of available beds was reached.[22] While the govern-ment implemented different strategies to increase available ICU beds, the measures taken were a linear response and were not enough to keep up with the exponential growth at hand. By March 17, 2020, more than 1,000 ICU beds were required, and COVID-19 patients occupied 50% of all ICU beds in the Lombardy region.[22] On February 26, 2020, schools and uni-versities closed in Lombardy, with the rest of Italy following suite on March 5, 2020; as well, a lockdown was imposed on the entire nation on March 9, 2020. However, it was too late to prevent saturation of the hos-pitals. On March 19, 2020, Italy recorded 3,405 deaths and passed China for the highest global COVID mortalities.[22]

The saturation of hospitals in Italy, specifically the Lombardy area, was unexpected at the time, but could have been predicted. One study performed a log-linear regression of the number of ICU patients.

This regression was used retrospectively to predict the ICU bed saturation timeline. Saturation depends greatly on the connectivity of a population, where a higher connectivity means COVID-19 will diffuse at a faster rate. Therefore, regions that are more connected have a higher risk of ICU saturation.[22] Lombardy is one of the most connected regions of Italy. The incubation period of COVID-19 as well as the degree of adherence of the population to restrictions also influences ICU saturation time. Based on the characteristics of the Lombardy region, the model predicted the ICU beds would reach 50% capacity on a date shortly before what actually happened (refer to Figure 3).[22] Based on the model, a much earlier lockdown date was identified, which could have avoided the saturation of hospitals. Although the lockdowns on March 9th and 21st prevented the collapse of the national healthcare system, they were much too late to avoid the saturation of ICU beds.[22]

A similar situation was observed in California. In December of 2020, there had been more than 1.7 million cases of COVID-19 since March

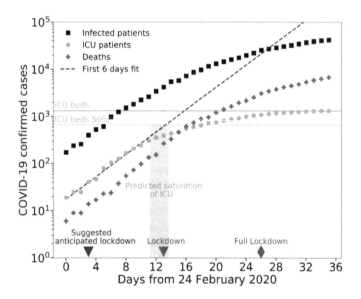

Figure 3:   Model predictions for ICU saturation versus actual data.[22] Note that the *y*-axis measures the log of confirmed cases, and that exponential curves appear linear in a log plot. Therefore, the growth is much steeper than indicated by first glance at the figure.

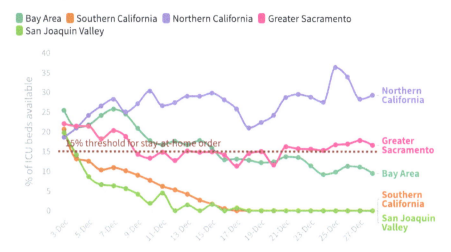

Figure 4:   Adjusted ICU capacity by region in California, December 2020.[26]

2020 in California.[23] and over 21,000 deaths[24]. COVID patients occupied over 21,000 hospital beds,[25] and models were predicting more than 33,000 hospitalisations by mid-January of 2021.[23] COVID-19 patients filled so many hospital beds that many had 0% ICU bed availability and field hospitals were being opened (refer to Figure 4). In Orange County, the ICU was at 105% capacity.[24] The overwhelming of the hospitals could have been predicted, especially after observing the effects in Italy; however strict enough restrictions were not put in place to bring the effective reproduction number below one.

3. Overdispersion

The reproductive number and its implications on the transmissibility of COVID-19 have been discussed in depth in the previous section. However, many countries observe fewer secondary cases than would be expected with the predicted high value for R_0; this suggests that not all cases cause secondary transmission.[8] Since the basic reproductive number is the average number of secondary cases resulting from one initial patient, it is not surprising that some patients will infect more, and others will infect few than average. Because of this underlying heterogeneity in transmission, individuals infect differently and at different rates. Without considering individual variation in infection, emerging disease outbreaks cannot be fully understood.

Dispersion refers to the heterogeneity of disease transmission. High dispersion means a high variation in transmission. With high dispersion, many individuals cause zero infections, while a few individuals cause many infections.[27] When the level of variation is very high in individual transmission, it is referred to as overdispersion. Overdispersion often refers to the small proportion of infected individuals who cause 80% of transmission. The heterogeneity in transmission can be estimated by describing the distribution of secondary cases.[28]

3.1 *The overdispersion parameter*

The overdispersion parameter, k, describes how variable the spread of infection can be. A low k value indicates high variation in transmission; a small number of people are responsible for a large amount of disease transmission, and a large proportion of the infected population has zero secondary transmission. As the value of k increases, a larger proportion of the population become responsible for the spread of disease, and the proportion who do not pass on infection shrinks. Several studies have estimated the k value of COVID-19 to be around 0.1–0.2.[8,9,27] Using this estimated k value, it is predicted that 80% of secondary transmission is caused by about 10–20% of infected individuals.[8,9,27] For example, based on estimates of the reproductive number and the overdispersion parameter, a group of 10 individuals infected with COVID-19 would be expected to cause 25 secondary infections. Within that group, one individual would be responsible for 20 secondary transmissions, while the other nine infected individuals would cause a combined five infections.[8,9,27]

3.2 *Super-spreading events*

With overdispersion, because many initial infections produce zero new cases, there is an increased die-out probability. Therefore, it is likely that COVID-19 has to be introduced into a susceptible population multiple times before an outbreak actually occurs.[27] For this reason, the early dynamics of COVID-19 must be largely a result of super-spreading events.[29]

When an event leads to a COVID-19 outbreak, sometimes due to only one infected individual, it is classified as a super-spreading event. A super-spreader is any individual that causes more infections than predicted by R.[30] There are many characteristics that contribute to an individual becoming a super-spreader. Super-spreaders often have high viral loads. The viral load is the amount of virus particles in an infected person's blood; therefore, a higher viral load increases infectivity.[30] The environment is another factor can increase the risk of super-spreading. Areas with high population density have been associated with higher rates of COVID-19 infection.[30] Additionally, super-spreading is more likely to occur in environments where air is being expelled with high velocity[30]; some examples include individuals participating in physical activity, or a setting where voices are being projected, such as yelling or singing. New variants of COVID-19 may also play a role in super-spreading. Because some variants are estimated to have different transmissibility's, those that are highly transmissible can result in super-spreading.[30]

One major superspreading event that occurred early on in the pandemic took place in Skagit County, Washington. In March of 2020, a symptomatic index patient attended a choir practise of 61 individuals, resulting in 32 confirmed and 20 probable secondary cases of COVID-19. Of these cases, three were hospitalised and two died.[31] One individual was the cause for 52 additional infections, a number tens of times larger than the R_0 value, making this a prime example of the heterogeneity of transmission.

Super-spreading events continue to be detrimental towards the end of an epidemic, when the disease is close to elimination. Because one person can initiate many new cases in a short period of time, progress can be reverted, and the epidemic can rebound. The "second-wave" of COVID-19 experienced in Canada in the fall of 2020 was largely influenced by super-spreading events. In October of 2020, a COVID-19 outbreak linked to a super-spreader occurred in Hamilton, ON. One infected individual attended spin classes over the course of a week, resulting in 85 additional cases. Direct transmission in the spin classes resulted in 54 primary cases among staff and other members, followed by 31 secondary cases linked to those primary cases.[32]

3.3 *Targeting overdispersion to reduce transmission*

While super-spreaders are a negative aspect of overdispersion, a low k value can be positive because so few people actually transmit COVID-19; most cases resolve without causing an outbreak. Reducing transmission may be easier than predicted by the reproduction number if the correct intervention methods are used to reduce super-spreaders. These intervention methods, however, cannot be properly identified without understanding factors determining individual infectiousness. Transmission is concentrated among the most active members of the population,[33] meaning that interventions should be targeted towards these individuals to most effectively prevent COVID-19 spread. Interventions to control super-spreading events include rapid identification and isolation, contact tracing, screening, and infection control.[29] Contact tracing is often used in COVID-19 investigations, but backward contact tracing is very valuable when targeting super-spreaders.[34] Since most individuals only transmit from zero to a few new cases, little is found with forward contact tracing. Using backward contact tracing is more useful because many people are infected as the result of a super-spreading event. Primary cases with high levels of transmission can be identified through this method, thereby increasing the number of subsequent cases averted.[34]

3.4 *Overdispersion and herd immunity*

Another positive effect of overdispersion is the potential impact on herd-immunity. As the COVID-19 pandemic progresses, the susceptible population is depleted and therefore the incidence of new cases declines. Variation in individual susceptibility and transmission amplify this effect.[35,36] This effect continues until the susceptible population is so reduced that herd immunity occurs. Based on the current reported reproductive number for COVID-19, herd immunity is predicted to be achieved at 50–75% immunity,[1–9] however the estimates are brought down by transmission variation. Based on reasonable estimates for the coefficient of variation of COVID-19, the actual HIT has been estimated to be as low as 10–40%.[33,35,36]

4. Contacts, Networks, and Venues of Transmission

4.1 *Characteristics of contacts*

Since the spread occurs from one infected person to others, characteristics of contacts and networks influencing transmission and susceptibility are important to the disease dynamics. Two characteristics that are frequently associated with transmission are gender and age. The gender ratios observed in COVID-19 infection are similar, indicating that gender does not impact transmission and susceptibility.[37,38] However, age plays a large role in the spread. The reported transmission rate from children has been observed to be low overall. However, it is especially low between children; they more commonly infect their parents than other children.[37] It has been observed that susceptibility increases with age, meaning adults are also more likely to infect other adults than to infect children.[37] While older adults are particularly vulnerable to COVID-19, they do not tend to be very active. The effect of increased susceptibility competes with reduced activity in the transmission within older populations.[37]

4.2 *Venues of transmission*

Networks are influenced not only by the characteristics of their individuals, but also by the location of occurrence. Since behaviours differ between settings, venue specific transmission of COVID-19 varies. Social distancing has impacted the number of contacts per person, as well as the venues in which interaction can occur. Outside of the household, contact between individuals typically occurs in schools, workplaces, social settings, and casual encounters.[39,40] Three venues commonly studied are households, schools, and workplaces because they are frequented in day-to-day life.

4.2.1 *Household transmission*

Household transmission plays a large role in the spread of COVID-19, especially with lockdown measures in place. When looking at the contribution of household cases to total transmission, households have been identified as the most common setting for transmission to occur, making up 20–60% of identified clusters.[40–42] The overall secondary attack rate of COVID-19 for close-contacts has been estimated at about 5%,[38] compared to the secondary attack rate within households of about 16%.[38] The secondary attack rate within households is more than three times greater than the rate for all close contacts, due to the high interactions within the house. For the same reason, household crowding increases transmission,[38] and different relationships within the house influence risk of transmission. For example, a spousal relationship with an infected individual increases likeliness of transmission.[38]

4.2.2 School transmission

Transmission of COVID-19 in schools has been a very controversial topic. Children are reported to have contributed to between 1% and 5% of total COVID-19 cases,[43] even though they make up significantly more than 5% of the entire population. Because there is limited evidence of child transmission, children are assumed to have minimal contribution to the spread, therefore many are unconcerned about transmission in schools. This is reaffirmed by several studies which have estimated less than 5% of total outbreaks to be linked to schools.[40,41,44] However, it is estimated that 20–50% of children are asymptomatic,[43] and since current testing mainly focuses on the unwell, there may be significant undercounting of child cases. The potential for unnoticed asymptomatic spread means the transmission in schools may actually be higher than observed.

4.2.3 Workplace transmission

Within the workplace, different work environments allow for varying risks of transmission. The transmission of illnesses in general is higher when work tasks involve interacting with customers, patients, and co-workers, or food preparation[45]. A few studies have estimated that work-related outbreaks contribute to about 5% of COVID-19 clusters and less than 15% of linked cases.[40,41,46] Occupations that have been identified with the highest percentages of exposure include healthcare workers; protective services such as police officers, firefighters, and transportation security screeners; drivers and transport workers; office and administrative support such as patient representatives, couriers, and medical secretaries; and cleaning and domestic workers.[45,46]

4.2.4 *Clustering*

There are also venues which are more prone to major clusters, including nursing homes, religious gatherings, and meat processing and packaging facilities.[37] In nursing homes where the demographic is older adults, when one case occurs, an outbreak often follows. Although the spread of infection in elderly care centres is rapid, it is relatively contained and therefore typically has a short path.[37,47,48] Cases in elderly care centres have been estimated to contribute to about 10% of all clusters.[40,49] Because of the increased susceptibility and weakened immune response of the elderly, the fatality rate of COVID-19 outbreaks is higher than across the entire population. In June of 2020, 80% of fatalities in Canada were in long-term facilities.[50] In March of 2021 in the United States, an estimated 40% of all COVID-19 fatalities are from nursing homes, even though less than 0.5% of the population lives in them.[51,52] In Ontario, about 80% of the nursing homes were either currently in or had previously experienced an outbreak as of March 2021.[53]

While religious clusters have been estimated to make up less than 10% of clusters,[40] their impact on their specific regions has been more severe. This is because cluster groups, such as religious gatherings, consist of more young and middle-aged adults, so the path of transmission can be long and hard to contain.[37] Earlier in the epidemic, religious gatherings were responsible for large proportions of cases in many countries. From February 27 to March 3, 2020, there was a Tablighi Jamaat meeting in Malaysia. This resulted in 1,545 cases[54] making up nearly 35% of all cases in Malaysia at the time.[55] A religious congregation held in Nizamuddin, Delhi in March of 2020 brought more than 5,000 people to the area and was responsible for 1,080 of the total 1,561 cases of COVID-19.[56,57]

Cluster groups have been a frequent occurrence in meat packaging and processing plants mainly because of the work environment. COVID-19 favours lower temperatures and either very high or relatively low humidity, which can be found in meat plants.[58] Additionally, social distancing is hard to maintain, and the loud machinery causes workers to speak louder, releasing more droplets.[58] Outbreaks in food processing plants have been estimated to account for about 5% of COVID-19 clusters.[40] Canada has seen numerous outbreaks in meat plants. Most notably, in April 2020 an outbreak occurred at the Cagrill meat-packaging plant in southern Alberta. Of 2,000 employees, 949 tested positive, and a total of 1,560 cases were linked back to the plant.[59] In March 2020 in South Dakota, there were 644 confirmed cases among Smithfield employees, accounting for 55% of the state caseload at the time.[60] Meat plant outbreaks have also been occurring all across the globe, including one in Germany with more than 1,500 positive cases among 7,000 workers and another at a slaughterhouse in Portugal with 129 cases among 300 workers.[58]

5. Other Disease Characteristics

Other important characteristics for transmission of COVID-19 include the incubation period, the latent period, the infectious period, the serial interval, and the contact period.

The incubation period is the interval between initial infection and the onset of clinical symptoms. For COVID-19, the incubation period is estimated to have a mean of about 5.2 days.[2,61]

The latent period is the time from initial infection to infectiousness, which is estimated to be in the range of 2–6 days.[4,62,63]

The infectious period is the period during which an infected person can transmit a pathogen to a susceptible host. The infectious period for COVID-19 is estimated to fall in the range of 3–18 days.[3,4,62,63]

The serial interval is the time between equivalent stages of two successive cases in a chain of transmission, usually between onset of symptoms or dates of transmission. The serial interval for COVID-19 has been estimated to be about 7.5 days.[2]

The contact period describes patterns of contacts within the population, where contact periods are behaviour specific. The contact period is estimated for COVID-19 to be in the range of 1.4–3.4.[63]

6. Modelling Transmission Dynamics of COVID-19

Once the epidemiologic characteristics of COVID-19 are known and the transmission between individuals is understood, this information can be combined with collected statistics to mathematically model the transmission dynamics. Mathematical models have been used to study the transmission of COVID-19 in a variety of ways. Models have been used to: estimate parameters; make predictions on the future growth patterns; and evaluate effects of parameter changes including interventions and restrictions, vaccination strategies, and variants of concern.

An important parameter that is a product of mathematical modelling is the reproduction number. Regardless of whether it is the basic or effective reproduction number, most R values are estimates of mathematical modeling. The resultant values depend on the type of model constructed, the parameters used in the model, and any other modeling assumptions, and therefore can vary depending on these inputs. In a systemic review of various estimates for R_0, it was found that exponential growth models predict a value ranging between 2.2 and 3.6, while compartmental models predict a value ranging between 4.1 and 6.5.[3]

As the pandemic progresses and more data are collected, models can be adapted to become more accurate. At the onset of COVID-19, limited information meant many models did not consider heterogeneity of transmission, however, time has shown that patterns of COVID-19 spread are highly heterogeneous. Without incorporating overdispersion into COVID-19 models, there is a large uncertainty in outbreak size.[28] Therefore, early models of COVID-19 transmission may have grossly underestimated the final size of the epidemic.[64,65]

6.1 *The SEIR model*

One model commonly used to model the dynamics of COVID-19 is the Susceptible-Exposed-Infectious-Recovered (SEIR) compartmental model [1]. Individuals are assumed to be either susceptible, exposed, infectious, or recovered, and move between compartments at rates governed by specific characteristics of COVID-19 (refer to Figure 5). The transition from susceptible to exposed is usually described as the contact rate beta, where

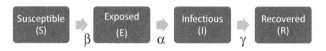

Figure 5: Flow diagram for SEIR compartmental model.

beta is the inverse of the contact period, and is influenced by the size of susceptible and infectious populations.[65,66] The reproductive number R is scaled by beta, so the higher the contact rate, the higher the reproductive number. Thus, mitigation strategies are targeted to reduce the contact rate beta and thereby lower the reproduction number.[65,66] Individuals move from the exposed compartment to infectious based on the incubation period, alpha. The incubation period alpha can also be described as the inverse of the latent period.[65,66] Individuals move from infectious to recovered by the recovery rate gamma, where gamma can be represented by the inverse of the infectious period.[65,66]

There are many variations of the SEIR model used in the analysis of COVID-19. One commonly seen is the SE_1E_2IR model, where E_1 includes pre-transmissive individuals and E_2 includes transmissive but not symptomatic individuals. Another adaptation is the SEIQR model, where Q represents individuals in quarantine, and theoretically not interacting with the susceptible population. Since age influences transmission and susceptibility, another variation is age structure SEIR models, where each age category has its own set of compartments. Age structure models are prominently used when analyzing vaccination strategies. As the pandemic progresses, evidence shows that reinfection is possible. Therefore, it is predicted that S_1EIS_2 models will become increasingly popular, where S_2 refers to individuals previously infected and susceptible to reinfection. Individuals in the S_1 and S_2 compartments become infected at different rates because those previously infected are less susceptible to the COVID-19 virus.

7. Discussion

7.1 *Summary*

The basic reproduction number is estimated to be in the range of 2.2–3.9, indicating high initial exponential growth, and a HIT of 50–75%.

The effective reproduction number can be reduced if targeted correctly, but the change in reproduction number will depend on the severity of restrictions and will experience a time delay. Many COVID-19 outbreaks have been due to insufficient reactions to exponential growth. If closer attention is paid to exponential growth patterns, outbreak sizes can be reduced.

Individual transmission of COVID-19 has high heterogenicity; 80% of secondary transmission is thought to be caused by 10–20% of infected individuals. This overdispersion often leads to superspreading events. However, if intervention methods are targeted to prevent super-spreading, transmission of COVID-19 is lower than predicted; the actual HIT may be as low as 10–40%.

Transmission is higher among adults than children, and susceptibility is the highest among older adults. Households are the most common setting for secondary transmission to occur. Clustering of cases has been reported at several venue types, including elderly care centres, religious gatherings, and meat processing plants.

Using knowledge on underlying transmission of COVID-19, mathematical models can be constructed. Modelling is used to estimate the reproduction number and the overdispersion parameter. Modelling is also useful for evaluating intervention methods, vaccination strategies, and variants of concern. The most common model used to represent COVID-19 spread is the SEIR model.

7.2 *Implications*

Given the high R_0 and potential for superspreading events, the dynamics of COVID-19 if left unattended would be explosive. However, interventions can be used to reduce the spread by appropriately targeting different factors (refer to Table 2).

The contact rate between individuals is mainly targeted through the use of non-pharmaceutical infections (NPIs). Social distancing reduces the number of contacts per person, and stay-at-home orders further restrict interactions outside of the household. Having a smaller social network reduces the number of contacts per person, thereby limiting opportunities for infection.

Table 2:   Strategies for targeting various aspects of COVID-19 transmission.

| | Targeted factor to reduce spread | | | |
	Contact rate	Risk of transmission	Infectious contact period	Importation of new cases
Diagnostics			✓	
NPIs	✓	✓	✓	✓
Therapeutics		✓		
Vaccines		✓		

For situations where contact occurs, the risk of transmission can be reduced; NPIs, therapeutics, and vaccines are various techniques for targeting this risk. A common NPI for reducing transmission risk is non-medical masking. Therapeutics are currently used in hospitals but could help lessen household transmission if the reach was expanded. Vaccines reduce both severe COVID-19 symptoms, and susceptibility to infection. Although the efficacy is not 100%, an infected individual has a significantly reduced risk of transmitting to the vaccinated population.

Tools can also be used to reduce the duration of infectious contact, such as diagnostics and NPIs. With an infectious period of up to 18 days, an infected individual has plenty of time to come in contact with susceptible populations. If diagnostic equipment and strategies are efficient, infected cases can be identified, reducing unknown transmission. Contact tracing is an NPI that has a similar effect. The infectious contact period can be lessened by identifying unknown cases through this method.

Finally, the importation of new cases can be reduced, mainly through the use of NPIs. With a constant introduction of outside individuals into a population, it can be assumed that a proportionate number are infected with COVID-19. National and regional travel restrictions minimise the flow of new individuals into a population, preventing any cases of COVID-19 present in the outside communities.

7.3 *Conclusion*

The purpose of this paper was to provide an overview on the transmission dynamics of COVID-19. By summarising the key factors and implications of the disease, the goal was to provide the audience with a general knowledge of how COVID-19 spreads; the information in this paper could be used to inform policy recommendations, to influence personal behaviour, or simply to improve understanding of transmission dynamics.

References

1. Linka K, Peirlinck M, Kuhl E. The reproduction number of COVID-19 and its correlation with public health interventions. *Computational Mechanics*. 2020;66(4):1035–1050.
2. Li Q, Guan X, Wu P, Wang X, Zhou L, Tong Y, *et al*. Early transmission dynamics in Wuhan, China, of novel coronavirus-infected pneumonia. *New England Journal of Medicine*. 2020;382(13):1199–1207.
3. Liu Y, Gayle AA, Wilder-Smith A, Rocklöv J. The reproductive number of COVID-19 is higher compared to SARS coronavirus. *Journal of Travel Medicine*. 2020;27(2):taaa021.
4. Park SW, Bolker BM, Champredon D, Earn DJD, Li M, Weitz JS, *et al*. Reconciling early-outbreak estimates of the basic reproductive number and its uncertainty: Framework and applications to the novel Coronavirus (SARS-CoV-2) outbreak. *medRxiv* 2020:2020.01.30.20019877.
5. Musa SS, Zhao S, Wang MH, Habib AG, Mustapha UT, He D. Estimation of exponential growth rate and basic reproduction number of the Coronavirus disease 2019 (COVID-19) in Africa. *Infectious Diseases of Poverty*. 2020;9(1):96.
6. Alimohamadi Y, Taghdir M, Sepandi M. Estimate of the basic reproduction number for COVID-19: A systematic review and meta-analysis. *Journal of Preventive Medicine and Public Health = Yebang Uihakhoe chi* 2020; 53(3):151–157.
7. Ahammed T, Anjum A, Rahman MM, Haider N, Kock R, Uddin MJ. Estimation of novel Coronavirus (COVID-19) reproduction number and case fatality rate: A systematic review and meta-analysis. *medRxiv* 2020:2020. 09.30.20204644.
8. Endo A, Centre for the Mathematical Modelling of Infectious Diseases COVID-19 Working Group, Abbott S, Kucharski AJ, Funk S. Estimating the overdispersion in COVID-19 transmission using outbreak sizes outside China. *Wellcome Open Res*. 2020;5:67.
9. Hasan A, Susanto H, Kasim MF, Nuraini N, Lestari B, Triany D, *et al*. Superspreading in early transmissions of COVID-19 in Indonesia. *Scientific Reports*. 2020;10(1):22386.

10. (10) COVID-19 situation update worldwide, as of Week 7, updated 25 February 2021. Available at: https://www.ecdc.europa.eu/en/geographical-distribution-2019-ncov-cases [Accessed 3 March 2021].

11. COVID-19 Data Repository by the Center for Systems Science and Engineering (CSSE) at Johns Hopkins University, 2021. Available at: https://github.com/CSSEGISandData/COVID-19.

12. Khailaie S, Mitra T, Bandyopadhyay A, Schips M, Mascheroni P, Vanella P, *et al.* Development of the reproduction number from coronavirus SARS-CoV-2 case data in Germany and implications for political measures. *BMC Medicine.* 2021;19(1):32.

13. Volz E, Mishra S, Chand M, Barrett JC, Johnson R, Geidelberg L, *et al.* Assessing transmissibility of SARS-CoV-2 lineage B.1.1.7 in England. *Nature.* 2021.

14. Davies NG, Abbott S, Barnard RC, Jarvis CI, Kucharski AJ, Munday JD, *et al.* Estimated transmissibility and impact of SARS-CoV-2 lineage B.1.1.7 in England. *Science.* 2021;372(6538):eabg3055. doi: 10.1126/science.abg3055. Epub 2021 Mar 3.

15. Stefanelli P, Trentini F, Guzzetta G, Marziano V, Mammone A, Poletti P, *et al.* Co-circulation of SARS-CoV-2 variants B.1.1.7 and P.1. *medRxiv.* 2021: 2021.04.06.21254923.

16. Shi A, Gaynor S, Li X, Lin X, Li H, Li Z, *et al.* Visualizing COVID-19's Effective Reproduction Number (Rt), 2021. Available at: http://metrics.covid19-analysis.org/.

17. A timeline of events in Canada's fight against COVID-19, 2020. Available at: https://www.cp24.com/news/a-timeline-of-events-in-canada-s-fight-against-covid-19-1.5231865?cache=jhiggtiw%3FclipId%3D104070.

18. Tracking every case of COVID-19 in Canada, 2021. Available at: https://www.ctvnews.ca/mobile/health/coronavirus/tracking-every-case-of-covid-19-in-canada-1.4852102.

19. d'Onofrio A, Manfredi P. Information-related changes in contact patterns may trigger oscillations in the endemic prevalence of infectious diseases. *Journal of Theoretical Biology.* 2009;256(3):473–478.

20. Lauer SA, Grantz KH, Bi Q, Jones FK, Zheng Q, Meredith HR, *et al.* The incubation period of Coronavirus disease 2019 (COVID-19) from publicly reported confirmed cases: Estimation and application. *Annals of Internal Medicine.* 2020;172(9):577–582.

21. Supino M, d'Onofrio A, Luongo F, Occhipinti G, Dal Co A. The effects of containment measures in the Italian outbreak of COVID-19. *BMC Public Health.* 2020;20(1):1806.

22. Melley B. COVID-19 models plot dire scenarios for California hospitals, 2020. Available at: https://abcnews.go.com/Health/wireStory/covid-19-models-plot-dire-scenarios-california-hospitals-74795007 [Accessed 3 March 2021].

23. Ellis R. COVID forces California to open field hospitals, 2020. Available at: https://www.webmd.com/lung/news/20201217/covid-forces-california-to-open-field-hospitals [Accessed 3 March 2021].

24. Moon S, Mossburg C. California hospitals stressed to the 'BRINK of catastrophe' by the coronavirus surge, 2020. Available at: https://www.cnn.com/2020/12/31/health/california-covid-hospitals-catastrophe/index.html [Accessed 3 March 2021].

25. Webeck E, Rowan HB. Adjusted ICU capacity in California, by region, 2021. Available at: https://flo.uri.sh/visualisation/4798065/embed.

26. Großmann G, Backenköhler M, Wolf V. Epidemic overdispersion strengthens the effectiveness of mobility restrictions. *medRxiv*. 2021:2021.01.22. 21250303.

27. Kucharski AJ, Althaus CL. The role of superspreading in Middle East respiratory syndrome coronavirus (MERS-CoV) transmission. *Eurosurveillance*. 2015;20(25):14–18.

28. Hébert-Dufresne L, Althouse BM, Scarpino SV, Allard A. Beyond R0: Heterogeneity in secondary infections and probabilistic epidemic forecasting. *Journal of The Royal Society Interface*. 2020;17(172):20200393.

29. Lee D. COVID-19: The truth about super-spreaders 2021. Available at: https://www.openaccessgovernment.org/covid-19-the-truth-about-super-spreaders/103490/.

30. Hamner L, Dubbel P, Capron I, Ross A, Jordan A, Lee J, *et al*. High SARS-CoV-2 attack rate following exposure at a choir practice — Skagit County, Washington, March 2020. Morbidity and Mortality Weekly Report 2020 May 15.

31. Frketich J. SpinCo Hamilton COVID outbreak is over, but questions remain on how it could have been prevented, 2020. Available at: https://www.thespec.com/news/hamilton-region/analysis/2020/10/27/spinco-hamilton-covid-outbreak-is-over-but-questions-remain-on-how-it-could-have-been-prevented.html [Accessed 3 March 2021].

32. Britton T, Ball F, Trapman P. A mathematical model reveals the influence of population heterogeneity on herd immunity to SARS-CoV-2. *Science*. 2020;369(6505):846–849.

33. Endo A, Leclerc QJ, Knight GM, Medley GF, Atkins KE, *et al*. Implication of backward contact tracing in the presence of overdispersed transmission in COVID-19 outbreak. *medRxiv*. 2020:2020.08.01.20166595.

34. Gomes MGM, Corder RM, King JG, Langwig KE, Souto-Maior C, Carneiro J, *et al*. Individual variation in susceptibility or exposure to SARS-CoV-2 lowers the herd immunity threshold. *medRxiv*. 2020:2020.04.27.20081893.

35. Neipel J, Bauermann J, Bo S, Harmon T, Jülicher F. Power-law population heterogeneity governs epidemic waves. *PLOS ONE*. 2020;15(10):e0239678.

36. Kim Y, Jiang X. Evolving transmission network dynamics of COVID-19 cluster infections in South Korea: A descriptive study. *medRxiv: The Preprint Server for Health Sciences*. 2020.

37. Madewell ZJ, Yang Y, Longini IM,Jr, Halloran ME, Dean NE. Household transmission of SARS-CoV-2: A systematic review and meta-analysis. *JAMA Network Open*. 2020;3(12):e2031756.

38. Nande A, Adlam B, Sheen J, Levy MZ, Hill AL. Dynamics of COVID-19 under social distancing measures are driven by transmission network structure. *medRxiv*. 2020:2020.06.04.20121673.

39. Leclerc QJ, Fuller NM, Knight LE, Funk S, Knight GM. What settings have been linked to SARS-CoV-2 transmission clusters? [version 2; peer review: 2 approved]. *Wellcome Open Research*. 2020;5(83).

40. Wong NS, Lee SS, Kwan TH, Yeoh E. Settings of virus exposure and their implications in the propagation of transmission networks in a COVID-19 outbreak. *The Lancet Regional Health — Western Pacific*. 2020;4.

41. COVID-19: Monthly Update, 2020. Available at: https://news.gov.bc.ca/files/ COVID19_Monthly_Update_Nov_2020.pdf.

42. Boast A, Goldstein H, Munro A. An evidence summary of Paediatric COVID-19 literature. *Don't Forget the Bubbles*. 2020.

43. Falk A, Benda A, Falk P, Steffen S, Wallace Z, Høeg TB. COVID-19 Cases and Transmission in 17 K–12 Schools — Wood County, Wisconsin, August 31–November 29, 2020. *MMWR Morbidity Mortality Weekly Report*. 2021 January 29.

44. Baker MG, Peckham TK, Seixas NS. Estimating the burden of United States workers exposed to infection or disease: A key factor in containing risk of COVID-19 infection. *PLOS ONE*. 2020;15(4):e0232452.

45. Lan F, Wei C, Hsu Y, Christiani DC, Kales SN. Work-related COVID-19 transmission. *medRxiv*. 2020:2020.04.08.20058297.

46. Edwards CH, Tomba GS, de Blasio BF. Influenza in workplaces: Transmission, workers' adherence to sick leave advice and European sick leave recommendations. *European Journal of Public Health*. 2016 Jun;26(3):478–485.

47. Webster RK, Liu R, Karimullina K, Hall I, Amlôt R, Rubin GJ. A systematic review of infectious illness Presenteeism: Prevalence, reasons and risk factors. *BMC Public Health*. 2019;19(1):799.

48. All Ontario: Case numbers and spread, 2021. Available at: https://covid-19.ontario.ca/data [Accessed 6 March 2021].
49. Webster P. COVID-19 highlights Canada's care home crisis. *Lancet* (London, England) 2021;397(10270):183.
50. Chen MK, Chevalier JA, Long EF. Nursing home staff networks and COVID-19. National Bureau of Economic Research Working Paper Series 2020; No. 27608.
51. Grabowski DC, Mor V. Nursing home care in crisis in the wake of COVID-19. *JAMA*. 2020;324(1):23–24.
52. COVID-19 — Long-term care homes, 2021. Available at: https://covid-19.ontario.ca/data/long-term-care-homes [Accessed 6 March 2021].
53. Daim N. Tabligh gathering cluster contributes highest positive Covid-19 figures, 2020. Available at: https://www.nst.com.my/news/nation/2020/04/581317/tabligh-gathering-cluster-.
54. Che Mat NF, Edinur HA, Abdul Razab M, Khairul Azhar, Safuan S. A single mass gathering resulted in massive transmission of COVID-19 infections in Malaysia with further international spread. *Journal of Travel Medicine*. 2020;27(3):taaa059.
55. Yezli S, Khan A. COVID-19 pandemic: It is time to temporarily close places of worship and to suspend religious gatherings. *Journal of Travel Medicine*. 2020;28(2):taaa065.
56. Sharma P, Anand A. Indian media coverage of Nizamuddin Markaz event during COVID-19 pandemic. *Asian Politics & Policy*. 2020:10.1111/aspp.12561.
57. Middleton J, Reintjes R, Lopes H. Meat plants — a new front line in the covid-19 pandemic. *BMJ*. 2020;370:m2716.
58. Dryden J, Rieger S. North America's biggest COVID-19 outbreak happened here — look inside, 2020. Available at: https://newsinteractives.cbc.ca/longform/cargill-covid19-outbreak [Accessed 6 March 2021].
59. Lussenhop J. Coronavirus at Smithfield pork plant: The untold story of America's biggest outbreak, 2020. Available at: https://www.bbc.com/news/world-us-canada-52311877.
60. Iyer AS, Jones FK, Nodoushani A, Kelly M, Becker M, Slater D, *et al.* Dynamics and significance of the antibody response to SARS-CoV-2 infection. *medRxiv: The Preprint Server for Health Sciences*. 2020.
61. Prem K, Liu Y, Russell TW, Kucharski AJ, Eggo RM, Davies N, *et al.* The effect of control strategies to reduce social mixing on outcomes of the COVID-19 epidemic in Wuhan, China: A modelling study. *The Lancet Public Health*. 2020;5(5):e261–e270.

62. Linka K, Peirlinck M, Kuhl E. The reproduction number of COVID-19 and its correlation with public health interventions. *Computational Mechanics.* 2020;66(4):1035–1050.

63. Tkachenko AV, Maslov S, Elbanna A, Wong GN, Weiner ZJ, Goldenfeld N. Time-dependent heterogeneity leads to transient suppression of COVID-19 epidemic, not herd immunity. *medRxiv.* 2020:2020.07.26.20162420.

64. Meyers LA, Pourbohloul B, Newman ME, Skowronski DM, Brunham RC. Network theory and SARS: Predicting outbreak diversity. *Journal of Theoretical Biology.* 2005;232(1):71–81.

65. Kermack WO, McKendrick AG, Walker GT. A contribution to the mathematical theory of epidemics. *Proceedings of the Royal Society of London Series A.* 1927;115(772):700–721.

66. Li MY, Muldowney JS. Global stability for the SEIR model in epidemiology. *Mathematical Biosciences.* 1995;125(2):155–164.

Part 3

Diagnostics and the
Role of Laboratories

Chapter 5

The Role of Nucleic Acid Amplification and Sequencing

Frederick Lam* and Inna Sekirov[†,‡]

*School of Population and Public Health, University of British Columbia, Vancouver, Canada

†Medical Microbiologist, Public Health Laboratory, BC Centre for Disease Control, Vancouver, Canada

‡Department of Pathology and Laboratory Medicine, Vancouver, Canada

Key Message

- The early identification of the whole genome sequence of SARS-CoV-2 allowed for the development of a reliable diagnostic standard in the reverse-transcriptase polymerase chain reaction (RT-PCR) test for COVID-19, which quickly became the clinical standard for diagnosis.
- Diagnostic methods played a critical role in the initial and ongoing response, informed transmission strategies and thereby reducing the reproductive rate (R_t) of COVID-19 infections.
- Diagnostic accuracy was a point of focus, and clinical studies of diagnostic accuracy of the available testing modalities was conducted, which were important given the profound implications of both positive and negative test results.

- In the early stages of the pandemic, the absence of definitive evidence of the impact of testing resulted in a range of different testing strategies employed in different jurisdictions. While some of the considerations were logistic, it has created useful case studies for understanding the potential positive benefits of scalable, mass-testing.
- The rise to prominence of different variants of interest of SARS-CoV-2 has kept whole genome sequencing relevant, and the focus needs to shift from an active to sentinel surveillance strategy to ensure the timely identification and response to clinically impactful variant strains.

1. Introduction

The earliest recognised patient with COVID-19 was hospitalised on December 12, 2019 in Wuhan, China presenting with a constellation of symptoms such as fever, severe cough, and dyspnoea. The initial cluster of index patients with a pneumonia-like illness did not respond to antibiotic therapies, nor were cultures returning a culpable pathogen. On further investigation for an etiological agent, bronchoalveolar lavage samples from these index patients were subjected to deep metatranscriptomic sequencing, which on January 10, 2020 yielded the first complete genomic sequence of what would eventually be named severe acute respiratory syndrome coronavirus 2 (SARS-CoV-2).[1,2] The genomic sequence of this novel virus was found to share 89.1% of its genetic sequence with severe acute respiratory syndrome (SARS)-like coronaviruses in bats, and phylogenetically belonged to the same genus as the coronavirus responsible for the SARS pandemic of 2003.[3] Not yet known at the time, these would be the initial cases that would quickly circumnavigate the globe resulting in the most impactful global pandemic in over 100 years.

2. Reverse Transcription Polymerase Chain Reaction (RT-PCR) Tests

Laboratories around the world were able to quickly develop polymerase chain reaction based diagnostic tests, in some cases, even before the publication of the viral genome on January 11, 2020 by targeting sequences common across all coronaviruses.[4] PCR quickly became the standard for diagnosing cases of SARS-CoV-2. The test utilises small nucleic acid sequences called *primers* that are engineered to bind specific, identified sequences in the RNA genome of the virus. Samples collected for these tests reflect the distribution of the protein receptor that SARS-CoV-2 preferentially binds, the angiotensin converting enzyme 2 protein (*ACE2*). The presence of *ACE2* receptors in the mucosa of the nasopharynx and oropharynx allows for samples to be obtained through a simple swab, as opposed to requiring a bronchoalveolar lavage for every test, and this remains the primary method of sample acquisition for RT-PCR diagnostic tests for SARS-CoV-2. The timing of testing can affect the test sensitivity. More often than not, the first point of contact with the virus occurs in the nasopharynx or oropharynx, and viral loads peak by day 5 and drops off after,[5] however the time course of viral load from lower respiratory tract samples may peak in an independent fashion, often later in the course of illness. This is demonstrated by some patients who are RT-PCR negative on nasopharyngeal swabs, but positive with samples from bronchoalveolar lavage,[6] and has implications on the impact of timing of testing on the test characteristics of PCR.

2.1 *Test accuracy and sensitivity*

The test characteristics have been a major point of interest, as there were initial concerns over the sensitivity of the RT-PCR tests. In a scoping review, Axell-House *et al.*[7] reviewed published testing characteristics for many of the available testing modalities including RT-PCR. In three studies comparing RT-PCR to clinically confirmed cases, the positive agreement rate ranged only between 38.42% and 59%. Further studies that have compared initial RT-PCR tests with subsequent repeat tests report sensitivity ranges from 57.9–94.6%. Only one of these studies reported specificity, which was 100%. Some of the limitations noted of these studies were significant heterogeneity, especially since studies conducted earlier in the pandemic had to contend with comparisons with evolving case definitions. Additionally, the diagnostic accuracy of tests does vary with time following onset of symptoms, with a large scale study of 1113 RT-PCR tests conducted showing positivity rates of 97.9% (for confirmed cases) for samples collected 0–7 days following symptom onset, diminishing to 68.8% for samples collected at 8–14 days post-symptoms onset, and an ongoing decline from there.[8]

One of the early issues that healthcare systems faced during the SARS-CoV-2 pandemic was the need to appropriately scale up the testing capacity. Although confirmed cases would not represent all the true cases in the population, modelling required accurate numbers. Differences in confirmed cases varied during different time points during the pandemic given differences in true community transmission, testing protocols and testing resources. This is especially true in regions that were facing rapid transmission of SARS-CoV-2, as the influx of demand for testing provided the dual concerns of reducing the interpretability of figures such as positivity rate, but also prevented laboratories from allocating resource to scaling up testing capacity. It is estimated that only 14% of true cases were officially documented early in the pandemic in China.[9] Similarly, early on in the pandemic in the United States, it was estimated that only approximately 4.2–16.7% of true cases were identified through testing and reporting.[10] However, estimates for modelling can remain reliable if the proportion of tests to the true case rate remains relatively constant.[11] One of the key estimates in consideration that heavily informs epidemic management strategies is the rate of transmission at each time point (R_t).

2.2 The impact of RT-PCR testing on reproductive rate (R_t)

The likely role of robust testing programs, which were enabled by the scalability and relatively quick turnaround time of RT-PCR, is the ability to quickly identify and isolate infected cases, thus reducing their potential for further transmission. One common framework used to model the dynamics of COVID-19 is the SEIR model[12,13], and is depicted in Figure 1. The SEIR model provides a deterministic framework for flow of individuals susceptible within a population, and the coefficients β, α, and γ are model parameters that characterise the infectious profile of the disease.

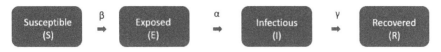

Figure 1:   The SEIR model, where β describes the probability of infection given contact, α describes the latent period of infection, and γ rate of recovery.

The value of the rapid implementation and scaling of RT-PCR is in the modulation of the parameter β. β denotes the probability of moving from the Susceptible compartment to the Exposed, and is a product of the number of contacts and the probability of transmission.[14,15] Timely diagnosis allows for the reduction of number of contacts by prompting isolation of diagnosed individuals, thus lowering β. R_t is proportional to β, therefore reductions in β is one avenue towards reduction of R_t in the overall pandemic control strategy. Early in the pandemic, public health administrations around the world emphasised the importance of quarantine for individuals with potential exposures and isolation of those who became symptomatic,[16] the non-specific nature and variable severity of presentation often meant incomplete adherence to these policies. Access to diagnostic testing helped to mitigate this risk, with laboratory case confirmation often triggering formal isolation recommendations, which for most individuals effectively ended the window of infectiousness. Unfortunately, one characteristic of SARS-CoV-2 is transmission in the absence of symptoms, either asymptomatic individuals (those who never go on to develop symptoms) or pre-symptomatic transmission (a period of infectivity prior to symptom onset).[17]

This can be visualised above in an expounded flow diagram of the SEIR model in Figure 2. Testing programs that focus on symptom triggered testing will only be able to reduce contacts from the symptomatic infectious compartment (I_s), whereas reduction of contacts from the other two contingent compartments (I_p and I_a) would require screening and contact tracing interventions.

These temporal dynamics of viral replication following infection mediates the effect of diagnosis. The SARS-CoV-2 virus has a median incubation of 5.7 days (with a range from 2 to 14 days), and infected individuals who eventually go on to develop symptoms will usually develop

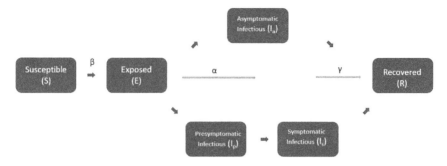

Figure 2: SEIR model where the Infectious compartment is shown to include Asymptomatic Infectious (I_a), Pre-symptomatic (I_p), and Symptomatic Infectious (I_s) individuals.

symptoms at 12 days following infection (with a range of 8–16 days).[18,19] Early epidemiological evidence provided estimates of a median serial interval of 5.2 days with a 95% confidence interval between 4.1 and 6.4 days. Looking at confirmed transmission pairs within their data, they found that approximately 7.6% of transmission links demonstrated a negative serial interval (shorter serial interval than incubation period). Through their model, they estimate that 37–48% of infection events occurred prior to symptom development, with a peak of infectiousness that spans 2 days before and 1 day after symptom onset.[20] However, newer estimates of the serial interval place it at 4 days, which would further increase the estimated duration of asymptomatic transmission.[19] Given that testing criteria in many jurisdictions is focused on symptomatic individuals, there is a high possibility for up to 50% of transmission events to have already occurred. However, that the peak of infectiousness spans until 1 day following onset of symptoms highlights the importance of having the testing capacity to test symptomatic individuals promptly.

Early in the pandemic, before the effects of public health interventions could be detected, R_o rates were estimated in Wuhan, China at a rate between 2.2 and 2.5.[21] In the United States, estimates of R_o during the initial wave of infections was 3.45, varying across states from 1.92 to 5.17.[11] The capability to accurately identify cases in a timely manner has made a large impact on the ability to manage the patients and effectively mitigate the risk of ongoing spread. One important implication of this is that it allowed for separation and management of the capacity of COVID-19 wards, in order to reduce the risk of unprotected exposure of healthcare staff to infectious individuals. One of the most devastating sequelae of an uncontrolled local epidemic occur when healthcare resource capacity is exceeded, which promptly results in both direct and indirect morbidity and mortality. Examples of this were demonstrated early in the pandemic in areas such as Northern Italy and the state of New York,[22,23] and as of writing (April 2021) appear to be unfolding in Brazil.[24,25]

2.3 *Impact and limitations of mass testing*

By March 12, 2020, approximately 2 months since the whole genome sequence of SARS-CoV-2 was published, South Korea had conducted nearly 250,000 tests, second behind China, and nearly 3 times the number of tests conducted by Italy, the next nation on the list.[26] Previous experience with Middle-East respiratory syndrome (MERS) virus in South Korea had primed them for the potential role of mass testing in attempts to contain an epidemic. By April 2020, the testing rate was at 992.8 tests per 100,000 population.[27] The initial testing in South Korea relied predominantly on RT-PCR, quickly approving 4 assays to aggressively scale up testing.[28] Diagnostic testing will always be one of many parts of effective epidemic management of communicable diseases, and the prompt South Korean reaction along with capacity to scale up testing likely led to its ability to very effectively bring down the reproductive rate (R_t) early on in its initial wave of infections. Estimates for South Korea approximate R_t were 2.9 in February 2020, reducing to 2.6 in March 2020, and eventually reaching approximately 1.0 before April 2020.[29] Differences in initial testing capacity can be seen when comparing with jurisdictions with a less robust testing approach. Japan reported its first confirmed case of COVID-19 on January 16, 2020.[30] Compared with South Korea, by April 30, 2020, Japan was only testing at a rate of approximately 3 tests per 100,000 population.[31] What initially appeared as linear growth of active cases, was rapidly uncovered to be exponential, following policy changes on March 4, 2020 when testing dramatically increased.[32] It is implausible that true community cases dramatically rose coincidentally with the increase in testing, and more likely an indication of diagnosing previously missed existing cases due to improved capacity, while the true extent of community cases was previously masked by testing limitations.

Although there have been examples of mass testing being incorporated in successful transmission management responses, there are challenges associated with implementing it on a large scale, and the predominant strategy worldwide has not included wide-scale mass testing. Testing of symptomatic individuals provides a clear inclusion criterion about who needs to be tested, but as mentioned, this comes with the limitation that a significant proportion of infectious individuals will be missed utilising this strategy. The question of to whom to expand testing requires operational considerations, as it is impractical to test everyone given that reagents and capacity for RT-PCR presents a logistic bottleneck that limits testing capacity.[33] An additional limitation presented by large scale testing requires consideration of what you do with the information. For example, screening type testing has been proposed for some special populations such as healthcare workers.[34] However, given the variable sensitivity of the tests, it does not provide enough confidence to be able to impact other transmission control in place and the additional information by this screening for many areas does not strike the appropriate balance between resource allocation and positive benefit.

2.4 *Alternate testing modalities*

Despite rapid development of diagnostic tests, the magnitude of the pandemic has produced great strains on laboratory testing capacity. Many concurrent efforts were undertaken to develop further assays and alternative testing methodologies. As of writing, there are 7 assay protocols provided by the WHO, with different gene sequence targets.[35] The effectiveness of the different assays appear comparable and this has been supported in *in vitro* comparisons.[36] Other similar molecular diagnostic tests exist including reverse transcription loop-mediated isothermal amplification (RT-LAMP), reverse transcription recombinase aided amplification (RT-RAA), droplet digital PCR (ddPCR), and Triplex real-time RT-PCR (rRT-PCR), these methods have been found to have reported sensitivities ranging from 82.8% to –100% (comparing to RT-PCR as opposed to true cases) and reported specificities ranging from 95.6% to –100%.[7]

Nucleic acid based tests are not the only diagnostic modality available, as increasingly, point of care tests are being developed based on detection of antigens that can be resulted in minutes, and their utility profile may be useful in addressing the gaps left by RT-PCR testing alone. These modalities will be discussed in the next chapter.

3. Viral Genomics

Genomic information and sequencing techniques have provided foundational knowledge that contributed in two different responses to the pandemic: outbreak investigation and ongoing surveillance.

3.1 *Outbreak investigation*

Early management strategies and efforts focused on characterisation of both the SARS-CoV-2 virus with a focus on outbreak investigation. The identification and dissemination of the genomic sequence of SARS-CoV-2 provided the information needed to develop diagnostic tests. Global response was rapid following the release of the whole genome sequence allowing for the development of nucleic acid based diagnostic tests such as reverse transcription polymerase chain reaction (RT-PCR). These assay protocols allowed for public health systems to use laboratory confirmed case definitions to organise the initial epidemic control responses. As well, the genetic information identified similarities with previously characterised coronaviruses, providing useful data for generating hypotheses on elements such as the likely mode of transmission, portal of entry, target receptors, as well as potential targets for therapies. The 16 non-structural proteins and at least 10 structural proteins have contributed to the understanding of the basis of infectiousness of the virus, as well as possible targets for vaccine development.[37,38]

Whole genome sequencing (WGS) helped to establish probable chains of transmission in cases with sparse/missing epidemiological links[39] by allowing public health agencies to correctly group case clusters, supplementing conventional epidemiological methods, and helped to select transmission-mitigating policies to implement. Genomic data was effectively collected and shared internationally through GISAID,[40] and it was seen that SARS-CoV-2 was undergoing genetic diversification in its global spread,[41–43] During the early stages of the pandemic a D614G substitution emerged;[44,45] this mutation in a coding region of the S (spike) protein is thought to have contributed to increased infectivity and subsequent spread.[46] Viruses in the *Coronaviridae* family use the spike protein to bind to the receptor on the host cells and SARS-CoV-2 spike protein with D614G substitution shows approximately 10–20 times higher affinity for *ACE2* compared to the wild-type spike protein of the original Wuhan strain of SARS-CoV-2.[38] D614G-containing strains have become the dominant strains of SARS-CoV-2 in world-wide circulation.[44]

3.2 *Ongoing surveillance*

More recently, as strain divergence has become a key issue, the focus of sequencing laboratories is shifting towards surveillance for the identification of emerging variants of SARS-CoV-2. The risk for the development of variants that confer a survival advantage to the virus, like the D614G substitution exists, and analytical frameworks have been established to classify identified variants that focus on the following factors: potential for further zoonotic emergence, transmissibility between humans, infection severity, susceptibility to adaptive immunity, response to vaccines, and response to therapeutics.[47] Evaluated against these factors, the Centre for Disease Control (CDC) differentiates strains as variants of interest (VOI), variants of concern (VOC), and variants of high consequence (VOHC, of which there are currently none).[48] Typically, a variant is classified as a VOI when there is clinical suspicion and/or limited evidence that the variant shows advantageous adaptations with respect to the factors listed above compared to the wild-type SARS-CoV-2. As evidence increases for adaptations, particularly with respect to diagnostic interference, increased transmissibility, increased disease severity, and interference with adaptive immunity including vaccine efficacy, the variant will be classified as a VOC. Finally, the label of VOHC is reserved for variants that have been associated with demonstrable failure of diagnostics, therapeutics, and/or significant increase in severe disease.

One of the earliest VOI was identified in Denmark, and labelled "Cluster 5" variant.[49] This variant arose in the setting of infected mink on mink farms. While there was earlier evidence of the human to mink to human transmission of SARS-CoV-2 virus,[49,50] the concern upon emergence of "Cluster 5" was related to the observed impacts of the accumulated mutations on susceptibility to antibody neutralisation,[51] although there were conflicting observations in this regard.[52] The concern for the creation of a potential new viral reservoir[53] prompted massive culls on mink farms. Other more notable variants, colloquially known by the name of the regions in which they were first identified, include SARS-CoV-2 B.1.1.7 (UK), SARS-CoV-2 B.1.351 (South Africa), and SARS-CoV-2 P.1 (Brazil),[54–56] and two variants B.1.427 and B.1.429 first detected in California.[48] Currently, there are 3 identified VOI and 5 VOC, which are summarised below in Table 1. Given the potential for variants to develop characteristics that reduce effectiveness of pandemic control measures such as diagnostics or vaccination, there is need for ongoing surveillance strategies.[57,58]

In terms of surveillance efforts, a gap exists between countries that have undertaken strong genomic surveillance such as the UK, where approximately 6–8% of positive samples are sequenced[59] compared to the United States where approximately 0.3% of positive samples are sequenced.[60] There is room for debate on what constitutes an ideal proportion of positive samples to sequence for monitoring for genetic variants, however a benchmark of 5% has been discussed as a feasible target.[56] Using the United States as an example, a strategy that implements increased sequencing will correspondingly require efficient coordination amongst laboratories in different states to identify potential new VOC. With ongoing high volume of active infections, network sensitivity will become an important feature in order to be able to identify and respond to variations in infectivity, evasion of diagnostic tests, or — particularly salient amidst the current vaccination efforts — reduced vaccine efficacy. To facilitate the coordination required, some researchers at Johns Hopkins University suggest replicating federal surveillance systems that countries such as the UK and Denmark have.[56]

The continued implementation of WGS faces several challenges as healthcare systems continue to adapt to the evolving pandemic. Some countries, such as Canada, have identified the use of sequencing as an important element and have invested resources to create an integrated

Table 1:   Variants of interest (VOI) and variants of concern (VOC) of SARS-CoV-2 that have been identified by the US CDC.[48]

Classification	Variant	Country/Region of initial discovery	Potential implications
(None)	"Cluster 5"	Denmark	(1) Mink serving as viral reservoir and/or new vector of transmission
VOI	SARS-CoV-2 B.1.526	New York/USA	(1) Potential reduction in neutralisation by Monoclonal Antibody Treatments (2) Potential reduction in neutralisation by convalescent and post-vaccination sera
VOI	SARS-CoV-2 B.1.525	New York/USA	(1) Potential reduction in neutralisation by monoclonal antibody treatments (2) Potential reduction in neutralisation by convalescent and post-vaccination sera
VOI	SARS-CoV-2 P.2	Brazil	(1) Potential reduction in neutralisation by monoclonal antibody treatments (2) Potential reduction in neutralisation by convalescent and post-vaccination sera
VOC	SARS-CoV-2 B.1.1.7	United Kingdom	(1) Increased Transmissibility (~50%) (2) Likely increased severity
VOC	SARS-CoV-2 B.1.351	South Africa	(1) Increased Transmissibility (~50%) (2) Moderate impact on neutralisation by monoclonal antibody treatments (3) Moderate reduction on neutralisation by convalescent and post-vaccination sera
VOC	SARS-CoV-2 P.1	Brazil/Japan	(1) Moderate impact on neutralisation by monoclonal antibody treatments (2) Reduced neutralisation by convalescent and post-vaccination sera (3) Likely increased severity
VOC	SARS-CoV-2 B.1.427	California/USA	(1) Increased Transmissibility (~20%) (2) Significant impact on neutralisation by monoclonal antibody treatments (3) Moderate reduction on neutralisation by convalescent and post-vaccination sera
VOC	SARS-CoV-2 B.1.429	California/USA	(1) Increased Transmissibility (~20%) (2) Significant impact on neutralisation by monoclonal antibody treatments (3) Moderate reduction on neutralisation by convalescent and post-vaccination sera

Notes: Variants of interest are characterised by potential impact to transmissibility, diagnosis, disease severity, response to vaccinations, and response to therapeutics. Variants of concern are characterised by evidence in support of impact to the same factors.

approach at regional and federal levels.[61] Adequate resource and capacity allows for a balance between outbreak investigation, where it can inform travel-restriction strategies and outbreak investigations at a more granular level,[62,63] and sentinel surveillance which requires random sampling without *a priori* detection biases.[56] Creating efficient data sharing pipelines that connect regional, national, and international databases, standardised definitions for classifying variants, and coordinated monitoring strategies will all be instrumental in early recognition for further VOC and prevention of VOHC.

4. Conclusion

In this section we started off by describing the first developed and still gold standard for diagnosing COVID-19, which is RT-PCR. We discussed how it plays a role in reducing R_t by helping to identify, confirm positive cases and appropriately recommend isolation in order to break the links of transmission. The foundation for the development of the nucleic acid diagnostic methods was based on whole genome sequence information. Initial COVID-19 management responses were facilitated by the identification of the WGS, and having a platform for information sharing. As much as it has played a key role in the early stages of the pandemic response, WGS remains an important part of pandemic response in identifying and responding to emerging VOC. Many regions around the world are shifting the focus of WGS from active outbreak investigations towards establishing adequate surveillance systems to ensure timely identification of potential VOC. Although, nucleic acid test diagnostic tests remain an important element of the COVID-19 response, other identified gaps in the real of diagnostics such as point-of-care testing and identification of post-infection status are in the purview of other diagnostic modalities, which will be addressed in the next chapter.

References

1. Wu F, Zhao S, Yu B, Chen YM, Wang W, Song ZG, *et al*. A new coronavirus associated with human respiratory disease in China. *Nature*. 2020;579 (7798):265–269.

2. Jiang G-M, Ren X, Liu Y, Chen H, Liu W, Guo Z, *et al.* Application and optimization of RT-PCR in diagnosis of SARS-CoV-2 infection. *Lancet Infectious Disease.* 2020.

3. Yang Y, Peng F, Wang R, Guan K, Jiang T, Xu G, *et al.* The deadly coronaviruses: The 2003 SARS pandemic and the 2020 novel coronavirus epidemic in China. *Journal of Autoimmunity.* [Internet]. 2020;109(March 2020): 102434. Available from: https://doi.org/10.1016/j.jaut.2020.102434.

4. Mahase E. Coronavirus: NHS staff get power to keep patients in isolation as UK declares "serious threat." *BMJ* [Internet]. 2020;368(February):m550. Available from: http://dx.doi.org/doi:10.1136/bmj.m550.

5. Wölfel R, Corman VM, Guggemos W, Seilmaier M, Zange S, Müller MA, *et al.* Virological assessment of hospitalized patients with COVID-2019. *Nature.* 2020;581(7809):465–469.

6. Little BP. False-negative nasopharyngeal swabs and positive bronchoalveolar lavage: Implications for chest CT in diagnosis of COVID-19 pneumonia. *Radiology.* 2021;298(3).

7. Axell-House DB, Lavingia R, Rafferty M, Clark E, Amirian ES, Chiao EY. The estimation of diagnostic accuracy of tests for COVID-19: A scoping review. *Journal of Infection.* [Internet]. 2020;81(5):681–697. Available from: https://doi.org/10.1016/j.jinf.2020.08.043.

8. Xiao AT, Tong YX, Gao C, Zhu L, Zhang YJ, Zhang S. Dynamic profile of RT-PCR findings from 301 COVID-19 patients in Wuhan, China: A descriptive study. *Journal of Clinical Virology.* 2020;127(March):0–6.

9. Li R, Pei S, Chen B, Song Y, Zhang T, Yang W, *et al.* Substantial undocumented infection facilitates the rapid dissemination of novel coronavirus (SARS-CoV-2). *Science.* (80-). 2020;368(6490):489–493.

10. Noh J, Danuser G. Estimation of the fraction of COVID-19 infected people in U.S. states and countries worldwide. *PLoS One* [Internet]. 2021;16(2): e0246772. Available from: http://dx.doi.org/10.1371/journal.pone.0246772.

11. Pitzer VE, Chitwood M, Havumaki J, Menzies NA, Perniciaro S, Warren JL, *et al.* The impact of changes in diagnostic testing practices on estimates of COVID-19 transmission in the United States. *medRxiv.* 2020.

12. Linka K, Peirlinck M, Kuhl E. The reproduction number of COVID-19 and its correlation with public health interventions. *Computational Mechanics.* [Internet]. 2020 [cited 2021 Apr 17];66:1035–1050. Available from: https://doi.org/10.1007/s00466-020-01880-8.

13. Carcione JM, Santos JE, Bagaini C, Ba J. A simulation of a COVID-19 epidemic based on a deterministic SEIR model. *Frontiers in Public Health.* 2020;8(May).

14. Tang Z, Li X, Li H. Prediction of New Coronavirus Infection Based on a Modified SEIR Model. [cited 2021 Apr 17]; Available from: https://doi.org/10.1101/2020.03.03.20030858.

15. Jones JH. Notes On R 0 1 The Basic Reproduction Number in a Nutshell. 2007.

16. WHO. Considerations for quarantine of contacts of COVID-19 cases. World Heal Organ [Internet]. 2020;(August):19082020. Available from: https://www.who.int/publications/i/item/considerations-for-quarantine-of-individuals-in-the-context-of-containment-for-coronavirus-disease-(covid-19).

17. Wu Z, Mcgoogan JM. Asymptomatic and pre-symptomatic COVID-19 in China. [cited 2021 Apr 17]; Available from: https://doi.org/10.1186/s40249-020-00679-2.

18. Weissleder R, Lee H, Ko J, Pittet MJ. COVID-19 diagnostics in context. *Science Translational Medicine*. 2020;12(546):1–7.

19. Salzberger B, Buder F, Lampl B, Ehrenstein B, Hitzenbichler F, Holzmann T, *et al*. Epidemiology of SARS-CoV-2. *Infection* [Internet]. 2020;(0123456789). Available from: https://doi.org/10.1007/s15010-020-01531-3.

20. He X, Lau EHY, Wu P, Deng X, Wang J, Hao X, *et al*. Temporal dynamics in viral shedding and transmissibility of COVID-19. *Nature Medicine*. 2020; 26(5):672–675.

21. Li Q, Guan X, Wu P, Wang X, Zhou L, Tong Y, *et al*. Early transmission dynamics in Wuhan, China, of novel Coronavirus-infected pneumonia. *New England Journal of Medicine*. 2020,382(13):1199–1207.

22. Gibertoni D, Adja KYC, Golinelli D, Reno C, Regazzi L, Lenzi J, *et al*. Patterns of COVID-19 related excess mortality in the municipalities of Northern Italy during the first wave of the pandemic. *Heal Place* [Internet]. 2021;67(May 2020):102508. Available from: https://doi.org/10.1016/j.healthplace.2021.102508.

23. Branas CC, Rundle A, Pei S, Yang W, Carr BG, Sims S, *et al*. Flattening the curve before it flattens us: Hospital critical care capacity limits and mortality from novel coronavirus (SARS-CoV2) cases in US counties. *medRxiv*. 2020;1–14.

24. Reuters T. Brazil COVID-19 deaths top 66,000 in March alone [Internet]. Canadian Broadcast Corporation. 2021 [cited 2021 Apr 2]. Available from: https://www.cbc.ca/news/world/brazil-covid-deaths-1.5973426.

25. Phillips T. Brazil stares into the abyss as Covid intensive care units fill up everywhere [Internet]. *The Guardian*. 2021 [cited 2021 Apr 2]. Available from: https://www.theguardian.com/world/2021/mar/19/brazil-coronavirus-intensive-care-unit-capacity.

26. Balilla J. Assessment of COVID-19 mass testing: The case of South Korea. *SSRN Electronic Journal.* 2020;(March).
27. Sen-Crowe B, McKenney M, Elkbuli A. COVID-19 response and containment strategies in the US, South Korea, and Iceland: Lessons learned and future directions. *American Journal of Emergency Medicine.* 2020;38(7):1537–1539.
28. Chang MC, Baek JH, Park D. Lessons from South Korea regarding the early stage of the COVID-19 outbreak. *Healthcare.* 2020;8(3):229.
29. Shim E, Tariq A, Chowell G. Spatial variability in reproduction number and doubling time across two waves of the COVID-19 pandemic in South Korea, February to July, 2020. *International Journal of Infectious Disease* [Internet]. 2021;102:1–9. Available from: https://doi.org/10.1016/j.ijid.2020. 10.007.
30. Schnirring L. Japan has 1st novel coronavirus case; China reports another death [Internet]. Center for Infectious Disease Research and Policy, 2020. Available from: https://www.cidrap.umn.edu/news-perspective/2020/01/ japan-has-1st-novel-coronavirus-case-china-reports-another-death.
31. Hasell J, Mathieu E, Beltekian D. A cross-country database of COVID-19 testing [Internet]. Our World in Data. 2021 [cited 2021 Mar 15]. Available from: https://ourworldindata.org/coronavirus-testing.
32. Omori R, Mizumoto K, Chowell G. Changes in testing rates could mask the novel coronavirus disease (COVID-19) growth rate. *International Journal of Infectious Disease* [Internet]. 2020;94:116–118. Available from: https://doi. org/10.1016/j.ijid.2020.04.021.
33. Smyrlaki I, Ekman M, Lentini A, Rufino de Sousa N, Papanicolaou N, Vondracek M, *et al.* Massive and rapid COVID-19 testing is feasible by extraction-free SARS-CoV-2 RT-PCR. *Nature Communications* [Internet]. 2020 Dec 1 [cited 2021 Apr 17];11(1):1–12. Available from: https://doi. org/10.1038/s41467-020-18611-5.
34. Henderson CE, Jackman JM, Md S. Covid-19 testing of asymptomatic individuals-no benefit but consequential false sense security. *Neurology and Therapeutics.*
35. World Health Organization. WHO Summary of Diagnostic Assays [Internet]. 2020 [cited 2021 Mar 15]. Available from: https://www.who.int/docs/default-source/coronaviruse/whoinhouseassays.pdf.
36. van Kasteren PB, van der Veer B, van den Brink S, Wijsman L, de Jonge J, van den Brandt A, *et al.* Comparison of seven commercial RT-PCR diagnostic kits for COVID-19. *Journal of Clinical Virology* [Internet]. 2020;128(April):104412. Available from: https://doi.org/10.1016/j.jcv. 2020.104412.

37. Cagliani R, Forni D, Clerici M, Sironi M. Coding potential and sequence conservation of SARS-CoV-2 and related animal viruses. *Infection, Genetics and Evolution* [Internet]. 2020;83(March):104353. Available from: https://doi.org/10.1016/j.meegid.2020.104353.

38. Uddin M, Mustafa F, Rizvi TA, Loney T, Al Suwaidi H, Al-Marzouqi AHH, *et al.* SARS-CoV-2/COVID-19: Viral genomics, epidemiology, vaccines, and therapeutic interventions. *Viruses.* 2020;12(526):81–88.

39. Rockett RJ, Arnott A, Lam C, Sadsad R, Timms V, Gray KA, *et al.* Revealing COVID-19 transmission in Australia by SARS-CoV-2 genome sequencing and agent-based modeling. *Nature Medicine* [Internet]. 2020;26(9): 1398–1404. Available from: http://dx.doi.org/10.1038/s41591-020-1000-7.

40. GISAID. Tracking of Variants [Internet]. 2021 [cited 2021 Mar 15]. Available from: https://www.gisaid.org/hcov19-variants/.

41. Yuan F, Wang L, Fang Y, Wang L. Global SNP analysis of 11,183 SARS-CoV-2 strains reveals high genetic diversity. *Transboundary and Emerging Disease.* 2020;(August):1–17.

42. Phan T. Genetic diversity and evolution of SARS-CoV-2. *Infection, Genetics and Evolution* [Internet]. 2020;81(February):104260. Available from: https://doi.org/10.1016/j.meegid.2020.104260.

43. van Dorp L, Acman M, Richard D, Shaw LP, Ford CE, Ormond L, *et al.* Emergence of genomic diversity and recurrent mutations in SARS-CoV-2. *Infection, Genetics and Evolution* [Internet]. 2020;83(April):104351. Available from: https://doi.org/10.1016/j.meegid.2020.104351.

44. Plante JA, Liu Y, Liu J, Xia H, Johnson BA, Lokugamage KG, *et al.* Spike mutation D614G alters SARS-CoV-2 fitness. *Nature* [Internet]. 2020; (September). Available from: http://dx.doi.org/10.1038/s41586-020-2895-3.

45. Hou YJ, Okuda K, Edwards CE, Martinez DR, Asakura T, Dinnon KH, *et al.* SARS-CoV-2 reverse genetics reveals a variable infection gradient in the respiratory tract. *Cell.* 2020;182(2):429–446.e14.

46. Korber B, Fischer WM, Gnanakaran S, Yoon H, Theiler J, Abfalterer W, *et al.* Tracking changes in SARS-CoV-2 spike: Evidence that D614G increases infectivity of the COVID-19 Virus. *Cell.* 2020;182(4):812–827.e19.

47. Public Health England. SARS-CoV-2 variants of concern and variants under investigation in England technical briefing 7. 2021;(March).

48. Center for Disease Control. SARS-CoV-2 Variant Classifications and Definitions [Internet]. 2021 [cited 2021 Apr 4]. Available from: https://www.cdc.gov/coronavirus/2019-ncov/cases-updates/variant-surveillance/variant-info.html#:~:text=Variants of concern might require,vaccines and treatments against the.

49. Larsen HD, Fonager J, Lomholt FK, Dalby T, Benedetti G, Kristensen B, *et al.* Preliminary report of an outbreak of SARS-CoV-2 in mink and mink farmers associated with community spread, Denmark, June to November 2020. *Eurosurveillance.* 2021;26(5).

50. Boklund A, Hammer AS, Quaade ML, Rasmussen TB, Lohse L, Strandbygaard B, *et al.* SARS-CoV-2 in Danish mink farms: Course of the epidemic and a descriptive analysis of the outbreaks in 2020. *Animals.* 2021;11(1):1–16.

51. Hayashi T, Yaegashi N, Konishi I. Effect of RBD (Y453F) mutation in spike glycoprotein of SARS-CoV-2 on neutralizing IgG affinity. Preprint. 2021.

52. Bayarri-Olmos R, Rosbjerg A, Johnsen LB, Helgstrand C, Bak-Thomsen T, Garred P, *et al.* The SARS-CoV-2 Y453F mink variant displays a pronounced increase in ACE-2 affinity but does not challenge antibody neutralization. *Journal of Biological Chemistry* [Internet]. 2021;100536. Available from: https://doi.org/10.1016/j.jbc.2021.100536.

53. Koopmans M. SARS-CoV-2 and the human–animal interface: Outbreaks on mink farms. *Lancet Infectious Disease* [Internet]. 2021;21(1):18–9. Available from: http://dx.doi.org/10.1016/S1473-3099(20)30912-9.

54. Naveca F, Souza V, Costa C. COVID-19 epidemic in the Brazilian state of Amazonas was driven by long-term persistence of endemic SARS-CoV-2 lineages and the recent emergence of the new Variant of Concern P. 1. Pre-Print. 2021;1–21.

55. Plante JA, Mitchell BM, Plante KS, Debbink K, Weaver SC, Menachery VD. The variant Gambit: COVID's next Move. *Cell Host Microbe* [Internet]. 2021; Available from: https://doi.org/10.1016/j.phrs.2020.104743.

56. Warmbrod KL, West R, Frieman M, George D, Martin E, Rivers C. Staying ahead of the variants: Policy recommendations to identify and manage current and future variants of concern staying ahead of the variants: Policy recommendations to identify and manage current and future variants of concern. Johns Hopkins Cent Heal Secur. 2021;(February).

57. Bal A, Destras G, Gaymard A, Stefic K, Marlet J, Eymieux S, *et al.* Two-step strategy for the identification of SARS-CoV-2 variant of concern 202012/01 and other variants with spike deletion H69-V70, France, August to December 2020. *Eurosurveillance.* 2021;26(3):1–5.

58. Stephenson J. Report outlines strategy for surveillance of emerging corona-virus variants. *JAMA Heal Forum* [Internet]. 2021 Feb 23;2(2):e210246–e210246. Available from: https://doi.org/10.1001/jamahealthforum.2021.0246.

59. COVID-19 Genomics UK Consortium. Summary Report: COG-UK geographic coverage of SARS-CoV-2 sample sequencing. 2020.

60. Stevens H, Berger M. U.S. ranks 43rd worldwide in sequencing to check for coronavirus variants like the one found in the U.K. [Internet]. *The Washington Post*. 2020 [cited 2021 Mar 15]. Available from: https://www. washingtonpost.com/world/2020/12/23/us-leads-world-coronavirus-cases-ranks-43rd-sequencing-check-variants/.

61. Public Health Agency of Canada. Government of Canada invests $53 million to address COVID-19 virus variants of concern [Internet]. 2021 [cited 2021 Apr 5]. Available from: https://www.newswire.ca/news-releases/government-of-canada-invests-53-million-to-address-covid-19-virus-variants-of-concern-884120129.html.

62. Meijer SE, Harel N, Ben-Ami R, Nahari M, Yakubovsky M, Oster HS, *et al*. Unraveling a nosocomial outbreak of COVID-19: The role of whole genome sequence analysis. *Open Forum Infectious Disease*. 2021.

63. Park AK, Kim I-H, Kim J, Kim J-M, Kim HM, Lee CY, *et al*. Osong public health and research perspectives genomic surveillance of SARS-CoV-2: Distribution of clades in the republic of Korea in 2020. *Osong Public Health and Research Persepctives*. 2021;12(1):37–43.

https://doi.org/10.1142/9789811249723_0006

Chapter 6

Antigen and Antibody Testing

Margaret Lin[*] and Mohammad Morshed[†,‡]

[*]*School of Population and Public Health, University of British Columbia, Vancouver, Canada*

[†]*Public Health Laboratory, BC Centre for Disease Control, Vancouver, Canada*

[‡]*Department of Pathology and Laboratory Medicine, Vancouver, Canada*

Key Message

- Antigen tests detect current infection with the virus similar to reverse transcription quantitative polymerase chain reaction (RT-qPCR).
- Antibody tests use blood samples to detect the presence of anti-SARS-CoV-2 IgM, IgG or a combination of IgM and IgG, which determines previous exposure.
- Point of care (POC) antigen tests are delivered via lateral flow assays on cassettes and can give results within minutes compared to RT-qPCR; however, the lack of an amplification step decreases the sensitivity of these tests to low viral titers.
- POC antibody tests can be used in seroprevalence studies and to evaluate the efficacy of vaccines, but caution must be taken when interpreting the results in the context of return to work.

- POC testing is insufficient alone to curb the spread of SARS-CoV-2; any rapid testing programs must be combined with social preventative measures.

1. Protein-based Testing

As the innate and adaptive immune system mount a response to SARS-CoV-2 infection, specific tests can identify the presence of COVID-19 antigens and antibodies. While the gold standard for COVID-19 detection is real time quantitative polymerase chain reaction (RT-qPCR) with samples from the nasopharynx, throat or saliva,[1] there is a delay between testing and informing the individual due to the time it takes to perform RT-qPCR and return results to individual. Rapidly disseminated tests to detect COVID-19 infection are thus necessary to help control the spread of infection.

Point of care (POC) testing can be defined as decentralised testing that can be performed with minimal training, requires minimal equipment, easily transportable, and provide results within two hours.[2,3] The results can be more rapidly disseminated than those of molecular testing, often while the individual being tested is still present. While antigen and antibody testing may also have a place as diagnostic tools within COVID care units, the higher sensitivity of RT-qPCR[4] will likely keep molecular methods as the test of choice within healthcare institutions. An individual with a negative SARS-CoV-2 antigen test may have a positive RT-qPCR result, and thus it is important to consider where the individual may be in the course of infection when evaluating if further diagnostic testing is required.[5]

Encounters between SARS-CoV-2 and immune cells fragment viral proteins into antigens for immune recognition. SARS-CoV-2 antigens can be detected during current infection, though a certain titer is needed before most tests can detect antigens. The presence of antigens serves as a marker for active infection, and thus can be used for diagnostics. Antibodies develop later in the course of the immune response once the body has mounted a defence, and thus can be used to determine previous exposure to infection. However, it should be noted that differing severities of COVID-19 infection mount different antibody responses, and quickly

Table 1:   Summary of COVID-19 protein-based testing.

	Antibody test	**Antigen test**
Target	Human-produced antibodies towards COVID-19: IgM, IgG, potentially IgA	COVID-19 component proteins: spike protein, nucleocapsid protein Less sensitive in tests: envelope protein, membrane protein[7]
Time for sampling	IgA and IgM: detectable at least 5 days since symptom onset[7] IgG: detectable at least 14 days since symptom onset[7] Lab test: Theoretically can capture as soon as antibody response is initiated, but likelihood of detection is increased during peak antibody titers	POC test: While antigen tests can be performed at any time, may only return a positive result with high viral load, such as the first 7 days post-symptom onset[8,9] Lab test: Theoretically, could capture at any time, but lab antigen tests are not generally performed
Site sampled	Blood, plasma, serum[10]	Nasopharyngeal swab, saliva, urine, gargle lavage, throat swab, nasal vestibule swab, sputum, tracheal aspirate[1,11]
Use	Test for past infection, seroprevalence study	Diagnose active infection

resolved infections may not confer the same level of protection as that from a severe disease course.[6] Viral load and antibody titers follow curves that influence the reproduction number of the virus. Therefore, serology tests can be used for an epidemiological perspective and an immunity perspective of the COVID-19 pandemic. The major differences between tests are summarised in Table 1.

1.1 *Antigen tests*

1.1.1 *Antigen test structure*

Diagnostic tests for COVID-19 primarily use the viral RNA to define the presence of absence of SARS-CoV-2. The single stranded RNA is vulnerable to heat and degradation by ribonucleases in the environment, which necessitates additional precautions to preserve samples. While proteases are also present in the environment, the stability of proteins makes them an alternate target for testing.

Lab-based testing, such as enzyme-linked immunosorbent assay (ELISA) is the gold standard for detection of COVID-19 proteins.[12] The primary interest in antigen testing lies in POC testing for rapid dissemination of results. POC antigen tests use lateral flow immunoassays (LFA) with either colloidal gold-labeled antibodies (CGIA) or fluorescent-labeled antibodies (LFIA).[3] Rapid antigen test strips are loaded onto a cassette,[3] similar to a home pregnancy test, for ease of distribution and use. The sample moves along the test strip to the lines of anti-antigen antibodies; if viral antigens are present, the antibodies will attach to the antigens and trigger the signal. Colloidal gold-based tests produce a visible line on the test strip, while immunofluorescent antibody tests require an immunofluorescence analyzer to identify a positive result.[3] The reaction happens within minutes, which permits individuals with positive results to be rapidly notified.

1.1.2 *Utility of antigen testing*

While vaccines for COVID-19 are generally targeted towards spike proteins,[13] antigen tests generally have antibodies for nucleocapsid proteins[10] as there is less variability and mutation in this region. Commercially produced antigen tests examined in the literature base include products from Beijing Savant, Shenzhen Bioeasy, Coris BioConcept, Liming Bio-Products and RapiGEN Inc.[3] While the early pandemic saw COVID-19 testing primarily by molecular methods, as of 2021 governments have rolled out an antigen testing program alongside a robust RT-qPCR program. The Canadian public health system, for example, has provided guidance for the implementation of the Abbott Panbio™ COVID-19 rapid antigen test across provinces.[14]

Antigen tests allow for infectious individuals at their peak viral titers to be identified and isolated. However, a certain threshold of antigen titer must be present in the individual's sample for the test to work. SARS-CoV-2 viral loads appear to peak in the upper respiratory tract during the first week of illness, but the viral peak also occurs just before or at the onset of symptoms.[15] While antigen testing may assist in identifying asymptomatic individuals, it may not capture individuals with low level viral shedding. Antigen tests also cannot determine the stage of infection, and whether the individual is resolving the infection or has newly acquired SARS-CoV-2. Antigen test results must be interpreted cautiously rather than an absolute determination of an individual's infection state.

1.2 *Antibody tests*

1.2.1 *Humoral immune response*

The kinetics of humoral response in COVID-19 are under investigation in cohorts across the world. Humoral response activates B cells and helper T-cells to generate antibodies that will neutralise, mark for opsonisation, or activate the complement system to help fight the pathogens.

Immunoglobulins (Ig), also known as antibodies, are classified as IgM, IgG, IgA, IgD, or IgE based on their structure and immunological properties. Antibodies can also be classified by function. Binding antibodies, upon attaching to a pathogen, make a pathogen easier for the immune system to detect. Neutralising antibodies stop a pathogen's ability to infect or divide, and can confer life-long immunity.[16] While infection with SARS-CoV-2 will generate both types of antibodies, research in rhesus macaques suggests that neutralising antibodies against spike proteins may prevent infection by rapidly initiating immunologic control rather than by providing sterilising immunity.[17]

Antibodies are also generated in progressive waves. IgM is the first indication of the body's response to an infection, but these antibodies tend be shorter lasting and less specific.[18] Class-switching then leads to a rise in IgG and IgM titers as the immune response progresses.[18] IgG for SARS-CoV infection have been documented to peak 4 months after infection, while IgM titers peaked 4 weeks after symptom onset.[19] Individuals with SARS-CoV2 infection seroconvert as early as 2 days after symptom onset, and 44–56% of patients have IgG by day 7 after symptom onset.[20] Anti-nucleocapsid IgM increase early but decline to undetectable levels by 2 months, while anti-spike protein IgG and anti-nucleocapsid IgG persist even 4 months after diagnosis.[20] The waves of antibody response must be considered when interpreting an antibody test's results.

Further research into the antibody profile of SARS-CoV-2 infection has revealed that the type of humoral response confers different lengths of immunity.[6] Asymptomatic and milder disease courses tend to be associated with lower antibody titers; these antibodies also remain in the body for a shorter period of time compared to individuals with more severe disease.[6] Lower IgM titers in particular have been seen in patients with milder disease.[21] The significance of antibody titers, in particular IgM, generally requires clinical experience to interpret.

1.2.2 *Antibody test structure*

The gold standard for antibody testing is ELISA; however, the materials needed for ELISA are not portable and the 2–5 hour long time to results is not conducive to POC testing.[10,22] Neutralisation assays may also be used to evaluate the presence of anti-SARS-CoV-2 antibodies, but these tests generally need three to five days before results are available.[22] ELISA, chemiluminescence immunoassay (CLIA), or LFA can be used for rapid antibody tests.[3] Most antibody tests evaluate IgG, IgM or a ratio of IgG/IgM,[23] though it is possible to target IgA. POC testing for antibodies is performed in a similar manner to that of antigen testing, using cassettes enclosing a LFA. Positive results for antibodies may be visualised through colour particles, alkaline phosphatase, colour latex, or platinum-gold colloids.[1] The specific visualisation method differs based on the manufacturer of the rapid antibody test. Commercial antibody tests are less common than antigen tests, and many studies that compare the performance of these tests to gold standard RT-qPCR have issues with biases.[23]

1.2.3 *Utility of antibody testing*

As the COVID-19 pandemic progressed, political and social factors pushed for interventions that would permit reopening locations to pre-pandemic use.[22] At the time, the political interest in antibody testing was its use to evaluate if individuals could safely return to work.[10] However, as news of reinfections and questions regarding the length of immunity arose, antibody tests as passports to reopening seemed less feasible. From an immunological perspective, antibody tests can be used to understand the dynamics of how the body responds to COVID-19 and what immunity may be gained from different levels of infection.[10] However, a positive antibody test result does not mean the individual will be permanently safe from further SARS-CoV-2 infection.

While some political authorities have advocated the development of herd immunity by infecting individuals, the immunity conferred by infection can differ from that of vaccines. Ideally, individuals would develop sterilising immunity and thus not be at risk of reinfection.[20] While it is theoretically possible to develop antibody tests that identify neutralising immunoglobulins, it may not be practical to roll out these tests when vaccination records are available.

1.3 *Real life considerations for POC testing*

Sensitivity measures how often a test correctly classifies individuals with a condition as positive, while specificity measures how often a test correctly classifies individuals without the condition as negative.[24] The sensitivity and specificity of protein-based testing versus molecular methods of detecting SARS-CoV-2 determine which test should be used in a particular scenario. However, as protein-based testing does not contain an amplification step to increase the amount of detectable viral material within a sample, both antigen and antibody testing are inherently less sensitive than RT-qPCR. This drawback also specifies time periods in which POC antigen and antibody tests may be best deployed: they must occur during peak antibody or antigen titers for the greatest likelihood of giving a correct positive result.

A Cochrane review found the average sensitivity of rapid RNA-based methods was 95.2% (95% CI: 86.7%, 98.3% from 11 studies) versus the average sensitivity of 56.2% (95% CI: 29.5%, 79.8% across 15 studies) of rapid antigen tests.[3] The average specificity was similar across molecular methods (98.9%, 95% CI: 97.3%, 99.5%) and antigen testing (99.5%, 95% CI: 98.1%, 99.9%).[3] While all but one of the antigen tests in the Cochrane review were commercial tests, the academic test had decent sensitivity (68%) and specificity (100%).[3] Table 2 summarises the sensitivity and specificity of antigen tests from select reviews.

When deploying POC tests, pre-test probability must also be considered when evaluating the results in an epidemiological framework. Pre-test probability is defined as the likelihood that a patient has a disease before the test is performed.[26] While sensitivity and specificity are not affected by disease prevalence, the positive predictive value (PPV) and the negative predictive value (NPV) are affected by prevalence.[24] The PPV describes the ability of a clinical test to correctly identify individuals who are positive for the condition, while the NPV describes the probability that an individual who tests negative does not in fact have the disease. In situations with high prevalence of SARS-CoV-2 infection, the PPV is inflated as it describes the percentage of individuals with a positive test who does have SARS-CoV-2 infection, which is higher in this scenario. Thus, it may become more difficult to assess which individuals are negative for the virus. When the prevalence of SARS-CoV-2 infection is low, a test with a higher specificity may help in ruling out who is not infected. Similar issues are found in rapid antibody testing. A Cochrane meta-analysis of hospitalised patients found that commercial antibody tests may have inflated positive results in high-risk scenarios, thus overestimating the immunity in high-risk scenarios and potentially exposing patients to healthcare workers with latent infection.[22,23] The different specificities and sensitivities of rapid tests will be best utilised according to the prevalence of circulating SARS-CoV-2.

Quality assurance is essential to any COVID-19 surveillance program, as the performance of tests is affected by their quality. The majority of antigen and antibody tests used in the literature are commercially produced, although meta-analyses have incorporated in-house tests developed by research institutions.[3,11,23] In the United States, authorisation from the Food and Drug Administration (FDA) is required before the tests can be marketed[27]; however, as the decisions of the FDA often impact policy making globally, FDA authorisation can influence how other countries approve or deny specific protein-based tests. As of October 2020, 80% of the tests that received emergency use authorisation from the FDA were molecular method based, with the remaining subset belonging to immunoassays for antigen and antibodies.[27] As seen in Table 2, the differences between tests'

Table 2:   Rapid tests evaluated by Deeks et al. 2020[23] and Bastos et al. 2020.[25]

Antigen test[23]	Detection method	Number of studies	Sensitivity range (95% CI)	Specificity range (95% CI)
Beijing Savant	LFIA	1	0.17 (0.09, 0.27)	1.0 (0.89, 1.00)
Coris Bioconcept	CGIA	2	0.50 (0.40–0.60)– 0.58 (0.49,0.65)	0.99 (0.97, 1.00)– 1.00 (0.92, 1.00)
In-house Diao 2020	LFIA	1	0.68 (0.61, 0.74)	1.00 (0.89,1.00)
Liming Bio-Products	CGIA	1	0.00 (0.00, 0.34)	0.90 (0.88, 1.00)
HapiGEN Inc	CGIA	1	0.85 (0.75, 0.92)	1.00 (0.89,1.00)
Shenzhen Bioeasy	LFIA	2	0.94 (0.86, 0.98)	1.00 (0.92, 1.00)

Serological test[25]	Number of samples among SARS-CoV-2 infected	Pooled sensitivity (95% CI)	Number of samples among SARS-CoV-2 non-infected	Pooled specificity (95% CI)
ELISA (IgG or IgM target)	766 (9 studies)	0.843 (0.756, 0.909)	1109 (6 studies)	0.976 (0.932, 0.994)
LFIA (IgG or IgM target)	2660 (11 studies)	0.660 (0.493, 0.793)	2874 (11 studies)	0.966 (0.943, 0.982)
CLIA (IgG or IgM target)	375 (2 studies)	0.978 (0.462, 1.00)	2804 (9 studies)	0.978 (0.629, 0.999)

performances can greatly impact their utility in the field. Organisations using widespread antigen or antibody testing in their workplaces must also implement proper training for test use to ensure optimal test performance.

Sampling site heavily impacts the performance of protein-based tests. Research on the precise impact of sampling from oropharynx versus the nasopharynx on antigen testing is ongoing. However, evidence from qRT-PCR studies suggests that oropharyngeal swabs have a decreased ability to pick up viral load than nasopharyngeal swabbing.[28] Saline mouth rinse/gargle may be a collection method for individuals who cannot tolerate swabbing or in the outpatient setting.[29] As detection of viral RNA in this setting had a sensitivity of 98%,[29] and saline rinse/gargle was used in the first SARS pandemic for antigen testing,[30] alternative methods of sample collection may be considered when implementing rapid antigen testing.

While the lab performance of antigen and antibody testing is generally high, the performance in the real world setting may vary drastically. A 2021 evaluation of three rapid POC LFAs for SARS-CoV-2 antibodies compared sensitivity for IgG and IgM in venous blood, obtained for laboratory testing, versus capillary blood obtained during field testing.[31] Sensitivity for venous blood IgG or IgM ranged between 91.1% (IgM, BioCan) to 94.9% (IgM, Artron), and specificity ranged from 93.5% (IgM, Artron) to 100% (IgM and IgG, BioCAN; IgG, Artron; IgM, BTNX Inc).[31] However, field tests of the Artron LFA demonstrated sensitivity of 66.7% and 91.5% specificity for IgM, while IgG performance showed 82.9% sensitivity and 99.4% specificity.[31] The drastic decrease in sensitivity for the antibody associated with long term immune response[20] in the Morshed *et al.* (2021) study is problematic for the application of rapid antibody tests in the workplace. If rapid antibody tests were applied to the evaluation of vaccine efficacy in the real world setting, the decrease in sensitivity may underestimate the protection provided by vaccination and lead to unnecessary expenditure or paradigm shifting. Further rigorous studies on the real world performance of COVID tests are needed.

2. Conclusion

As of 2021, the lockdowns and social measures to decrease transmission have been enacted for a year. Pressure to quickly identify infected individuals and determine those who are able to rejoin the workforce with decreased risk has incentivised the use of antigen and antibody tests. While the beginning of the COVID-19 pandemic saw primarily molecular-based testing, protein-based testing has been rolled out for field usage.

Molecular methods and protein-based testing ultimately occupy two different niches within the spectrum of public health tools. While rapid molecular method tests do exist and appear to have better performance than antigen tests the bulk of literature does not follow test manufacturers' instructions for usage, which may impact their findings.[3] Rapid molecular tests such as the Cepheid Xpert Xpress also require incubation in order to perform the amplification step,[3] as they are performed similarly to RT-qPCR. It is unlikely that non-medical personnel would be able to perform a rapid molecular test to the standards needed for accurate COVID-19 surveillance. However, rapid antigen tests may be crucial to evaluating infection control strategies in the epidemiological setting, as their ease of use permits widespread application in different sectors of the population.[1,3,32]

In the clinical care setting, RT-qPCR will likely remain the dominant test when establishing a confirmed case of COVID-19. While literature reviews have found the percent agreement between nucleic amplification test methods alone is dismal,[33] further research is needed to compare the concordance between molecular methods and protein based testing. Antigen tests may supplement clinical care by assisting in rapid triage of individuals who present at the emergency room, while antibody tests may be used to determine if patients have had prior COVID-19 infections.

Protein-based testing trades performance for speed of results. In the workplace setting, the use of antigen testing may distinguish between individuals with the common symptoms of respiratory ailments such as allergies and those who are actively infected with SARS-CoV-2. Mildly ill patients viral RNA shedding peaks on the day of symptom onset, and remains high for a week post-symptom onset before declining.[32,34] Positive antigen tests are generally seen with positive RT-qPCR results in real world studies of POC antigen testing,[32] which suggest that antigen tests may be used in lieu of molecular methods for rapid testing in workplaces. Whether it is sufficient to identify the most infectious individuals with antigen tests remains to be seen, as these individuals should ideally remain isolated under current COVID-19 paradigms.

Ultimately, the results of protein-based testing and molecular methods must be conveyed to patients. Emphasis should be placed on informing individuals that the presence of SARS-CoV-2 antibodies does not ensure life-long protection from reinfection, and that a negative RT-qPCR result does not mean lack of infection.[33] While rapid antigen testing can identify individuals at their peak infectiousness, and rapid antibody testing can identify individuals with some level of immunity, these testing methods must be used in conjunction with existing public health measures to curb the spread of SARS-CoV-2.

References

1. Yamayoshi S, Sakai-Tagawa Y, Koga M, Akasaka O, Nakachi I, Koh H, *et al*. Comparison of Rapid Antigen Tests for COVID-19. *Viruses*. 2020;12(12):1420.
2. Organization WH. *In vitro* diagnostic medical devices (IVDs) used for the detection of high-risk human papillomavirus (HPV) genotypes in cervical cancer screening. 2018.
3. Dinnes J, Deeks JJ, Adriano A, Berhane S, Davenport C, Dittrich S, *et al*. Rapid, point-of-care antigen and molecular-based tests for diagnosis of SARS-CoV-2 infection. *The Cochrane Database of Systematic Reviews*. 2020;8:Cd013705.
4. Sethuraman N, Jeremiah SS, Ryo A. Interpreting diagnostic tests for SARS-CoV-2. *JAMA*. 2020;323(22):2249–2251.
5. Control CfD, Prevention. Interim guidance for antigen testing for SARS-CoV-2. Updated December 16, 2020.
6. Röltgen K, Powell AE, Wirz OF, Stevens BA, Hogan CA, Najeeb J, *et al*. Defining the features and duration of antibody responses to SARS-CoV-2 infection associated with disease severity and outcome. *Science Immunology*. 2020;5(54):eabe0240.
7. Tantuoyir MM, Rezaei N. Serological tests for COVID-19: Potential opportunities. *Cell Biology International*. 2020.
8. Gremmels H, Winkel BM, Schuurman R, Rosingh A, Rigter NA, Rodriguez O, *et al*. Real-life validation of the Panbio™ COVID-19 antigen rapid test (Abbott) in community-dwelling subjects with symptoms of potential SARS-CoV-2 infection. *EClinicalMedicine*. 2021;31:100677.
9. Linares M, Pérez-Tanoira R, Carrero A, Romanyk J, Pérez-García F, Gómez-Herruz P, *et al*. Panbio antigen rapid test is reliable to diagnose SARS-CoV-2

infection in the first 7 days after the onset of symptoms. *Journal of Clinical Virology*. 2020;133:104659.

10. La Marca A, Capuzzo M, Paglia T, Roli L, Trenti T, Nelson SM. Testing for SARS-CoV-2 (COVID-19): A systematic review and clinical guide to molecular and serological in-vitro diagnostic assays. *Reproductive Biomedicine Online*. 2020;41(3):483–499.

11. Diao B, Wen K, Chen J, Liu Y, Yuan Z, Han C, *et al.* Diagnosis of acute respiratory syndrome coronavirus 2 infection by detection of nucleocapsid protein. *MedRxiv*. 2020.

12. Kyosei Y, Yamura S, Namba M, Yoshimura T, Watabe S, Ito E. Antigen tests for COVID-19. *Biophysics and Physicobiology*. 2021:bppb-v18. 004.

13. Dai L, Gao GF. Viral targets for vaccines against COVID-19. *Nature Reviews Immunology*. 2021;21(2):73–82.

14. Group CPHLNLDCatCPHLNRVIW. Interim guidance on the use of the Abbott Panbio™ COVID-19 Antigen Rapid Test. *Canada Communicable Disease Report*. 2021;47(1):17–22.

15. Cevik M, Tate M, Lloyd O, Maraolo AE, Schafers J, Ho A. SARS-CoV-2, SARS-CoV, and MERS-CoV viral load dynamics, duration of viral shedding, and infectiousness: A systematic review and meta-analysis. *The Lancet Microbe*. 2021;2(1):e13–e22.

16. Dutta A, Huang C-T, Lin C-Y, Chen T-C, Lin Y-C, Chang C-S, *et al.* Sterilizing immunity to influenza virus infection requires local antigen-specific T cell response in the lungs. *Scientific Reports*. 2016;6:32973–.

17. Yu J, Tostanoski LH, Peter L, Mercado NB, McMahan K, Mahrokhian SH, *et al.* DNA vaccine protection against SARS-CoV-2 in rhesus macaques. *Science*. 2020;369(6505):806–811.

18. Kim DS, Rowland-Jones S, Gea-Mallorquí E. Will SARS-CoV-2 infection elicit long-lasting protective or sterilising immunity? Implications for vaccine strategies (2020). *Frontiers in Immunology*. 2020;11(3190).

19. Liu W, Fontanet A, Zhang P-H, Zhan L, Xin Z-T, Baril L, *et al.* Two-year prospective study of the humoral immune response of patients with severe acute respiratory syndrome. *The Journal of Infectious Diseases*. 2006;193(6): 792–795.

20. Randolph HE, Barreiro LB. Herd immunity: Understanding COVID-19. *Immunity*. 2020;52(5):737–741.

21. Wang Y, Zhang L, Sang L, Ye F, Ruan S, Zhong B, *et al.* Kinetics of viral load and antibody response in relation to COVID-19 severity. *Journal of Clinical Investigation*. 2020;130(10):5235–5244.

22. Kopel J, Goyal H, Perisetti A. Antibody tests for COVID-19. *Baylor University Medical Center Proceedings*. 2021;34(1):63–72.
23. Deeks JJ, Dinnes J, Takwoingi Y, Davenport C, Spijker R, Taylor-Phillips S, *et al*. Antibody tests for identification of current and past infection with SARS-CoV-2. *Cochrane Database of Systematic Reviews*. 2020(6).
24. Sackett DL, Haynes RB, Tugwell P. Clinical epidemiology: A basic science for clinical medicine: Little, Brown and Company; 1985.
25. Bastos ML, Tavaziva G, Abidi SK, Campbell JR, Haraoui L-P, Johnston JC, *et al*. Diagnostic accuracy of serological tests for COVID-19: Systematic review and meta-analysis. *BMJ*. 2020;370:m2516.
26. Parikh R, Parikh S, Arun E, Thomas R. Likelihood ratios: Clinical application in day-to-day practice. *Indian Journal of Ophthalmology*. 2009;57(3): 217–221.
27. Vandenberg O, Martiny D, Rochas O, van Belkum A, Kozlakidis Z. Considerations for diagnostic COVID-19 tests. *Nature Reviews Microbiology*. 2021;19(3):171–183.
28. Wang X, Tan L, Wang X, Liu W, Lu Y, Cheng L, *et al*. Comparison of nasopharyngeal and oropharyngeal swabs for SARS-CoV-2 detection in 353 patients received tests with both specimens simultaneously. *International Journal of Infectious Diseases*. 2020;94:107–109.
29. Goldfarb DM, Tilley P, Al-Rawahi GN, Srigley JA, Ford G, Pedersen H, *et al*. Self-collected saline gargle samples as an alternative to health care worker-collected nasopharyngeal swabs for COVID-19 diagnosis in outpatients. *Journal of Clinical Microbiology*. 2021;59(4):e02427-20.
30. Liu IJ, Chen P-J, Yeh S-H, Chiang Y-P, Huang L-M, Chang M-F, *et al*. Immunofluorescence assay for detection of the nucleocapsid antigen of the severe acute respiratory syndrome (SARS)-associated coronavirus in cells derived from throat wash samples of patients with SARS. *Journal of Clinical Microbiology*. 2005;43(5):2444–2448.
31. Morshed M, Sekirov I, McLennan M, Levett PN, Chahil N, Mak A, *et al*. Comparative analysis of capillary versus venous blood for serologic detection of SARS-CoV-2 antibodies by RPOC lateral flow tests. *Open Forum Infectious Diseases*. 2021;8(3):ofab043-ofab.
32. Kotsiou OS, Pantazopoulos I, Papagiannis D, Fradelos EC, Kanellopoulos N, Siachpazidou D, *et al*. Repeated antigen-based rapid diagnostic testing for estimating the coronavirus disease 2019 prevalence from the perspective of the workers' vulnerability before and during the lockdown. *International Journal of Environmental Research and Public Health*. 2021;18(4):1638.

33. Axell-House DB, Lavingia R, Rafferty M, Clark E, Amirian ES, Chiao EY. The estimation of diagnostic accuracy of tests for COVID-19: A scoping review. *Journal of Infection*. 2020;81(5):681–697.

34. Rajgopal T. Antibody testing in the context of COVID-19 and return to work. *Indian Journal of Occupational and Environmental Medicine*. 2020; 24(2):51–54.

Part 4

Public Health Measures in the Community

Chapter 7

Contact Tracing, Screening, Self-Isolation and Quarantine

Anne Lesack* and Veronic Clair*,†

*School of Population and Public Health, University of British Columbia, Vancouver, Canada

†Communicable Diseases and Immunization Services, BC Centre for Disease Control, Vancouver, Canada

Key Message

- Non-pharmaceutical interventions are integral to the control of communicable diseases particularly in the absence of robust pharmaceutical interventions. The non-pharmaceutical interventions of screening, contact tracing, quarantine and isolation have been adapted to suit the context and nature of the pandemic, including widespread access to digital technologies, the length of the latency period, and the overdispersion parameter of COVID-19.
- Screening, contact tracing, quarantine and isolation are implemented with the intention of lowering the reproductive number of COVID-19 and are most effective in reducing viral transmission when implemented simultaneously. Additionally, the combined use of approaches to screening and contact tracing result in a more robust system which counteracts the limitations of using approach in isolation.

- Each intervention has benefits, limitations, and unintentional consequences to consider in the timing, length, and extent of implementation. Considerations to the population and context of interest are crucial for implementing interventions that minimise consequences while supporting adherence by the population.

1. Introduction

Non-pharmaceutical interventions have been used to successfully control the spread of communicable diseases for centuries. In the 1918–1919 influenza pandemic, interventions including quarantine and isolation were used in concert to limit the spread of the virus. The early implementation, sustained use and combination of interventions resulted in lower total mortality burden.[1] Screening, contact tracing, quarantine and isolation have played an integral role in the COVID-19 pandemic and have demonstrated their continued importance in transmission control. These strategies build off each other, with the robustness of one strategy affecting the efficacy of the following strategy: for example, the sensitivity of screening methods will determine how many exposed or infected individuals need to be quarantined or isolated. Countries have taken different approaches to these four interventions depending on their resources, governance and population density with these factors playing a role in their implementation and management. The theory and rationale behind each of these practices are grounded in the epidemiology of communicable diseases with each implemented with the goal of lowering the reproductive number of COVID-19. Each intervention has strengths and limitations that affect their ability to reduce the reproductive number, but together remain an important mitigating strategy for the spread of the virus.

2. Screening

Screening is a systematic approach to identify at risk individuals by detecting an agreed upon prognostic factor in a presumptively healthy individual with the intention that detection of the factor will lead to immediate intervention.[2] Screening can be used to detect both cases and exposed individuals at risk for disease development, therefore the "agreed upon prognostic factor" can be either an underlying symptom or a risk factor such as exposure to a diagnosed case.[2] When screening for cases, screening is a means of detecting asymptomatic individuals or symptoms in an individual who doesn't recognise they are displaying symptoms of COVID-19.[3] This strategy is a means of presumptively identifying COVID-19 infection by asking or testing for symptoms or active infection in a rapid manner.[4] Screening is a secondary prevention method and has the potential to lower the effective reproductive number (R_t) through the early detection of infected individuals and the implementation of isolation measures earlier than in the absence of screening.[2] Screening is not a diagnostic tool. Therefore, if screening results indicate potential infection, in most cases, individuals will be directed to receive diagnostic testing to confirm screening outcomes.[4]

2.1 *Screening methods*

There are both subjective and objective methods of ascertaining probable underlying infection. Subjective measures ask individuals about their experience of symptoms, as objective methods measure the potential for disease onset through temperature checks or rapid test-based approaches. The ability to detect an infected or probable case of COVID-19 relies on multiple factors, including: the incubation period of the disease, sensitivity of tools used, the proportion of individuals that are aware that they have been exposed, the proportion of subclinical cases and the proportion of infected individuals who truthfully answer screening questions.[5] Different screening methods can capture different subsets of the population. For example, methods which assess symptomology are unable to capture cases who are in the incubation period or who are sub-clinical, but contact and travel history may capture individuals who are in the incubation period through the identification of a direct exposure.[3] COVID-19 has a median incubation period of 5 days (period between infection and symptom onset), thus, methods which assess symptomology (e.g. temperature checks, symptom assessment questionnaires) will not capture individuals who are in the incubation period.[6] Additionally, these methods will not capture sub-clinical cases. It has been estimated that 16% of COVID-19 cases are asymptomatic throughout the course of infection with certain subsets of the population particularly likely to experience sub-clinical manifestation (i.e. children).[7]

Individuals who both do not know their exposure history (i.e. are not aware they were exposed) and are not displaying symptoms (i.e. in latent phase, asymptomatic or subclinical) will be fundamentally undetectable using symptom or contact history questionnaires.[5] In Figure 1, Viswanathan *et al.* depict the relationship between screening methods and where on the disease trajectory they are able to capture cases of COVID-19.

Screening strategies have been implemented widely, with various methods applied in school, workplace, and medical contexts. Different methods have benefits and drawbacks in terms of their sensitivity, how early in the disease history they can detect infection and the resource allocation required. Table 1 outlines the different screening approaches used to detect cases.

2.2 *Proposed solutions and conclusions*

In assessing the appropriateness of screening methods it is important to consider their ability to identify the greatest number of underlying

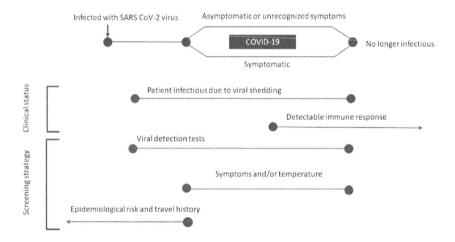

Figure 1:   Role of screening in identifying people with COVID-19.[3]

Table 1:   COVID-19 screening approaches, methods, benefits, and limitations.

Approach	Method to trigger isolation	Benefits and limitations
Methods to detect cases		
Symptom assessment questionnaires	Capture cases who are displaying symptoms and may not be aware of disease risk.	• The breadth of symptoms listed will determine who is captured by the tool; narrow criteria may miss individuals experiencing less common manifestations of COVID-19.[8] • The ways in which a tool measures symptom presence (e.g. length of time a symptom has been present) will affect the tools sensitivity and specificity. • Questionnaires will not capture individuals who are in the incubation period (i.e. asymptomatic but shedding the virus) or those who have subclinical manifestation.[5] • The threshold set for symptom presence may create unintentional consequences (e.g. psychological and financial) if individuals are required to isolate unnecessarily. • Screening tools require truthful disclosure of information. Trust within the government and policies may affect willingness to accurately disclose symptoms and may support some individual's defence of non-disclosure or rule breaking.[9]
Temperature checks	Measure core body temperature: >38.0 °C indicates the body is producing an immunological response.	• Non-contact infrared thermometers have been widely used as a rapid and non-invasive means of measuring temperature with reduced cross-infection risk.[10] • Efficacy of case detection relies on scanners sensitivity and specificity; scanners measuring temperature at the forehead have been detected to have an average sensitivity of 0.808 and specificity of 0.920.[10]

(Continued)

Table 1: *(Continued)*

Approach	Method to trigger isolation	Benefits and limitations
		• Temperature checks are fundamentally unable to detect pre-symptomatic or non-symptomatic patients.[10] The CDC has reported only 43.1% of cases presented with fever.[11]
		• Temperature screening has been shown to lack sensitivity in hospital patients, demonstrating lower sensitivity in earlier stages compared to later stages of illness.[12]
		• Using a temperature cut-off of 38°C only captured 18% of positive COVID-19 cases in a cohort of young, predominantly male military recruits on the first day they presented with symptoms. A cut-off of 37.1°C detected 63% of positive cases.[13]
Rapid lab testing	Identify active cases through presence of COVID-19 virus or antigens.	• Effectiveness of lab testing as a screening tool will depend on test sensitivity as well as the prevalence of COVID-19 within the population.[14]
		• Real-time reverse transcriptase polymerase chain reaction (RT PCR) has appropriate sensitivity to assist in screening, although this method risks eliciting false negative and false positive responses in part due to the viral load of the patient and issues with specimen collection, handling, and technical procedures.[15]
		• Rapid Antigen Detection Tests often contain areas coated in anti-SARS-CoV-2 antibody and will detect the presence of an antigen produced by the virus in a nasopharyngeal or nasal swab.[16]

| | | • Rapid Antigen tests have a lower sensitivity than RT PCR methods, although test sensitivity may be less important in screening than in diagnostic testing with factors such as frequency of testing and speed of reporting playing important roles in efficacy of screening measures.[17]
• Rapid lab testing can be resource intensive and expensive and may not be a viable option for resource constricted regions or countries. |

Methods to detect exposed individuals

Contact exposure history	Identify people who have been in contact with a case and are at risk of developing or have developed COVID-19 symptoms.	• May be useful in detecting asymptomatic or subclinical cases; as exemplified in a study on returning travellers, known exposure history identified 2 out 114 travellers who were positive but asymptomatic.[18] • Exposure history may fail to detect individuals who choose not to disclose known exposure.[5]
Travel history	Capture individuals who have travelled from a country with active COVID-19 transmission; identify individuals for quarantine.	• A study conducted in Iceland at the beginning of the pandemic (April 2020) indicated 65% of cases had recently travelled; this proportion decreased to 15.5% in a later phase of the study.[19] • As the pandemic progresses and outbreaks emerge in all countries, selectively isolating based on country of travel is no longer feasible as all countries present risk of exposure. • Most countries have imposed mandated quarantine for travels coming from any country, making this no longer an effective method of selectively isolating individuals.

COVID-19 cases, while minimising the unintended consequences of the screening, both on the individual subjected to the screen, and the organisation implementing the screening measures. As outlined in Table 1 the objectives, benefits and limitations of each method vary; based on these factors it is proposed that the type of screening method is decided based on the specific context and demographic of interest. For example, as children and youth are more likely to experience sub-clinical manifestation, temperature checks and symptom assessment will be less effective in identifying underlying cases. Therefore, contact exposure history and/or rapid lab testing may act as the most effective way of identifying cases in children. For adult workplaces, symptom screening and contact history may act as an efficient mechanism for determining infection. Temperature checks, although widely implemented, may not be an effective use or resources if resource constraints are present. In the use of symptom assessment questionnaires, broader criteria may more readily identify cases who present with less common symptoms, although this may increase the risk of unintended consequences such as unnecessary quarantine. For all contexts it is important to recognise that screening methods used on their own may lack sensitivity due to environmental or human factors, therefore the use of methods in combination may act as a protective measure against individual method limitations.[14]

3. Contact Tracing

Contact tracing is a means of exposure assessment and is the process of identifying, assessing, and managing individuals who have been exposed to COVID-19 to prevent further transmission of the virus.[20] The identification of contacts will reduce the R_t by removing exposed individuals from the general population (through quarantine) before they enter the latent phase. Onward spread of the virus will be prevented and public health workers will be afforded the opportunity to instruct contacts of additional precautions to take to decrease the risk of onward spread (for example, self-monitoring, testing if symptoms develop, and additional non-pharmaceutical interventions).

Individuals who have had contact with a confirmed case who was likely to be infectious, should be elicited via contact tracing. The WHO defines a contact as: "a person in any of the following situations from 2 days before and up to 14 days after the onset of symptoms in the confirmed or probable case of COVID-19:

- Face-to-face contact with a probable or confirmed case of COVID-19 within 1 meter and for more than 15 minutes.
- Direct physical contact with a probable or confirmed case of COVID-19.
- Direct care for an individual with probable or confirmed COVID-19 without using proper personal protective equipment.
- Other situations, as indicated by local risk assessments" (p. 3).[21]

The definition of a contact considers various aspects which affect the likelihood of transmission, including: the duration of interaction, proximity, symptomology, and timing of interaction in relation to a known infected case.[22] Specifically, the time frame in which case contacts are contacted is directly related to the infectious and latency period of the virus, these 2 periods determine the contact elucidation period.[22] There is variation in how countries and organisations define a contact, with the WHO's 14-day post-symptom guideline being fairly conservative. For example, the E.U. identifies a contact as an individual who has had contact with a confirmed case 2 days before to 10 days after the onset of symptoms in a case.[23] The amount of time (15 minutes) is recognised to be an arbitrary cut off point used as a means of eliciting a type of higher risk contact between individuals. Some countries, including those in the EU and the USA have specified contacts are those who have had 15 minutes of consecutive or non-consecutive time, over a 24 period, indicating that there may not be a clear cut exposure threshold and more of a dose-response relationship.[24] Lastly the distance parameter is influenced by studies indicating distancing under 1meter is associated with increased transmission of the virus and subsequent infection.[25] The 1 meter threshold is also arbitrary and many countries use 2 meters, as there is still likely significant infectious particulate that can reach a susceptible individual beyond 1 meter; loud conversations, signing, and heavy breathing all increase the expulsion of infectious particulate from the respiratory tract.[26]

3.1 *Process of contact tracing*

The process of contact tracing follows a similar pattern in most country contexts. There are two main approaches to contact tracing, forward tracing, and backward tracing. Forward tracing is the process of notifying and isolating individuals who have recently been exposed and may have become infected by a known case of COVID-19.[27] Backward or retrospective tracing attempts to identify the source of infection for the case under investigation as a means of identifying additional cases and contacts.[23] Japan and Singapore have integrated a bidirectional approach (the combination of forward and backward tracing) but this approach remains relatively uncommon, with most countries solely conducting forward tracing.[27] Countries have also implemented various measures to support effective contact tracing, including digital and manual personal information collecting at entry into establishments. These measures facilitate the contact tracing process in the event that patrons were exposed to someone else in attendance who was infectious at the time. These processes assist particularly in situations where cases have been in indoor spaces (e.g. restaurants, stores, bars, etc.) where they are near other individuals they do not know.

When a positive case is identified, contacts who fall within the contact elucidation period are contacted. Through manual tracing, a public health official contacts and interviews the case contact. When contacted by a public health worker the WHO recommends the sharing of the following information with the contact:

1. Process and rational for contact tracing.
2. Information on quarantine (i.e. proper conditions).
3. What symptoms to look for?
4. What they should do if they develop symptoms/feel unwell (i.e. who to contact, testing and treatment protocols)?
5. Information regarding privacy and data protection (i.e. how will the organisation use, process and store their personal information).
6. Answer questions raised by the contact.[20]

The manual interview acts as a mechanism to ascertain symptomology and relay information regarding quarantine procedures.[20] Regions vary in their protocols regarding follow-up testing, for example, in the E.U. all contacts that become symptomatic are tested, as in South Korea, contacts who fall in high risk groups are routinely tested as non-high risk contacts are only tested if they became symptomatic.[23,28] Lastly, confirmed cases will follow regional or national isolation guidelines, and suspected cases will follow regional or national quarantine guidelines. When a contact becomes a confirmed case (i.e. receives positive lab results) this triggers another round of contact tracing.

3.2 *Approaches to tracing*

The above process describes forward tracing, the process of identifying individuals who may have been infected by a confirmed case, to prevent further transmission through secondary cases.[27] Forward tracing is the approach most commonly implemented historically and throughout the COVID-19 pandemic.[29] Backward and bidirectional tracing are additional approaches to contact tracing. Backward tracing is the process of identifying the source of infection for a newly established case through the identification of their contacts prior to symptom development.[30] A large proportion of COVID-19 transmission is fuelled by superspreading events with high variability in onward transmission from one person to the next (i.e. overdispersion).[30] A high degree of dispersion means the identification of a super-spreader has the potential to significantly reduce the onward transmission of the virus, through the forward tracing of all the super-spreaders contacts.[27,30] By backward tracing, the source (parent) of infection is identified as the more infections (offspring) a source has produced the more likely they are to be identified as a contact in their offspring's contact tracing list.[31] Bradshaw *et al.* modelled the impact of bidirectional tracing, indicating that shifting from a forward to bidirectional approach, doubled the impact of contact tracing compared to forward tracing alone. Additionally, modelling conducted by Endo *et al.*, found that in the case of COVID-19, the use of backward tracing in combination with forward tracing increased the effectiveness of tracing by a factor of 2-3. Backward tracing is more resilient against fluctuations in COVID-19 test sensitivities, showing increased efficacy compared to forward tracing in situations of low-test sensitivity.[27] Currently most recommendations support identification of contacts 2 days before the onset of symptoms. As the mean incubation period is estimated to be 5.1 days, a reverse tracing system would need to widen their contact collection period to improve the efficacy of this method; this increased tracing window may put more resource burden on the system.[6,27]

4. Methods of Tracing

4.1 *Manual contact tracing*

Manual approaches to contact tracing mean a case contact is contacted through phone or email. Manual approaches are beneficial as they allow a contact to ask questions and receive context specific responses. Additionally, they are a lower barrier approach than phone application-based tracing as they reach individuals who do not have smart phones, are not technologically competent, or comfortable sharing their data via a telephone app.[32] Manual approaches have some limitations in their timeliness as each call to a contact can take around 20 minutes.[32] In addition, the effectiveness of manual tracing is highly dependent on the number of contacts correctly identified by a case during the contact tracing process.[33] There is a potential for recall issues or social desirability bias to be introduced if cases systematically underreport the number of contacts they have had prior to isolation particularly if they have broken local or regional guidelines regarding socialising practices. Manual tracing is also highly affected by the prevalence of COVID-19 within the community. In the situation the prevalence of cases exceeds the capacity of community resources there will be delay or absence of quarantine of exposed individuals increasing the risk of continued transmission.[34] Due in part to these limiting factors, there is an assumed 3-day delay between an index cases positive test results and the notification of their contacts using conventional methods identified in the literature.[35,36]

4.2 *Digital contact tracing*

Digital contact tracing approaches typically involve the use of personal smart phone applications which note the length of time spent within a certain distance to another smart phone. An alert is generated through the app if an individual's phone indicates they have been in close contact with an infected person in the previous days.[35] Phone applications have the potential to instantaneously notify contacts about an exposure, reducing the tracing delays associated with conventional methods such as phone calls.[35] In addition to improved timeliness, the use of phone apps can increase the number of contacts associated with a case as this method does not rely on the accurate recall of each contact. Due to the nature of tracing apps, the efficacy of this method depends on the proportion of the population who use the app as well as the duration in which the app is optimally in use.[36] As simulated by Kretzschmar *et al.* mobile tracing apps may speed up the process of identifying contacts but "in all cases, a contact could only be traced if both the index case and the contact were app users" (p. e455). Despite this, "app-based tracing on its own remains more effective than conventional tracing alone, even with 20% coverage, due to its inherent speed" (20 p. e457). An additional limitation of app-based tracing is the systematic exclusion of certain subsets of the population, including certain age groups who do not use the technology (young ~ <10 years old and old ~ >80), and populations that may not have access to smart phones (lower socio-economic status groups).[33]

5. Challenges of Contact Tracing Approaches

5.1 *Timeliness*

An important aspect of effective contact tracing is its ability to reach contacts within the recommended number of days during periods of high volume (i.e. timeliness). Kretzschmar *et al.* identified, to hold the effect reproductive number below one ($R_t = 0.80$), in a context with an R_t of 1.2, 80% of infectious individuals would need to be tested, with a testing delay (time between symptom onset and test results) and tracing delay (time to trace a contact) of 0 days, with 80% of contacts identified (p. e456). With an increase in testing delay to 2 days, a tracing coverage of 80% or tracing delay of ≤1 day needs to be maintained to hold R_t below 1. If testing is delayed ≥3 days, R_t will no longer be able to be maintained below 0 even with 100% contact tracing with no time delay. The reduction in testing delay was concluded by Kretzschmar *et al.* to be the most important factor in improving the effectiveness of contact tracing efforts. Achieving such high levels of testing and low levels of testing and tracing delays are likely not realistic in practice as factors effecting who gets tested, delays in test results, and delays in contacting cases and contacts all impact the ability to reach the identified optimal cut off points. A notable feature of COVID-19 disease history is the onset of infectivity before symptoms appear. Therefore, the rapid testing and receiving of results and quick identification of contacts will potentially lower the percentage of transmission that occurs during the latent phase as people will be notified earlier of potential infection. Additionally, the number of subclinical infections effects the ability to control an outbreak and efficacy of contact tracing measures. As modelled by Hellewell *et al.*, the difference between 0% and 10% subclinical infection results in a significant reduction in the ability to control an outbreak regardless of high percentage of contacts traced for each infected case.[37]

5.2 *Privacy concerns*

Public adoption of contract tracing apps, or other data collection measures require public trust and confidence that personal information will not be used for other purposes. Furthermore, for phone applications, users need to trust the technology. An identified barrier to contact tracing methods is concern regarding governmental surveillance and fear of continued use of data beyond the pandemic.[38] General concerns regarding the security of app technology and increased likelihood of hacking have also been expressed.[38] Ahmed *et al.* discuss aspects of contact tracing app's architecture which impact their susceptibility to nefarious actions, including how they use and store data.[39] Increased transparency may act as a means of dispelling concerns and can be fostered by making the app source code open as well as providing the public with a Privacy Impact Assessment of the technology being used and recommended.[39] Additionally, assurances of ethical data use, protections around personal data use and transparent oversight are aspects of this trust building that may work in concert to encourage participation in contact tracing measures.[36]

5.3 *Recommendations and conclusions*

Contact tracing is most effective when the system is robust and responsive, with the ability to handle large volumes. Certain methods indicate an increased capacity to handle fluctuations in volume in a timely manner, better attaining the goal of identifying and quarantining exposed individuals. Reverse contact tracing is highly impactful due to its ability to identify super-spreaders, the main driving force of viral spread, unlike more conventional forward tracing methods.[40] However, it is very challenging to implement well in practice, as recall biases for several days past hinder the effectiveness of backward tracing. Proposed solutions have been to ask people where they think they got their infection, or limiting the backward tracing to a section of the period where someone could have contracted COVID-19, focusing on the most likely timeline of exposure based on median incubation. Due to the high level of dispersion in the COVID-19 pandemic, a combination of forward and backward tracing into a bidirectional approach may act as a means of addressing the strengths and weaknesses of each approach simultaneously. Additionally, the combined use of manual and technological approaches to contact-tracing may similarly counteract the limitations of each method when used in isolation. Bradshaw *et al.*'s modelling concluded that combined approaches to bidirectional tracing was the most effective strategy in controlling an outbreak in a variety of scenarios. In periods of case surges, it may be most effective to focus on reverse tracing versus forward tracing due to limited and overwhelmed resources.

6. Quarantine and Isolation

Quarantine is the separation or restriction of movement of well individuals who may have been exposed to a confirmed or probable case of COVID-19. The objective of quarantine is to decrease the number of contacts of an exposed individual before they develop symptoms. As COVID-19 is transmissible before the development of symptoms, with a proportion of cases never manifesting symptoms (estimated to be 16–20%) this is an essential measure to reduce transmission.[7,41] Quarantine reduces R_t by separating those in quarantine from the general population between the end of the latent and beginning of the incubation period (period of asymptomatic transmission). The WHO recommends that contacts of confirmed or probable COVID-19 cases quarantine at home or in a designated quarantine facility for 14 days from their last exposure.[42] The WHO recommended length of quarantine aligns with the incubation period of COVID-19, which is 5.1 days, with 97.5% of cases showing symptoms within 11.5 days.[6] The 14-day cut off length of quarantine is selected due to the high unlikelihood of symptoms being detected 14-days after infection.[6] 14-days is a conservative cut off for length for quarantine, and countries have approached this cut off in different ways as rapid testing has become increasingly more available. For example, in the EU, a contact can take a test 10 days after exposure and can terminate quarantine measures if the test is negative, as India has maintained a 14-day quarantine period.[43] Additionally, modelling studies have indicated that reducing the length of quarantine to 7 or more days coupled with a test close to the end of the quarantine period is comparable in efficacy to a 14-day quarantine period with no test.[44] Waiting until the 7 day mark is important as it allows for enough time for viral load to build and become detectable through testing; testing at the 7 day timepoint has proven to be comparably effective to testing performed past 7 days.[44] During the recommended quarantine period, individuals are asked to remain at home or within a designated quarantine facility and not leave or interact with other individuals until the period is complete.

6.1 *Isolation*

Isolation is the separation of infected individuals (confirmed cases) from the healthy population. Isolation directly reduces R_t by removing confirmed cases of COVID-19 from the general population, eliminating their ability to transmit the virus to contacts.[37] All confirmed (through lab testing) or assumed cases (displaying symptoms) of COVID-19 must isolate. Similarly, to quarantine guidelines, the WHO recommended length of isolation aligns with the incubation period of COVID-19. There are differences in recommendations between regions regarding length of isolation period as well as for different subsets of the population. For example, in the EU, asymptomatic cases who have received a positive test result are recommended to isolate for a 10-day period from the date of sample collection.[43] Immunocompromised patients within the EU are recommended to receive 2 consecutive negative PCR test results in a 24-hour period; a similar approach is encouraged for severely ill patients. Comparatively, mild to moderate cases can discontinue quarantine 10 days after the onset of symptoms and clinical improvement of associated symptoms (including discontinuation of fever for ≥3 days).[43]

6.2 *Quarantine and isolation enforcement mechanisms*

In order to track adherence to quarantine and isolation guidelines countries have implemented different mechanisms. In some countries, regular phone calls by health professionals are used as a means of checking in on the patient.[45] In countries including South Korea and England, health professionals have additionally undertaken random visits to quarantining individuals.[46,47] The maintenance of monitoring measures may be stressed in times of resources scarcity; in such times it is possible that these mechanisms have limited efficacy, as in the 2003 SARS outbreak individuals felt little fear of getting caught when breaking quarantine due to spotty or inconsistent monitoring due to an overwhelmed health system.[48] Often, in addition to monitoring check-ups, fines or imprisonment are put in place to further discourage rule violations. In Spring 2020, South Korea implemented a one-strike out policy in conjunction with a maximum fine increase from 3 million to 10 million Korean Won (from $2,700 to $9,000 US) to discourage individuals from breaking quarantine.[46] Similarly, England, Indian states and Canada have also have implemented fines for breaking quarantine with fines ranging from around $27 US (2,000 Rs in India) to around $600, 000 US ($750,000 Canadian) depending on offense.[47,49,50] Ryu *et al.* have identified that stricter policy measures do not increase adherence or significantly decrease policy violations. These measures may have limited ability to alter adherence if the reasons for breaking rules are felt to be unavoidable by the individual.

7. Barriers to Effective Quarantine and Isolation Practices

7.1 *Appropriate settings*

For quarantine and isolation measures to be effective as possible, individuals require appropriate settings to quarantine; whether in the home or in a designated facility, individuals who are quarantining are recommend to be in an adequately ventilated room that allows the constant turnover of air within the space.[42] Specifically, quarantining or isolating within the home presents an opportunity for transmission between household members. Modelling by Kucharski *et al.* indicated by solely using quarantine as an intervention method, there would be a mean reduction in transmission by 29% if infected individuals quarantined within the home (i.e. with family members), and a reduction of 35% if individuals were quarantined outside of the home (i.e. not with family members).[33] The WHO guidelines for home quarantine recommend allocating a separate bedroom in the home to support the separation of household members from the quarantining individual.[42] If a separate room is not available, placing beds at least 1 metre apart is recommended. Use of a separate bathroom is encouraged and frequent hand washing/cleaning practices throughout the day.[42] These recommendations inherently require a large, uncrowded space to adequately adhere to the recommendations. Individuals who are limited in their ability to effectively quarantine in their home if they are living in small, shared spaces with other family or household members, thus increasing the likelihood of transmission to fellow members.

7.2 *Support*

Individuals may be unable to abide by quarantine rules if they lack a support system outside of the household who is able to carry out necessary tasks such as grocery shopping or purchasing of medications.[49] Individuals receiving support from outside of their household during isolation are reported to be more likely to adhere to isolation guidelines.[50] In South Korea, local health authorities distributed basic necessities to all individuals quarantining including sanitary products and basic necessities.[46] Measures such as these, likely act as preventative mechanisms to the breaking of quarantine rules.

7.3 *Financial compensation*

The ability to adhere to measures may be lower for individuals with financial resource constraints; although desire to comply may be high regardless of income, the ability to isolate is lower for those of lower socio-economic status.[50] Compliance with quarantining measures may be significantly improved with the guarantee of compensation for lost income due to absence from work due to quarantine or isolation. A study conducted by Bodas and Peleg in Israel at the beginning of the pandemic (February 2020) identified a 25% increase (from 71% to 96%) in intention to comply to a medical official instructed, 2-week quarantine if monetary compensation for lost wages were provided.[51] Implementing sick leave policies that are non-punitive and align with current healthcare recommendations may increase adherence to quarantine practices while preventing vulnerable populations from being disproportionately affected.[52]

8. Recommendations and Conclusions

As testing mechanisms becoming increasingly available, they are increasingly able to support the quarantine and isolation processes. There are large financial and psychological costs to quarantine and isolation, with studies indicating adherence to quarantine requirements decreasing as the length extends.[44] Due to these factors and the comparable efficacy of a 7-day quarantine with testing and a 14-day quarantine without testing (most widely implemented), a shorter quarantine is optimal if financially feasible by the country. As seen with quarantine, the incorporation of testing into isolation measures has the potential to reduce the length of isolation time and consequently the consequences of an extended isolation period particularly for mild and moderate cases of COVID-19. Additionally, if countries are financially able, providing compensation may decrease the burden and increase adherence to quarantine guidelines. In terms of resource allocation, the benefits of faster return to work and decreased psychological toll may outweigh the cost of extra testing even in resource restricted contexts.

9. Limitations

There are several limitations to this chapter. Due to the emerging nature of COVID-19 and various aspects of the disease that are unknown, findings reported at the beginning of the pandemic (early 2020) may differ significantly in their conclusions and understanding of the virus when compared to articles published in early 2021. An additional limitation is the amount of information and detail that could be provided in an introductory chapter. Each topic deserves a chapter of their own and therefore relevant aspects of each non-pharmaceutical approach could have been further expanded upon. The emerging nature of the virus means there are vast differences in the study populations, study sizes and contexts used and observed, often with natural experiments conducted as opportunities for inquiry presented themselves. This feature makes it challenging to compare results across studies. Lastly, all research articles read and reported on were written in English; this approach may have systematically excluded research from certain countries or regions presenting a different approach or conclusions. All of these factors play into the interpretation of recommendations and conclusions. As more information comes available and more is known about the virus, conclusions made within this chapter may no longer hold.

10. Summary Remarks

Screening, contact tracing, quarantine and isolation are all effective measures to slow and prevent the transmission of COVID-19. These four methods are effective especially when used in concert with each other as they build upon each other, often relying on the speed and thoroughness of the previous intervention to maximise the efficacy of the next. Each intervention method has benefits and limitations with varying efficacy in reducing R_t depending on how they are implemented, who they are used on and citizen's level of trust in the measures. In addition, capacity within health systems is crucial to scale these methods efficiently as well as support citizens in the full adherence of recommendations. These methods have been extremely impactful throughout the pandemic and especially in the absence of pharmaceutical interventions.[53] Although the dynamics of COVID-19 are rapidly changing and countries are increasingly vaccinating their populations, the early ascertainment of infected individuals and subsequent restriction of their contact with the healthy population through the maintenance of these mechanisms will be integral to control the spread of the virus until herd immunity is reached by all countries.[54]

References

1. Markel H, Lipman HB, Navarro JA, Sloan A, Michalsen JR, Stern AM, Cetron MS. Nonpharmaceutical interventions implemented by US cities during the 1918–1919 influenza pandemic. *JAMA* [Internet]. 2007 Aug 8 [cited 16 April 2021];298(6):644–654. Available from: https://jamanetwork.com/journals/jama/article-abstract/208354.

2. Speechley M, Kunnilathu A, Aluckal E, Balakrishna MS, Mathew B, George EK. Screening in public health and clinical care: Similarities and differences in definitions, types, and aims–a systematic review. *JCDR* [Internet]. 2017 Mar [cited 20 March 2021];11(3):LE01. Available from: https://www.ncbi.nlm.nih.gov/pmc/articles/PMC5427344/.

3. Viswanathan M, Kahwati L, Jahn B, Giger K, Dobrescu AI, Hill C, *et al.* Universal screening for SARS-CoV-2 infection: A rapid review. *Cochrane Library* [Internet]. 2020 [cited 20 March 2021];2020(9): CD013718–CD013718. Available from: https://www.cochranelibrary.com/cdsr/doi/10.1002/14651858.CD013718/full.

4. A Dictionary of Epidemiology [Internet]. New York: Oxford University Press; 2008. Screening. [cited 9 March 2021]; [1 page]. Available from: https://www-oxfordreference-com.ezproxy.library.ubc.ca/view/10.1093/acref/9780195314496.001.0001/acref-9780195314496-e-1699?rskey=raToaE&result=1.

5. Gostic K, Gomez AC, Mummah RO, Kucharski AJ, Lloyd-Smith JO. Estimated effectiveness of symptom and risk screening to prevent the spread of COVID-19. *Elife* [Internet]. 2020 Feb 24 [cited 15 March 2021];9:e55570. Available from: https://elifesciences.org/articles/55570.

6. Lauer SA, Grantz KH, Bi Q, Jones FK, Zheng Q, Meredith HR, *et al.* The incubation period of coronavirus disease 2019 (COVID-19) from publicly reported confirmed cases: Estimation and application. *Annals of Internal*

Medicine [Internet]. 2020 May 5 [cited 25 March 2020];172(9):577–582. Available from: https://www.acpjournals.org/doi/full/10.7326/M20-0504.

7. He J, Guo Y, Mao R, Zhang J. Proportion of asymptomatic coronavirus disease 2019: A systematic review and meta-analysis. *Journal of Medical Virology* [Internet]. 2021 Feb [cited 15 March 2021];93(2):820–830. Available from: https://onlinelibrary.wiley.com/doi/full/10.1002/jmv. 26326.

8. Chow EJ, Schwartz NG, Tobolowsky FA, Zacks RL, Huntington-Frazier M, Reddy SC, Rao AK. Symptom screening at illness onset of health care personnel with SARS-CoV-2 infection in King County, Washington. *JAMA* [Internet]. 2020 May 26 [cited 15 March 2021];323(20):2087–2089. Available from: https://jamanetwork.com/journals/jama/article-abstract/2764953.

9. Cairney P, Wellstead A. COVID-19: Effective policymaking depends on trust in experts, politicians, and the public. *Policy Design and Practice* [Internet]. 2020 Oct 23 [cited 15 March 2021]:1–4. Available from: https://www. tandfonline.com/doi/full/10.1080/25741292.2020.1837466.

10. Aggarwal N, Garg M, Dwarakanathan V, Gautam N, Kumar SS, Jadon RS, Gupta M, Ray A. Diagnostic accuracy of non-contact infrared thermometers and thermal scanners: A systematic review and meta-analysis. *Journal of Travel Medicine* [Internet]. 2020 Dec [cited 16 March 2021];27(8):taaa193. Available from: https://academic.oup.com/jtm/article/27/8/taaa193/5920642? login=true.

11. Stokes EK, Zambrano LD, Anderson KN, Marder EP, Raz KM, Felix SE, *et al*. Coronavirus disease 2019 case surveillance — United States, January 22–May 30, 2020. *Morbidity and Mortality Weekly Report* [Internet]. 2020 Jun 19[cited 16 March 2021];69(24):759. Available from: https://www.ncbi. nlm.nih.gov/pmc/articles/PMC7302472/.

12. Mitra B, Luckhoff C, Mitchell RD, O'Reilly GM, Smit DV, Cameron PA. Temperature screening has negligible value for control of COVID-19. *Emergency Medicine Australasia* [Internet]. 2020 Oct [cited 27 March 2021];32(5):867–869. Available from: https://onlinelibrary.wiley.com/doi/ full/10.1111/1742-6723.13578.

13. Bielecki M, Crameri GA, Schlagenhauf P, Buehrer TW, Deuel JW. Body temperature screening to identify SARS-CoV-2 infected young adult travellers is ineffective. *Travel Medicine and Infectious Disease* [Internet]. 2020 Aug [cited 25 March 2021]; 37:101832. Available from: https://www.ncbi. nlm.nih.gov/pmc/articles/PMC7403846/.

14. Alberta Health Services. Effectiveness of Screening Programs for Reducing the Spread of COVID-19 in Healthcare Settings. AHS; 2020 June 12, p. 24.

15. Tahamtan A, Ardebili A. Real-time RT-PCR in COVID-19 detection: Issues affecting the results. *Expert Review of Molecular Diagnostics* [Internet]. 2020 May 3 [cited 6 Apr 2021];20(5):453–454. Available from: https://www.tandfonline.com/doi/pdf/10.1080/14737159.2020.1757437.

16. Schwartz KL, McGeer AJ, Bogoch II. Rapid antigen screening of asymptomatic people as a public health tool to combat COVID-19. *CMAJ* [Internet]. 2021 Mar 29 [cited 6 Apr 2021];193(13):E449–E452. Available from: https://www.cmaj.ca/content/193/13/E449.short.

17. Larremore DB, Wilder B, Lester E, Shehata S, Burke JM, Hay JA, *et al.* Test sensitivity is secondary to frequency and turnaround time for COVID-19 screening. *Science Advances* [Internet]. 2021 Jan 1 [cited 14 Apr 2021]; 7(1):eabd5393. Available from: https://advances.sciencemag.org/content/7/1/eabd5393?ref=theprepping-com.

18. Hoehl S, Rabenau H, Berger A, Kortenbusch M, Cinatl J, Bojkova D, Behrens P, Böddinghaus B, Götsch U, Naujoks F, Neumann P. Evidence of SARS-CoV-2 infection in returning travelers from Wuhan, China. *New England Journal of Medicine* [Internet]. 2020 Mar 26 [cited 2 Apr 2021];382(13):1278–1280. Available from: https://www.nejm.org/doi/full/10.1056/nejmc2001899.

19. Gudbjartsson DF, Helgason A, Jonsson H, Magnusson OT, Melsted P, Norddahl GL, Saemundsdottir J, Sigurdsson A, Sulem P, Agustsdottir AB, Eiriksdottir B. Spread of SARS-CoV-2 in the Icelandic population. *New England Journal of Medicine* [Internet]. 2020 Jun 11 [cited 2 Apr 2021]; 382(24):2302–2315. Available from: https://www.nejm.org/doi/full/10.1056/NEJMoa2006100.

20. World Health Organization. Contact tracing in the context of COVID-19: Interim guidance. WHO; May 2020 May 10, p. 7.

21. World Health Organization. Public health surveillance for COVID-19: Interim Guidance. WHO; 2020 Aug 07, p. 10.

22. Centre of Disease Control. COVID-19 — Appendices [Internet]. CDC; 2021 [updated 2021 March 6; cited 7 March 2021]. Available from: https://www.cdc.gov/coronavirus/2019-ncov/php/contact-tracing/contact-tracing-plan/appendix.html#contact.

23. European Centre for Disease Prevention and Control. Contact tracing: Public health management of persons, including healthcare workers, who have had contact with COVID-19 cases in the European Union — third update. Stockholm: ECDC; 2020 Nov 18, p. 18.

24. Pringle JC, Leikauskas J, Ransom-Kelley S, Webster B, Santos S, Fox H, Marcoux S, Kelso P, Kwit N. COVID-19 in a correctional facility employee

following multiple brief exposures to persons with COVID-19 — Vermont, July–August 2020. *Morbidity and Mortality Weekly Report* [Internet]. 2020 Oct 30 [cited 3 Apr 2021];69(43):1569. Available from: https://www.ncbi.nlm.nih.gov/pmc/articles/PMC7640999/.

25. Chu DK, Akl EA, Duda S, Solo K, Yaacoub S, Schünemann HJ, *et al*. Physical distancing, face masks, and eye protection to prevent person-to-person transmission of SARS-CoV-2 and COVID-19: A systematic review and meta-analysis. *The Lancet* [Internet]. 2020 Jun 27 [cited 3 Apr 2021]; 395(10242):1973–87. Available from: https://www.sciencedirect.com/science/article/pii/S0140673620311429.

26. Jones NR, Qureshi ZU, Temple RJ, Larwood JP, Greenhalgh T, Bourouiba L. Two metres or one: What is the evidence for physical distancing in covid-19?. *BMJ* [Internet]. 2020 Aug 25 [cited 17 Apr 2021];370. Available from: https://www.bmj.com/content/370/bmj.m3223.

27. Bradshaw WJ, Alley EC, Huggins JH, Lloyd AL, Esvelt KM. Bidirectional contact tracing could dramatically improve COVID-19 control. *Nature Communications* [Internet]. 2021 Jan 11 [cited 1 Apr 2021];12(1):1–9. Available from: https://www.nature.com/articles/s41467-020-20325-7.

28. Park YJ, Choe YJ, Park O, Park SY, Kim YM, Kim J, *et al*. Contact tracing during coronavirus disease outbreak, South Korea, 2020. *Emerging Infectious Diseases* [Internet]. 2020 Oct [cited 8 Apr 2021];26(10):2465–2468. Available from: https://stacks.cdc.gov/view/cdc/94765/cdc_94765_DS1.pdf.

29. Kleinman RA, Merkel C. Digital contact tracing for COVID-19. *CMAJ* [Internet]. 2020 Jun 15 [cited 3 Apr 2021];192(24):E653–6. Available from: https://www.cmaj.ca/content/192/24/E653.short.

30. Endo A, Centre for the Mathematical Modelling of Infectious Disease COVID-19 Working Group, Leclerc QJ, Knight GM, Medley GF, Atkins KE, *et al*. Implication of backward contact tracing in the presence of overdispersed transmission in COVID-19 outbreaks [version 3]. *Wellcome Open Research* [Internet]. 2021 March 31 [cited 3 April], 5(239):1–17. Available from: https://wellcomeopenresearch.org/articles/5-239/v3.

31. Kojaku S, Hébert-Dufresne L, Mones E, Lehmann S, Ahn YY. The effectiveness of backward contact tracing in networks. *Nature Physics* [Internet]. 2021 Feb 25 [cited 23 March] 1:1–7. Available from: https://www.nature.com/articles/s41567-021-01187-2.

32. Baraniuk C. Covid-19 contact tracing: A briefing. *BMJ* [Internet]. 2020 May 13 [cited 23 March];369:m1859. Available from: https://www.bmj.com/content/bmj/369/bmj.m1859.full.pdf.

33. Kucharski AJ, Klepac P, Conlan AJ, Kissler SM, Tang ML, Fry H, *et al.* Effectiveness of isolation, testing, contact tracing, and physical distancing on reducing transmission of SARS-CoV-2 in different settings: A mathematical modelling study. *The Lancet Infectious Diseases* [Internet]. 2020 Oct 1 [cited 23 March 2021];20(10):1151–1160. Available from: https://www.sciencedirect.com/science/article/pii/S1473309920304576.

34. Public Health Agency of Canada. Evidence Brief of SARS-CoV-2 Contact Tracing [Internet]. Public Health Agency of Canada Emerging Science Summaries; 2021 Feb 10 [cited 31 March 2021], p. 17.

35. Kretzschmar ME, Rozhnova G, Bootsma MC, van Boven M, van de Wijgert JH, Bonten MJ. Impact of delays on effectiveness of contact tracing strategies for COVID-19: A modelling study. *The Lancet Public Health* [Internet]. 2020 Aug 1 [cited 31 March 2021];5(8):e452–e459. Available from: https://www.sciencedirect.com/science/article/pii/S2468266720301572.

36. Ferretti L, Wymant C, Kendall M, Zhao L, Nurtay A, Abeler-Dörner L, *et al.* Quantifying SARS-CoV-2 transmission suggests epidemic control with digital contact tracing. *Science* [Internet]. 2020 May 8 [cited 29 March]; 368(6491):9. Available from: https://science.sciencemag.org/content/368/6491/eabb6936.abstract.

37. Hellewell J, Abbott S, Gimma A, Bosse NI, Jarvis CI, Russell TW, *et al.* Feasibility of controlling COVID-19 outbreaks by isolation of cases and contacts. *The Lancet Global Health* [Internet]. 2020 Apr 1[cited 2021 March 12];8(4):e188 e496. Available from: https://www.thelancet.com/journals/langlo/article/PIIS2214-109X(20)30074-7/fulltext.

38. Megnin-Viggars O, Carter P, Melendez-Torres GJ, Weston D, Rubin GJ. Facilitators and barriers to engagement with contact tracing during infectious disease outbreaks: A rapid review of the evidence. *PloS One* [Internet]. 2020 Oct 29 [cited 9 March 2021];15(10):e0241473.Available from: https://journals.plos.org/plosone/article?id=10.1371/journal.pone.0241473.

39. Ahmed N, Michelin RA, Xue W, Ruj S, Malaney R, Kanhere SS, Seneviratne A, Hu W, Janicke H, Jha SK. A survey of covid-19 contact tracing apps. *IEEE Access* [Internet]. 2020 Jul 20 [cited 1 April 2021];8:134577–134601. Available from: https://ieeexplore.ieee.org/abstract/document/9144194.

40. Endo A. Centre for the mathematical modelling of infectious diseases Covid-19 working group, Abbott S, Kucharski AJ, Funk S. Estimating the overdispersion in COVID-19 transmission using outbreak sizes outside China. *Wellcome Open Research* [Internet]. 2020 Jul 10 [cited 4 April 2021];5 (67): 1–17. Available from: https://www.ncbi.nlm.nih.gov/pmc/articles/PMC7338915/.

41. Buitrago-Garcia D, Egli-Gany D, Counotte MJ, Hossmann S, Imeri H, Ipekci AM, *et al.* Occurrence and transmission potential of asymptomatic and presymptomatic SARS-CoV-2 infections: A living systematic review and meta-analysis. *PLoS Medicine* [Internet]. 2020 Sep 22 [cited 2021 Apr 18]; 17(9):e1003346. Available from: https://journals.plos.org/plosmedicine/article?id=10.1371/journal.pmed.1003346&fbclid=IwAR2Pu67FUJLESoE TBAL0KDWB_RmPUW_RPzFsfy_rOzzWQFYsgfbPgnFP_ZY.

42. World Health Organization. Considerations for quarantine of contacts of COVID-19 cases: Interim Guidance. WHO; 2020 Aug 19, p. 6.

43. European Centre for Disease Prevention and Control. Guidance for discharge and ending of isolation of people with COVID-19. Stockholm: ECDC: 2020 Oct 16, p. 7.

44. Public Health Agency of Canada. Emerging Evidence on COVID-19: Evidence Brief of COVID-19 quarantine length reduction strategies and effectiveness, Update 1. PHAC Emerging Sciences Summaries: 2020 Dec 3, p. 20.

45. Government of Canada. Mandatory quarantine or isolation [Internet]. *Government of Canada.* 2021 [updated 2021 April 08; cited 17 April 2021]. Available from: https://travel.gc.ca/travel-covid/travel-restrictions/isolation#exemptions.

46. Ryu S, Hwang Y, Yoon H, Chun BC. Self-Quarantine Noncompliance During the COVID-19 Pandemic in South Korea. *Disaster Medicine and Public Health Preparedness* [Internet]. 2020 Oct 12 [cited 1 April 2021]:1–4. Available from: https://www.cambridge.org/core/journals/disaster-medicine-and-public-health-preparedness/article/selfquarantine-noncompliance-during-the-covid19-pandemic-in-south-korea/44485280CA49B6C2B7A15F 289D4DEB8C.

47. Government of the UK. Guidance: Self-isolation compliance checks after international travel. Government of the UK; 2021 Apr 12 [cited 16 Apr 2021]:1. Available from: https://www.gov.uk/guidance/self-isolation-compliance-checks-after-international-travel.

48. DiGiovanni C, Conley J, Chiu D, Zaborski J. Factors influencing compliance with quarantine in Toronto during the 2003 SARS outbreak. *Biosecurity and Bioterrorism: Biodefense Strategy, Practice, and Science* [Internet]. 2004 Dec 1 [cited 15 Apr 2021]; 2(4):265–272. Available from: https://www.liebertpub.com/doi/abs/10.1089/bsp.2004.2.265.

49. Public Health Agency of Canada. Evidence brief on adherence to isolation and quarantine recommendations during COVID-19 [Internet]. Public Health

Agency of Canada Emerging Science Summaries; 2021 Jan 2 [cited 1 April 2021]:11.

50. Independent Scientific Pandemic Influenza Groups on Behaviours. Impact of financial and other targeted support on rates of self-isolation or quarantine. SPI-B; 2020 Sep 16, p. 11.

51. Bodas M, Peleg K. Income assurances are a crucial factor in determining public compliance with self-isolation regulations during the COVID-19 outbreak–cohort study in Israel. *Israel Journal of Health Policy Research* [Internet]. 2020 Dec [cited 14 Apr 2021]; 9 (54):1–10. Available from: https://ijhpr.biomedcentral.com/track/pdf/10.1186/s13584-020-00418-w.pdf.

52. Lewnard JA, Lo NC. Scientific and ethical basis for social-distancing interventions against COVID-19. *The Lancet Infectious Diseases* [Internet]. 2020 Jun 1 [cited 14 Apr 2021];20(6):631–633. Available from: https://ijhpr. biomedcentral.com/track/pdf/10.1186/s13584-020-00418-w.pdf.

53. Lai S, Ruktanonchai NW, Zhou L, Prosper O, Luo W, Floyd JR, *et al.* Effect of non-pharmaceutical interventions to contain COVID-19 in China. *Nature* [Internet]. 2020 Sep [cited 14 Apr];585(7825):410–413. Available from: https://www.nature.com/articles/s41586-020-2293-x?fbclid=IwAR2dya0pm bsHmo2Awftr1EGE9aqiucveRhtDQL8Wogx_aaFeKa2UzCwa4Xo.

54. Scudellari M. How the pandemic might play out in 2021 and beyond. *Nature* [Internet]. 2020 [cited 14 Apr]:22–25. Available from: https://pesquisa. bvsalud.org/portal/resource/fr/mdl-32760050.

Chapter 8

Restrictions on Travel

Ali Okhowat[*,†,‡], Bassel Bali[*], and Mark Lysyshyn[*,§]

[*]*School of Population and Public Health, University of British Columbia, Vancouver, Canada*

[†]*Department of Family Practice, Faculty of Medicine, University of British Columbia, Vancouver, Canada*

[‡]*Division of Global Health, Faculty of Medicine, University of British Columbia, Vancouver, Canada*

[§]*Vancouver Coastal Health, Vancouver, Canada*

Key Message

- The 2005 International Health Regulations (IHR) provide a legal framework outlining countries' rights and responsibilities in detecting, assessing and responding to public health events and emergencies that have the potential to cross borders.
- The spread of SARS-CoV-2 showed that countries' attainment of essential public health functions and health system readiness were not well correlated with limiting or preventing deaths from COVID-19. In response to COVID-19, reforms have been forwarded to strengthen IHR and other mechanisms to prevent the next pandemic.
- Reviews of international travel restrictions have found that policies focused on screening patients from regions of the world with COVID-19 epidemics or those that relied on symptom or sign

145

screening or lax quarantine requirements were likely to have missed SARS-CoV-2 positive persons.

- While symptom or exposure-based screening policies at points of entry may not be effective on their own, PCR testing at borders will likely lead to a significant reduction in false negatives.
- A risk-based approach to international travel means that countries must systematically and regularly undertake risk assessments to guide the introduction, refinement or cancellation of basic versus supplementary risk mitigation measures and travel-based restrictions based on consideration of factors relevant to the potential importation, exportation or onward transmission of SARS-CoV-2.
- The WHO publications of July 2021, *Policy considerations for implementing a risk-based approach to international travel in the context of COVID-19* and the technical annex, provide an important framework for implementing a risk-based approach to international travel restrictions.

1. Introduction

Can a cough in Cairo one week lead to lockdowns in London the next? Do pre-departure or post-arrival SARS-CoV-2 diagnostic tests help in reducing virus transmission? What about quarantine measures upon arrival — are they useful and, if so, what is the difference in effectiveness between seven versus ten days or longer? How should increasing vaccination rates or the spread of variants of concern (VOCs) inform policy decisions on risk mitigation measures? How do local transmission dynamics affect guidance regarding how many persons can safely gather in different spaces? How can countries most effectively protect their domestic populations against the spread of SARS-CoV-2 while facilitating the re-opening of borders and trade?

These are the questions that we must now contend with as we struggle to extinguish outbreaks in across a landscape of international travel that has been scorched by the pandemic. Per data from the International Civil Aviation Organization (ICAO), a review of 2019 versus 2020 international passenger flight data reveals a mean drop of 63% worldwide (Figure 1).

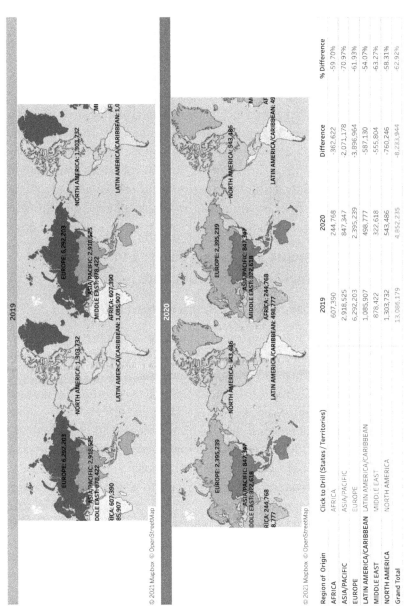

Figure 1:   Comparison of international passenger flights per region (2019 versus 2020).[1]

Region of Origin	Click to Drill (States / Territories)	2019	2020	Difference	% Difference
AFRICA	AFRICA	607,390	244,768	-362,622	-59.70%
ASIA/PACIFIC	ASIA/PACIFIC	2,918,525	847,347	-2,071,178	-70.97%
EUROPE	EUROPE	6,292,203	2,395,239	-3,896,964	-61.93%
LATIN AMERICA/CARIBBEAN	LATIN AMERICA/CARIBBEAN	1,085,907	498,777	-587,130	-54.07%
MIDDLE EAST	MIDDLE EAST	878,422	322,618	-555,804	-63.27%
NORTH AMERICA	NORTH AMERICA	1,303,732	543,486	-760,246	-58.31%
Grand Total		13,086,179	4,852,235	-8,233,944	-62.92%

Pre-pandemic practices related to travel are unlikely to resume without change. Our "new normal" for international and even domestic travel and large gatherings will likely include new policies and international agreements, standard public health and social measures, and a menu of administrative, engineering and personal protective equipment-related controls that will become commonplace. In the pandemic's current timeline, however, it is important to understand which measures could be the most helpful by implementing evidence-informed policy and applying precautionary principles that protect the most vulnerable. To this end, this chapter begins with a background on the International Health Regulations (IHR, 2005) and other global or regional infectious hazards coordination mechanisms before moving on to a review of preventive and mitigating measures relevant to travel (international and domestic) and quarantine.

2. Global Agreements and Goals Related to the Control of Disease Spread Between Countries

2.1 *The International Health Regulations (2005)*

In the aftermath of the severe acute respiratory syndrome (SARS) epidemic in 2003, increases in international travel and trade and the emergence of novel infectious and other health hazards, 196 countries agreed in 2005 to the IHR. This is a legal framework that outlines countries' rights and responsibilities in detecting, assessing and responding to public health events and emergencies that have the potential to cross borders. Specifically, the IHR (2005) seek to, "prevent, protect against, control and provide a public health response to the international spread of disease in ways that are commensurate with and restricted to public health risks, and which avoid unnecessary interference with international traffic and trade."[2] The IHR requires — among other commitments — that nations strengthen core surveillance and response capacities at the primary, subnational, and national levels and at designated international ports, airports, and ground crossings.[3]

The COVID-19 pandemic was an important test of the IHR. After COVID-19 emerged in January 2020, the WHO recommended some precautions for travelers and advised against any travel or trade restraints.

The WHO Director-General issued temporary recommendations under the IHR (2005) after declaring a public health emergency of international concern (PHEIC) on January 30. In contrast, most countries implemented differing degrees of international travel restrictions by the end of March 2020, and many countries closed their borders to most international travelers shortly thereafter. At the date of writing (July 2021), international travel restrictions are still in force in most countries with one-third of worldwide destinations partially closed. According to the latest data, the emergence of new variants of the COVID-19 virus has prompted many governments to reverse efforts to ease travel restrictions.

2.2 *The sustainable development goals (2015)*

In 2015, the UN General Assembly endorsed the 2030 Agenda for Sustainable Development. As an extension of a five-part holistic development paradigm based on, "People, Planet, Partnership, Peace and Prosperity," this vision articulated goals and monitoring activities that have been summarised in 17 sustainable development goals (SDGs), 169 targets and more than 230 indicators. Five core principles underpinned the development of the Agenda:

1. **Interconnectedness and indivisibility:** The 17 SDGs are interconnected and indivisible meaning that countries should focus on attaining all of them to truly achieve any one of them.
2. **Inclusiveness:** Participation using a whole-of-society approach is needed to achieve the goals.
3. **Leaving no one behind:** All people, especially those who are most vulnerable, should benefit from the attainment of these goals, hence the need for local, disaggregated data.
4. **Multi-stakeholder partnerships:** Partnerships should be established to share resources and collaborate on implementation.
5. **Universality:** The Agenda applies to all countries and contexts at all times.

SDG 3 seeks to ensure healthy lives and promote well-being for all at all ages but health-related targets can be found in all of the SDGs and

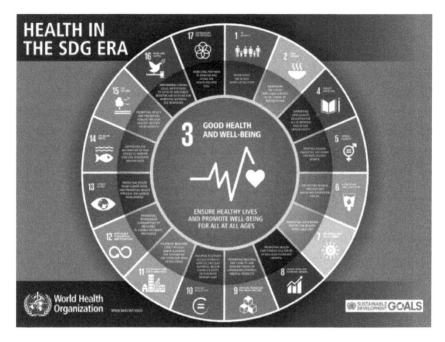

Figure 2:   SDG 3 interrelates with all other SDGs.

progress on one SDG affects and is affected by progress on other SDGs (Figure 2). While goals 3.3 and 3.B refer to communicable disease control and research and development targets, respectively, 3.D speaks most directly to the programs that all countries should have in place to protect epidemics from spreading out of control. The global target refers to, "[strengthening] the capacity of all countries, in particular developing countries, for early warning, risk reduction and management of national and global health risks." The strengthening of IHR at the national level has thus been formalised through the United Nations system via indicator 3.D.1 that each country should, theoretically, report on every year in its pursuit of the SDGs. The IHR self-assessment and reporting tool that each Member States undertake captures the level of self-assessed national capacities and is measured as a percentage fulfillment of essential public health capacities that States Parties are required to have in place through-out their territories (pursuant to Articles 5 and 12, and Annex 1A of the IHR (2005) requirements).[4]

Unfortunately, the spread of SARS-CoV-2 showed that countries' attainment of essential public health functions and health system readiness were not well correlated with limiting or preventing deaths from COVID-19 (see Chapter 17, Figure 1). While the reasons for this are complex, Member States are unanimous in agreeing upon the fact that the current international system cannot bring an end to the current pandemic nor prevent the next one. Additionally, while the policies and interventions will invariably be debated, the role of international travel and conveyance is one that is undeniably central to the discussion of pandemic preparedness, response and recovery.

2.3 *The need for international coordination*

As countries move forward with further adjustments of travel restrictions and strengthening of IHR capacities, a coordinated approach is essential. Harmonised screening, testing and immunisation requirements will be a necessary prerequisite to the reopening of travel without unnecessary difficulties for travelers and service providers.[5] Unfortunately, this pandemic laid bare the limitations of the global goals and agreements, as many countries undertook unilateral actions in an attempt to prevent or limit the transmission of disease.

In response, renewed calls for solidarity have emerged through the establishment of new councils and expert panels, such as the WHO Council on the Economics of Health for All, the COVID-19 Global Research and Innovation Forum, and the One Health High-Level Expert Panel, as well as countries' decisions to support temporary waivers on intellectual property rights for COVID-19 vaccines. As well, new initiatives and organisations have come to the fore in the leadup to the World Health Assembly and G20 Global Health Summit in May 2021, including the launch of the Global Pandemic Radar in the UK, the Germany-based WHO Hub for Pandemic and Epidemic Intelligence, and the first WHO BioHub Facility (as part of the WHO BioHub System) in Geneva. Lastly, several recent publications, including the reports of the Independent Panel on Pandemic Preparedness and Response, the Independent Oversight and Advisory Committee for the WHO Health Emergencies Programme, and the Review Committee on the Functioning of the IHR (2005) during the

COVID-19 Response, have outlined reforms that should happen to the IHR and wider detection, assessment and response mechanism in place globally to prevent the spread of the next epidemic. These are covered further in this volume's final chapter but include:

1. Prioritise pandemic preparedness as a top political and leadership priority.
2. Establish a new global pandemic surveillance system.
3. Launch a pandemic supply chain platform.
4. Institute rapid and sustained financing mechanisms for pandemic preparedness and response.
5. Empower a focused, independent and fully funded World Health Organization.

2.4 *Examples on preventing or mitigating SARS-CoV-2 transmission via travel-related policies*

Almost all governments have attempted to include within their response toolkit to the COVID-19 pandemic some form of travel-related and mass gathering restrictions that have sought to prevent or slow the virus's spread. Approaches and outcomes have been heterogeneous yet a review of specific countries' interventions is helpful in gleaning insights from some of the more effective interventions.

Thailand was the first country outside China that reported a new case of COVID-19 in Bangkok on January 13, 2020. In response, it formed a contact tracing platform to assess importation risk and monitor the spread of the virus via international tourists and Thais coming from high-risk countries. This data was collected from all domestic airports to facilitate tracking and strict follow up on quarantine requirements. These measures enabled Thailand to achieve reasonable control following the first wave (Figure 3).[6] These tracing applications were genuinely beneficial for preliminary screening of those people who traveled from outbreak locations, in addition to reducing the visits to public health service centers. Apart from the above measures, the government lockdown policy significantly reduced individual mobility, including cross-border movement.[7]

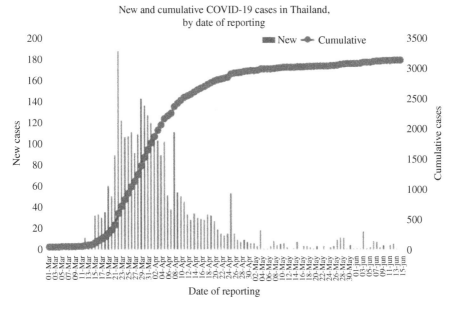

Figure 3: COVID-19 daily statistics in Thailand (March 01– June 15, 2020).[8]

Australia and New Zealand were also distinguished for employing aggressive public health measures with a view to reducing transmission to zero. Strict travel restrictions, quarantine and physical distancing measures, as well as early and widespread testing and contact tracing were credited with enabling the Australian and New Zealand governments to mitigate extensive community transmission of COVID-19.[9] Many high resource countries were, however, far less responsive to the threat of SARS-CoV-2 transmission until well into the community transmission phase of domestic spread. The United States, many European countries and parts of Canada initiated controls later and with a view to balancing public health controls with a desire to keep society and economies functioning. This led to a higher likelihood of introduction of virus from abroad and of facing importation risks of additional cases that would lead to a tipping point of exponential growth.

2.5 *A model of travel-related COVID-19 transmission*

Numerous articles have been published regarding travel-related modelling of COVID-19 transmission risks.[10–12] Several indicate that in early stages of local spread, travelers may edge transmission dynamics towards a tipping point and some suggest that they have worse health outcomes than domestic populations.[13,14] Under these circumstances, higher rates of introduction are naturally expected to increase the risk of a domestic epidemic. In the early stages of the pandemic, both international and domestic travel likely contributed to increasing risk within the domestic populations.[15] This model supports the value of quarantine as an early public health intervention and predicts lower risk of epidemic establishment with stronger limits on both domestic and international travel.[16]

Travel can contribute to epidemic spread in several ways:

1. Most modes of transportation create greater opportunities for close contact with many individuals, often in an enclosed environment.
2. Introductions from regions of the world with a higher burden of disease are a major source of epidemic seeding.

National and international guidance on control of travelers has been evolving. Unfortunately, policies that paid attention primarily to screening patients from parts of the world known to be experiencing epidemics frequently fell behind the rapid spread of the virus. Policies that relied only on insensitive methods like symptom or temperature screening were likely to miss people with few or no symptoms or who were pre-symptomatic or asymptomatic transmitters. Quarantine requirements were not strictly monitored or enforced were found to be permeable even into the third wave of the pandemic in countries like Canada.

2.6 *The case of Canada*

Early in the pandemic, data from many provinces in Canada (supported by whole genome sequencing results) indicated the importance of importation from abroad — especially from the United States — in initiating the first wave of the pandemic.[17] Consequently, Canadian health authorities

Table 1: Test volumes and positivity rates for SARS-CoV-2 via Canadian border testing results (February 21–June 24, 2021).

| | Air | | Land | | Overall |
Date	Tests completed	Percent positive (%)	Total tests completed	Percent positive (%)	percent positive (%)
Feb 21–28, 2021	10,117	1.4	2,534	0.2	1.2
Mar 1–31, 2021	125,828	1.6	43,876	0.3	1.3
Apr 1–30, 2021	173,667	2.1	90,741	0.4	1.5
May 1–31, 2021	141,659	0.4	141,432	0.2	0.3
June 1–24, 2021*	134,895	0.3	101,920	0.1	0.3
Totals	586,166	1.2	380,503	0.2	0.8

Note: *June 2021 results are incomplete as test results are still incoming.

have actively consulted an importation risk model since the early days of the pandemic.[18] This dynamic model provided estimates of the average weekly number of travelers arriving in Canada infected with COVID-19 with a focus on the mode of travel and positivity rates (Table 1).

Data from ArriveCAN, a digital tool used by the Government of Canada to collect contact and quarantine information from travellers upon and after entry into Canada, was used to discern the proportion of travelers exempt from pre-arrival testing for those using land versus air modes of transportation. Key inputs for both land and air travel and pre-arrival PCR testing within 72 hours for non-essential travelers included:

- The volume of travelers (by air and land).
- Country- and American state-specific weekly incidence rates.
- Temporal trends in infection dynamics.
- Border measures (pre-arrival testing within 72 hours for non-essential travelers).

More recently, with the rise of VOIs and VOCs, importation risk estimates have also been disaggregated by VOC type (see Table 2).

Table 2:   WHO designated VOC (as of June 30, 2021).[19]

WHO label	Pango lineages	GISAID clade	Nextstrain clade	Additional amino acid changes monitored*	Earliest documented samples	Date of designation
Alpha	B.1.1.7	GRY	20I (V1)	+S:484K +S:452R	United Kingdom, Sep-2020	18-Dec-2020
Beta	B.1.351 B.1.351.2 B.1.351.3	GH/501Y.V2	20H (V2)	+S:L18F	South Africa, May-2020	18-Dec-2020
Gamma	P.1 P.1.1 P.1.2	GR/501Y.V3	20J (V3)	+S:681H	Brazil, Nov-2020	11-Jan-2021
Delta	B.1.617.2 AY.1 AY.2	G/478K.V1	21A	+S:417N	India, Oct-2020	VOI: 4-Apr-2021 VOC: 11-May-2021

Note: *Only found in a subset of sequences.

Table 3:   Positive test sequencing results in Canada (February 22–June 18, 2021).[20]

Mode	Variant of concern (VOC) Total	Alpha VOC B.1.1.7	Beta VOC B.1.351	Delta VOC B.1.617.2	Gamma VOC P.1	Variants of interest (VOI) total
Border total	2,766	2,053	93	453	85	247
Land total	469	341	17	71	63	53
Air total	2,292	1,712	76	382	22	194

As of June 18, 2021, all VOCs have been imported to Canada and comprise a considerable proportion of isolates with a particularly concerning rise in the highly transmissible delta variant (Table 3).

Of note, these models estimated that there were 2,223 infected travelers expected to arrive in Canada, by air and land, during a single week (February 28–March 3, 2021). The US continued to be the primary source of importation risk to Canada, followed by Lebanon and India (Figure 4).

Likewise, Table 4 shows the mean number of infected travelers arriving at major Canadian airports for the same week (February 28–March 3, 2021). Also shown are the number of countries contributing infected travelers and the top country contributors.

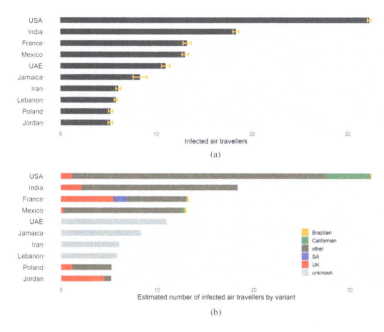

Figure 4: For the period February 28–March 3, 2021: (a) the top 10 countries expected to have contributed air travelers infected with SARS-CoV-2; (b) and the estimated distribution of variants from these travelers.[21]

Table 4: Mean number of infected travelers arriving at major Canadian airports and number of contributing regions (February 28–March 3, 2021).[22]

Airport	Mean Number of infected travellers	Number of contributing regions (countries and US states)	Top countries
Toronto Pearson	84	240	USA, India, UAE/Jamaica
Montréal-Trudeau	38	235	France, USA, Mexico
Vancouver International	23	222	USA, France, India
Calgary International	18	217	USA, Mexico, Netherlands

On January 7, 2021, non-essential travelers were required to have a PCR negative test result within 72 hours of departure. This intervention has had a significant impact, and since then, there is evidence for significant decreases that resulted in the number of travelers arriving who tested positive for SARS-CoV-2 (Figure 5, solid line).

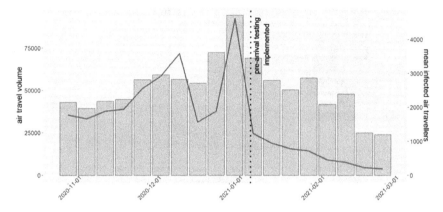

Figure 5:   Estimated number of air travellers arriving infected into Canadian airports over time (solid line), in comparison to the volume of air travellers (dotted stacks).[23]

Note: Data shown relative to the date when the pre-arrival test was implemented on January 7, 2021.

3. Considerations for a Risk-Based Approach to the Resumption of International Travel

The implementation of travel restrictions cascaded in March and April of 2020 as exponential spread of SARS-CoV-2 and overburdened health systems forced countries to seek out measures that would further prevent the spread of COVID-19. Despite the persistent use of this very important package of policy tools, the lack of "real world evidence" is a concern in studies that have sought to assess the impact of travel restrictions on the spread of COVID-19. These reviews have primarily relied on modelling simulations to estimate the effect of these interventions given the lack of a counterfactual scenario. A recent Cochrane review that examined 49 modelling and 13 observational studies focused on containing the spread of COVID-19 via international travel control measures grouped the interventions into the following four, non-mutually exclusive interventions:

1. Preventing entry across international borders to stop non-essential travellers from crossing international borders.
2. Limiting travel to and from specific countries — especially those with high rates of reported cases or dangerous transmission dynamic characteristics.

3. Testing travellers arriving to or departing from a country if they have symptoms or have been in contact with an infected person.
4. Quarantining incoming international or domestic travellers for a certain period of time.

Travel restrictions focused on reducing or stopping cross-border travel were reviewed in 31 modelling studies. The range in reductions of COVID-19 transmission were considerable — including some that found no beneficial effect. This likely resulted from differing assumptions about the stringency of travel restrictions, the destinations affected by these restrictions and baseline versus evolving transmission dynamics in the arrival versus departure countries. Of note, all studies predicted that while these restrictions could delay, from one to 85 days, the spread of COVID-19 in the arrival country.

Of the studies that examined pre-departure or point of entry screening measures (13 modelling studies and 13 observational studies), modelling studies found that symptom-based screening decreased from 1% to 53% importation or exportation of cases and had the added benefit of delaying outbreaks. Observational studies, however, reported an even wider range, from 0% to 100%, with most studies reporting less than 54% detected.

Of the 12 modelling studies examining the effectiveness of quarantine, all found it to be a beneficial measure, though the effect estimates varied widely with some studies reporting as few as 450 cases being prevented while other reported 64,000 fewer cases. This likely reflects different assumptions about baseline incidence rates, local transmission dynamic characteristics and assumed compliance rates with quarantine measures.

For the seven modelling and four observational studies that reviewed quarantine and screening measures, most found some benefit in reductions in cases, though there was a wide range with, for example, observational studies reporting from 68% to 92% of cases reportedly being detected. This likely reflected differences in baseline incidence of SARS-CoV-2 infection in incoming travellers and the frequency of testing.

Of note, investigators' confidence in the strength of the results was limited given that most were based on mathematical models and of those that derived from observational studies were not readily comparable given different specifications of travel-related interventions. Overall, restricting cross-border travel was deemed to be a potentially helpful measure. In contrast, symptom-based screening was found to likely to lead to many false negatives while testing at points of entry would find more but would still miss a large number of cases if only done once at border points. Lastly, quarantine lasting at least 10 days was found to be likely the most effective when combined with testing. An important point that was highlighted in their conclusion was that while travel-related restrictions are likely beneficial in reducing the spread of COVID-19 across borders, more studies should focus on both the benefits and risks of travel-related control measure — not only at the individual level but also at the level of societies at large.

3.1   *Considerations for implementing a risk-based approach to international travel in the context of COVID-19*

In December 2020, the WHO released a guidance document, *Policy considerations for implementing a risk-based approach to international travel in the context of COVID-19*, advising countries on measures related to COVID-19 and importation and exportation risks via international travel. Since then, three important developments occurred that necessitated updated recommendations to be issued on July 2, 2021.[24] First, the scale up of vaccination campaigns in countries around the world has led to a significant increase in vaccine-derived immunity (that has added population-level protections to rising levels of infection-derived immunity) and a concomitant decrease in transmission of SARS-CoV-2. Second, the spread of SARS-CoV-2 VOC — which may be more infective, virulent, or evade protections afforded from vaccine or prior infection-derived immunity — have forced countries to re-examine travel restrictions to and from specific countries and/or regions. Lastly, with vaccination rates rising and   case counts, generally, falling in most regions around the world, many countries are re-examining their travel restrictions and looking to a phased re-opening of international non-essential travel to and from their borders.

The focus on a risk-based approach means that countries must systematically and regularly undertake risk assessments to guide the introduction, refinement or cancellation of travel-based restrictions based on consideration of factors relevant to the potential importation, exportation or onward transmission of SARS-CoV-2. By mid-2021, this means including considerations of vaccination status, VOCs and variants of interest (VOIs) and the evidence of the effectiveness (or lack thereof) of specific risk mitigation measures related to international travel. Examples of three primary outcomes related to these interventions are:

1. Cases detected due to the measure.
2. Shift in epidemic development.
3. Cases avoided due to the measure.

Risk mitigation measures should focus on application of, at minimum, basic risk mitigation measures that may be targeted to or within the scope of individuals, organisations, and governmental authorities to reduce virus transmission. At the individual level, these measures include not allowing confirmed, probable, or suspect cases or their contacts to travel, implementing physical distancing and mask wearing policies, and considering deferral of travel for all persons at increased risk or who come from communities of increased risk of transmission. As well, international travellers should continue to self-monitor for signs or symptoms of influenza-like illness. At the organisational level, coordination between disease prevention and control, surveillance and case management entities at the subnational, national and international levels should continue. An important caveat to note is that contact tracing or related activities where patient-identifiable information may be shared (even in the aggregate) must be balanced with due consideration of stringent privacy protections. At the level of government managing ports of entry, environmental, administrative and personal protective equipment controls should be reinforced in order to ensure that undue transmission does not occur. This includes considerations of crowd control, engineering modifications to ensure physical distancing and adequate ventilation of closed spaces, as well as signage and other notifications to remind all persons to adhere to basic risk mitigation measures.

Supplementary risk mitigation measures may be guided by a risk assessment process that considers context-specific questions and the risk tolerance of the jurisdiction under consideration. Depending on the context, additional measures related to the following interventions may be deemed beneficial:

- Exit and entry screening for signs and symptoms of COVID-19.
- SARS-CoV-2 testing for international travellers.
- Quarantine for international travellers.
- Border closure or suspension of travel.
- Proof of COVID-19 vaccination in the context of international travel.

3.2 *Exit and entry screening for signs and symptoms of COVID-19*

With this in mind, it is helpful to consider the key questions for inbound versus outbound travel that may inform national and sub-national supplementary risk mitigation measures related to international travel in the context of COVID-19 (Table 5).

4. Conclusions

Reducing the spread of COVID-19 and alleviating overburdened healthcare systems has become an international priority. Disease modelling and evidence-based reviews have demonstrated that risk-mitigation measures for travel, quarantine and self-isolation policies are each helpful in different contexts to achieving this goal. While symptom or exposure-based screening policies at points of entry may not be effective on their own, polymerase chain reaction (PCR) testing at borders will likely lead to a significant reduction in false negatives. However, if performed only upon arrival, even PCR testing will likely omit a significant percentage of cases. Supplementing this with quarantine of at least 10 days will invariably improve the effectiveness of detection. Due consideration must be given though to baseline transmission dynamics, travel volumes, the implementation of other public health and social measures and the implementation characteristics of travel-related measures.

Table 5: Inbound versus outbound travel-related questions to consider for a risk-based approach to international travel in the context of COVID-19.

Inbound travel	Outbound travel
Will the number of cases to be imported from the country of departure likely have a significant impact on the current transmission level in the country of destination?	How likely are travellers to be infected in the country of destination compared to their likelihood of getting infected in the country of departure, taking into consideration the potential circulation of VOIs and/or VOCs in the country of destination?
What is the air, land and sea route-specific volume of travellers? What is the probability of individuals from the country of departure being infected?	What travel-related measures are implemented for inbound travellers in the country of destination, including the use of individualised public health measures based on a person's SARS-CoV-2 immunity status following COVID-19 vaccination or natural infection?
Are any variants classified by WHO as VOIs or VOCs that are not present in the country of destination predominant in the country of departure? Are there unexpected epidemiological trends or signals in the country of departure that may indicate the appearance of new VOCs or VOIs? Do variants that are present in the country of departure evade immunity? Or, if the country of departure has limited sequencing capacities, have VOCs or VOIs been widely detected among travellers arriving from this country?	Does the country of destination have sufficient response capacity to treat travellers who may need medical care while traveling?
Is an individualised approach to public health measures based on a person's SARS-CoV-2 immunity status being implemented in the country of destination?	Does the country of departure have sufficient capacity to enforce mandatory public health and social measures on return of travellers?
Are the current response capacities in the country of destination sufficient to cope with the potential rise of imported cases from the country of departure? This should include risk communication capacities to inform incoming travellers, in appropriate languages, about mechanisms for seeking care and public health and social distancing measures in place. Are such public health and healthcare capacities accessible to all travellers, including refugees, migrants and temporary or seasonal workers?	In line with the principle of shared responsibility for global health, national authorities should also consider measures to limit exportation of cases, particularly when new VOCs or VOIs emerge.

References

1. Comparison of international passenger flights 2019 versus 2020. International Civil Aviation Organization (ICAO). COVID-19 Air Traffic Dashboard. https://data.icao.int/coVID-19/operational.htm [Accessed 30 April 2021].

2. World Health Organization (WHO) Newsroom. Emergencies: International health regulations and emergency committees. https://www.who.int/news-room/q-a-detail/emergencies-international-health-regulations-and-emergency-committees [Accessed 04 May 2021].

3. Von Tigerstrom B, Halabi S, Wilson K. The International Health Regulations (2005) and the re-establishment of international travel amidst the COVID-19 pandemic. *Journal of Travel Medicine*. 2020;27(8).

4. SDG indicator metadata. UN Stats. United Nations. https://unstats.un.org/sdgs/metadata/files/Metadata-03-0D-01.pdf [Accessed 05 May 2021].

5. Von Tigerstrom B, Wilson K. COVID-19 travel restrictions and the International Health Regulations (2005). *BMJ Global Health*. 2020;5(5): e002629.

6. Haddawy P, Lawpoolsri S, Sa-ngamuang C, Su Yin M, Barkowsky T, Wiratsudakul A *et al*. Effects of COVID-19 government travel restrictions on mobility in a rural border area of Northern Thailand: A mobile phone tracking study. *PLOS ONE*. 2021;16(2):e0245842.

7. Mungaomklang A, Atsawawaranunt K, Kochakarn T, Batty E, Kaewmalang P, Kongklieng A *et al*. Pitfalls of exceptions for COVID-19 travel quarantine: Lessons from a dignitary visit to Thailand. *Journal of Travel Medicine*. 2021;28(2).

8. WHO Thailand situation report — COVID-19. World Health Organization Thailand Country Office. WHO Health Emergencies Programme. https://www.who.int/docs/default-source/searo/thailand/2020-06-15-tha-sitrep-92-covid19.pdf?sfvrsn=98499022_2 [Accessed 14 April 2021].

9. Shaban RZ, Li C, O'Sullivan MVN *et al*. COVID-19 in Australia: Our national response to the first cases of SARS-CoV-2 infection during the early biocontainment phase. *International Medicine Journal*. 2021;51(1):42–51. doi:10.1111/imj.15105.

10. Ogden NH, Fazil A, Arino J, Berthiaume P, Fisman DN, Greer AL *et al*. Artificial intelligence in public health: Modelling scenarios of the epidemic of COVID-19 in Canada. *Canada Communicable Disease Report* 2020; 46(8): 198.

11. Shah NH, Sheoran N, Jayswal E, Shukla D, Shukla N, Shukla J, Shah Y. Modelling COVID-19 transmission in the United States through interstate

and foreign travels and evaluating impact of governmental public health interventions. *Journal of Mathematical Analysis and Applications*, 2020: 124896.

12. Yang J, Li J, Lai S, Ruktanonchai CW, Xing W, Carioli A, *et al.* Uncovering two phases of early intercontinental COVID-19 transmission dynamics. *Journal of Travel Medicine* 2020;27(8):taaa200.

13. Bielecki M, Patel D, Hinkelbein J, Komorowski M, Kester J, Ebrahim S *et al.* Reprint of: Air travel and COVID-19 prevention in the pandemic and peri-pandemic period: A narrative review. *Travel Medicine and Infectious Disease* 2020;38:101939.

14. Gunthe SS, Patra SS. Impact of international travel dynamics on domestic spread of 2019-nCoV in India: Origin-based risk assessment in importation of infected travelers. Globalization and Health 2020;16:1–7.

15. Shah N, Sheoran N, Jayswal E, Shukla D, Shukla N, Shukla J *et al.* Modelling COVID-19 transmission in the United States through interstate and foreign travels and evaluating impact of governmental public health interventions. *Journal of Mathematical Analysis and Applications*. 2020;124896.

16. Burns J, Movsisyan A, Stratil JM, Biallas RL, Coenen M, Emmert-Fees KMF, Geffert K, Hoffmann S, Horstick O, Laxy M, Klinger C, Kratzer S, Litwin T, Norris S, Pfadenhauer LM, von Philipsborn P, Sell K, Stadelmaier J, Verboom B, Voss S, Wabnitz K, Rehfuess E. International travel-related control measures to contain the COVID-19 pandemic: A rapid review. *Cochrane Database of Systematic Reviews* 2021;3:Art. No.: CD013717. DOI: 10.1002/14651858.CD013717.pub2.

17. McLaughlin A, Montoya V, Miller RL, Mordecai G, Worobey M, Poon A, Joy J. Early and ongoing importations of SARS-CoV-2 in Canada. 2021. medRxiv.

18. Arino J *et al.* *Investigation of Global and Local COVID-19 Importation Risks*. Report to the Public Health Risk Science division of the Public Health Agency of Canada, 2020.

19. World Health Organization (WHO). Tracking SARS-CoV-2 variants. https://www.who.int/en/activities/tracking-SARS-CoV-2-variants/ [Accessed 30 June 2021].

20. Public Health Agency of Canada. COVID-19: Summary data about travellers, testing and compliance. Government of Canada. https://www.canada.ca/en/public-health/services/diseases/coronavirus-disease-covid-19/testing-screening-contact-tracing/summary-data-travellers.html#a3 [Accessed 28 June 2021].

21. National Microbiology Laboratory. COVID-19: PHAC modelling group report. Public Health Agency of Canada. Ottawa, Canada, pp. 19–20.

22. National Microbiology Laboratory. COVID-19: PHAC modelling group report. Public Health Agency of Canada. Ottawa, Canada, p. 22.
23. National Microbiology Laboratory. COVID-19: PHAC modelling group report. Public Health Agency of Canada. Ottawa, Canada, p. 20.
24. World Health Organization (WHO). Policy considerations for implementing a risk-based approach to international travel in the context of COVID-19. https://www.who.int/publications/i/item/WHO-2019-nCoV-Risk-based-international-travel-2020.1 [Accessed 02 July 2021].

Chapter 9

Non-Medical Masking, Hygiene and Social Distancing

Tina Cheng* and Michael Brauer*,†

*School of Population and Public Health, University of British Columbia, Vancouver, Canada

†Institute for Health Metrics and Evaluation, University of Washington, Seattle, USA

Key Message

- Non-pharmaceutical interventions (NPIs), actions apart from getting vaccinations and taking medications, include wearing non-medical masks, washing hands, and physical distancing and a variety of other measures which are the subject of other chapters in this book.
- NPI's protect individuals and communities by reducing the number of spreaders, reducing the reproductive number (growth function) and by providing decision-makers time to introduce additional definitive measures such as immunisation.
- Non-medical masks block virus-containing particles/droplets via mechanical and electrostatic filtration, and have proven up to 79% effective in reducing transmission in close contacts of primary cases. On a population level, countries and regions with mask mandates showed evidence of a decreased burden of COVID-19 cases and deaths.

- Hand washing is effective in reducing transmission of many infections. Soap and water work to trap and remove pathogens and have advantages over alcohol-based hand sanitisers and surface disinfectants when soiling is present.
- Physical distancing of at least 2 meters is better than 1 meter. Increased distances reduce the likelihood of exposure to a high viral load through droplets/air and on surfaces close to an infectious person.
- NPIs should be combined for optimum protection and tailored depending on the risk levels. NPIs should be practiced continuously during vaccine roll-out and tapered only slowly during the early post-pandemic era.

1. Introduction

1.1 *Wearing masks, washing hands, and watching your distance*

In order to effectively control the spread of COVID-19, all levels of society, from communities to individuals, must play their role. Understanding how the SARS-CoV-2 coronavirus spreads, knowing how to prevent illness, and taking care of mental and physical wellbeing are essential in controlling disease spread. Non-pharmaceutical interventions (NPIs), actions apart from immunisation and pharmacotherapy, can protect individuals and communities by reducing the number of spreaders, reducing the reproductive number (growth function), and providing decision-makers more time to stop the spread of disease.[1] Many factors contribute to the virus's reproductive number (R_0), which is defined as the average number of infections caused by an infected individual in a fully uninfected population. This R_0 is inherently associated with how contagious the virus is, the available viral load, individual susceptibility and the rate and duration of potential infectious contacts.[1] NPIs help by decreasing potential viral exposure and reducing the reproductive number, to ultimately flatten the curve (Figure 1).

Besides staying at home and isolating when feeling ill, there are multiple actions on the individual level one can take to help stop the virus's

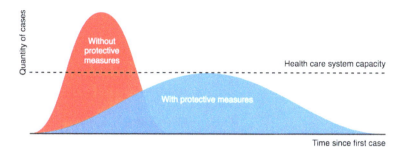

Figure 1: Pandemics and how to flatten the curve.[2]

spread, including wearing non-medical masks, practicing good hygiene, and social distancing. Each NPI measure alone may not be sufficient to control the spread; combined NPI measures allow optimal protection.

2. Viral Transmission

The transmission of coronavirus depends on the amount of viable viral particles expelled by one infected person; these liquid particles constitute a continuum that ranges from larger (>50 μm) respiratory droplets to smaller aerosols (Table 1). The number and size of droplets vary depending on factors such as activity, and the environment, while the percentage of infectious particles depends on viral load. For example, a cough produces more and larger droplets overall while a sneeze propels virus farther.[3] Viral load is proportional to infectiousness, and studies found viral load is the highest before or during early stages of symptoms.[4] Asymptomatic individuals commonly shed virus, thus transmitting infections unknowingly.[4] Environmental factors, such as good ventilation, can decrease the number of droplets in the air. Temperature and humidity affect the rate at which water evaporates from droplets, thus impacting the length of time particles remain in the air.[5] Survival of the viral particles depends on what surface it lands on. Virus remains viable for up to 72 hours on plastic and stainless steel and up to 24 hours on cardboard.[3] Longer survival on surfaces can contribute to transmission, but this is proportionally less relevant where much transmission is found to be airborne, as is the case with COVID-19.

Table 1:   Brief summary of viral droplets.[6]

General types of virus-containing particles	Features
Larger particles (50–100 μm)	Settle faster, fall to the ground within 2 meters
Smaller particles (0.52–2 μm)	Remain airborne for minutes to hours Travel farther Lower probability of each particle containing virus

3. Non-Medical Masks

Non-medical masks (NMMs) are those made of cloth or other materials and are not certified by Health Canada or other regulators as medical grade. They can act as a barrier to help stop the spread of droplets. Medical masks are recommended for individuals working in healthcare or infected individuals and their caregivers. Previously, masks have been shown to reduce primary and secondary transmission of respiratory infections such as influenza.[7,8]

Since viral particles range in size and masks physically block the particles, their effectiveness is based on the materials used and their fit. The laws of physics influence how particles interact with the masks' fibres and the masks' ability to capture particles. While larger particles are easier to trap, smaller particles have increased motion thus, also increasing their chance of being trapped.[6] Medium-size particles are the hardest to capture and filtration relies on electrostatic interactions with mask materials[3] (Figure 2). Masks are typically more effective in blocking particles during exhalation than inhalation, as the force of exhaling accelerates particles, increasing their chance of being caught by the masks' fibers[9] (Figure 3). The mask construction is not the only important factor in filtration. NMMs are most effective when fitted, worn, and handled correctly (Table 2).[10,11]

NMMs are recommended for the general public to wear indoors and outdoors, especially when physical distancing cannot be maintained.[10] Case studies have shown the effectiveness of wearing masks during close contact. In the United States, two hair stylists with COVID-19 spent at least 15 minutes with each of 139 clients. However, this resulted in no infections as everyone wore face coverings.[13] Looking at the transmission

Cloth Mask

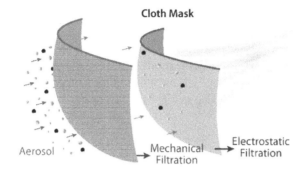

Aerosol   Mechanical → Electrostatic
            Filtration   Filtration

Figure 2: Mask mechanism.[9]

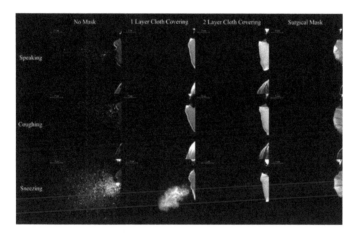

Figure 3: Effect of mask blocking exhalation.[12]

of COVID-19 within those living in the same household, masks played an indispensable role to prevent transmission. While the risk of household transmission was 18 times higher than other forms of close contact, face mask use by the primary case and family contacts prior to symptom development was 79% effective in reducing transmission (OR = 0.21, 95% CI: 0.06–0.79).[14]

On a population level, a comparison of 15 states in the United States and the District of Columbia found community mask mandates led to a slowdown in the daily COVID-19 case and death rates.[15] Simulations showed when 80% of the community used a mask, it would reduce

Table 2:   Guidelines on handling NMMs.[10,11]

Correct Handling of Non-Medical Masks
The ability to reduce particles largely depends on the materials used to create the mask and not the layers of materials (5). Filters such as non-woven polypropylene can be used in between layers (5). All NMMs, regardless of layers, should:
- Completely cover the nose, mouth, and chin without gaping. - Not contain an exhalation valve. - Fit securely to the head. - Fit comfortably to avoid frequent adjustments. - Maintain its shape after washing and drying.
Before putting on and taking off NMMs, one should wash or sanitize hands (5). NMMs should not be shared (6). Damage, fabric break down, or change in fit will reduce the protection of cloth masks (5). In order to safely reuse NMMs, NMMs should be washed after each use (5). NMMs are recommended to be washed in a washing machine, using the warmest temperature setting with regular laundry detergent, followed by thorough drying in a dryer at a high temperature if possible.

COVID-19 spread to an extent comparable to a strict lockdown.[16,17] The Institute of Health Metrics and Evaluation suggests that 129,574 (95% CI: 85,284–170,867) deaths were preventable from September 2020 to February, 2021, if 95% of the population wore masks.[18] Meta-analysis on the effectiveness of masks at preventing respiratory viral infections further showed the use of masks by non-healthcare workers decreased virus infection by 47% (OR = 0.53, 95% CI: 0.35–0.79).[19] The protective effect of wearing masks was interestingly influenced by culture, and the protective effect was higher in Asia (OR = 0.31), when compared to Western countries (OR = 0.55).[19]

However, NMMs are only source control measures and cannot be considered as Personal Protective Equipment (PPE).[10] Concerns have been raised for the possibility of NMMs leading to risk compensation, in which a false sense of security may be developed resulting in neglect of other essential measures such as hand hygiene practices.[20] However, on a population level, there is limited evidence on safety measures encouraging other risky behaviours.[20] A Thai study found that mask wearers were actually more likely to comply to other NPIs such as physical distancing and handwashing measures compared to non-mask wearers, despite having a higher likelihood of having longer duration of physical contact.[21] Therefore, it is important to encourage wearing masks correctly along with other NPIs.

4. Hygiene

4.1 *Hand washing*

While the primary route of COVID-19 transmission is via inhalation, droplets are released when a person coughs, speaks, or sneezes, and viral particles may land on frequently touched surfaces. Hygiene practices, including hand washing and surfaces disinfecting, can eliminate and decrease the viral load and droplets on surfaces, though it is not clear how large a role such efforts played for COVID-19. In general, hand washing is a strong tool to avoid getting sick and spreading germs to others. Previous studies for other pathogens support the effects of handwashing in reducing respiratory illnesses by 16–21% and limiting faecal–oral transmissions by up to 58%.[22,23] Handwashing at least three times per day was found to be statically significantly associated with reduced likelihood of household transmission in the last pandemic, influenza A (H1N1).[24] Meta-analysis further suggests the use of any soap combined with hand-hygiene education had an overall 21% (95% CI: 5%–34%) reduction in respiratory illnesses.[25] Given current public health efforts focus on pro-moting hand washing during the COVID-19 pandemic, maintaining awareness of hygiene should be continued during immunisation roll-out.

Our hands are common vectors for transmitting diseases, especially as unwashed hands can cause infection through the mouth, nose, and eyes. Hand washing with soap disrupts the virus's fatty layer and, therefore, disturbs viral functions.[26] Soap and water work together to trap and remove pathogens by forming micelles that trap the coronavirus, dirt and other harmful chemicals. At least 20 seconds are needed during hand washing to allow soap molecules to break the virus and ensure all areas of the hand have been cleaned.[27,28] Regular handwashing is recommended as a frequent activity, especially when one is likely to be in contact with germs, such as before touching the eyes, nose, mouth, or face, and before eating food. The steps on how to effectively wash hands are outlined below:[28]

1. Wet hands with running water.
2. Apply soap.
3. Lather and scrub hands with soap, covering all surfaces including the palm and backs of hands, between fingers, and under nails for at least 20 seconds.
4. Rinse hands well under clean, running water.
5. Dry hands using a clean towel.
6. Use a towel to turn off the tap (in public spaces).

The World's Health Organization suggests alcohol (at a concentration of at least 60% by volume) can work as a disinfectant on the skin if one cannot access clean water and soap.[23] However, concentrations of alcohol lower than 60% may not work equally well for a large range of pathogens and may only reduce growth instead of eliminating germs.[13] Alcohol-based hand rubs are less effective than washing hands with soap and water as the viral particles remain on the skin's surface rather than being rinsed away.[13] Homemade hand sanitisers may also present health risks such as skin irritation and lead to a false sense of security.[28] Hand sanitisers require caution when in reach of children, as ingesting even a small amount of sanitiser can be fatal.[29]

4.2 *Surface disinfecting*

Besides hand washing, disinfecting commonly used surfaces may be beneficial, as early studies suggested coronavirus can live on surfaces from a few hours to days.[16] However, disinfecting is less effective than hand washing, where germs are physically removed by soap and water.[30]

Disinfecting works by using chemicals to kill or inactivate germs but does not necessarily remove them. The Government of Canada provided an ongoing list of hard-surface disinfectants recommended for use.[31] However, transmission via environmental surfaces (fomites) of SARS-CoV-2 is considered relatively low compared to airborne transmission, as the interactions with environmental factors cause damage to virus particles and lower the efficiency of transferring virus from surfaces to mucous membranes.[32]

However, surface disinfectant can help limit the transfer of viral particles when the appropriate disinfectant is used, especially for surfaces in used by an infected individual. In a retrospective study looking at household infection for infected patients, daily use of chlorine or ethanol-based disinfectant in households was 77% effective at preventing infection (OR = 0.23, 95% CI 0.07–0.84).[14] Chemical disinfectants should be used safely by following instructions on the labels. Public settings and institutions like schools should develop a schedule for routine cleaning and training on correct use and storage of disinfection products for relevant staff.

5. Social Distancing

5.1 *Community interventions*

Physical distancing is deemed another important NPI in numerous jurisdictions to control the COVID-19 outbreak. While most cities have restrictions on gatherings and non-essential activities, physical distancing for essential activities is still necessary. By definition, physical distancing means to stay at least 2 metres from others in both indoor and outdoor spaces.[5] It is important to note that where airborne transmission occurs, such distancing would not be expected to prevent all transmissions. In community, interventions that may operate and ensure physical distancing include public facilities closure, cancellation of public events or school closure.

Droplets exist across a continuum of sizes and their distance travelled ranges depending on ventilation and airflow. Specifically, for SARS-CoV-2, evidence suggests the risk of transmission at 1 metre is 2–10 times higher than at 2 metres.[33] The World Health Organization (WHO) also indicated physical distancing of less than 1 metre has at least a 10% higher transmission risk than physical distancing of more than 1 metre.[34] Many jurisdictions concluded that physical distancing of at least 2 meters is better than 1 metre.

On average, implementation of any physical intervention (closure of workplaces, cancellation of public events, and public transport) was associated with an overall reduction in COVID-19 incidence in 149 countries across the globe by 13% (IRR = 0.87, 95% CI: 0.85–0.89).[35] Countries such as Singapore and China, with high population density, demonstrated that high community compliance to social distancing, masking and handwashing can contain the COVID-19 epidemic.[36] It is instructive that these jurisdictions were among the first to embrace widespread mask use. As we have reviewed above, the evidence for impact of nonmedical masking is very clear. In China, social distancing and masking measures reduced the value of effective reproduction number ($R = 2.5$) by up to 60%.[36]

Considering the multiple factors in effective social distancing, rules on distancing should reflect graded levels of risk. Jones *et al.* proposed a set of distance guidelines for different risk levels (Figure 4). In high-risk

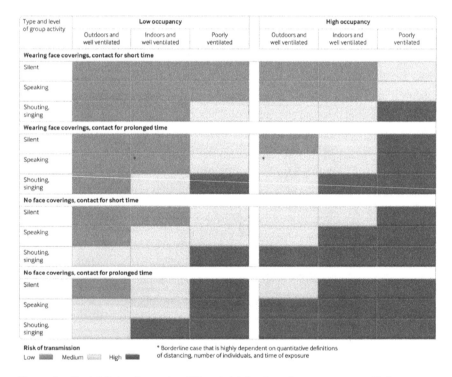

Figure 4:   Social distancing under different risk levels — low occupancy with face coverings for a short contact has the lowest risk.[37]

situations, such as indoor environments with poor ventilation, high levels of occupancy, prolonged contact time, and no face coverings, physical distancing beyond 2 metres and minimising occupancy time should be considered. Increased distances reduce the likelihood of exposure to a high viral load through droplets/air and on surfaces close to an infectious person.

5.2 *Individual interventions*

On an individual level, practices of social distancing also include:

- Avoiding crowded places and staying at home when possible.
- Avoid nonessential travel.
- Avoid common greetings such as shaking hands.
- Shop or take public transportation during off-peak hours.
- Whenever possible, use technology to keep in touch with friends and family.

Although physical distancing is needed, there are ways to stay socially connected. Research has highlighted physical distancing's impact on mental health including increased loneliness, anxiety and depression,[38] More effective strategies are needed to ensure and maintain connections with marginalised and vulnerable populations.

6. Conclusion

In general, wearing NMMs was the most effective strategy among the three discussed NPIs and requires minimal effort, especially when coming into close contact with others is unavoidable. However, masks alone do not protect against all COVID-19, and should be combined with physical distancing whenever possible and hand hygiene. NPIs are effective public health tools to contain communicable diseases and need to be continuously practiced during vaccine roll-out and into the early post-pandemic era. When a majority of the public follow appropriate guidelines on NPIs, their collective effort can reduce the risk of future waves of infection.[39]

Making sure everyone has the ability and support to utilise these NPIs requires collective effort. Consistent and continuous public messaging and public infrastructures are needed in helping the public safely practice NPIs. For example, the distribution of NMMs should be supported by the government, as well as building infrastructures to allow easy access to masks, clean running water, soap, and a way to dry hands. Other no-touch policies to consider include visual reminders, such as signs or posters in public spaces, to remind the public to wear masks, wash hands, and maintain distances. NPIs in combination with other measures including vaccines and prophylaxis will ultimately allow us to move forward towards normal life.

References

1. BCCDC. Prevention & Risks [Internet]. [cited 2021 Feb 20]. Available from: http://www.bccdc.ca/health-info/diseases-conditions/covid-19/prevention-risks.
2. BCCDC Foundation for Public Health. Pandemics & How to Flatten the Curve [Internet]. [cited 2021 Mar 12]. Available from: https://bccdcfoundation.org/pandemics-how-to-flatten-the-curve/.
3. Dhand R, Li J. Coughs and sneezes: Their role in transmission of respiratory viral infections, including SARS-CoV-2. *American Journal of Respiratory and Critical Care Medicine.* 2020;202(5):651–659.
4. Cevik M, Tate M, Lloyd O, Maraolo AE, Schafers J, Ho A. SARS-CoV-2, SARS-CoV, and MERS-CoV viral load dynamics, duration of viral shedding, and infectiousness: A systematic review and meta-analysis. *The Lancet Microbe.* 2021;2(1):e13–e22.
5. Mecenas P, Bastos RT da RM, Vallinoto ACR, Normando D. Effects of temperature and humidity on the spread of COVID-19: A systematic review. *PLOS ONE.* 2020;15(9):e0238339.
6. Prather KA, Wang CC, Schooley RT. Reducing transmission of SARS-CoV-2. *Science.* 2020;368(6498):1422–1424.
7. Larson EL, Ferng Y, Wong-McLoughlin J, Wang S, Haber M, Morse SS. Impact of non-pharmaceutical interventions on URIs and influenza in crowded, urban households. *Public Health Reports.* 2010;125(2):178–191.
8. Brainard J, Jones NR, Lake IR, Hooper L, Hunter PR. Community use of face masks and similar barriers to prevent respiratory illness such as COVID-19: A rapid scoping review. *Eurosurveillance.* 2020;25(49).

9.   Konda A, Prakash A, Moss GA, Schmoldt M, Grant GD, Guha S. Aerosol filtration efficiency of common fabrics used in respiratory cloth masks. *ACS Nano*. 2020;14(5):6339–6347.

10. Canada PHA of. About COVID-19 non-medical masks [Internet]. aem. 2020 [cited 2021 Feb 20]. Available from: https://www.canada.ca/en/public-health/services/diseases/2019-novel-coronavirus-infection/prevention-risks/about-non-medical-masks-face-coverings.html.

11. BCCDC. Masks [Internet]. 2021 [cited 2021 Feb 20]. Available from: http://www.bccdc.ca/health-info/diseases-conditions/covid-19/prevention-risks/masks.

12. Bahl P, Bhattacharjee S, Silva C de, Chughtai AA, Doolan C, MacIntyre CR. Face coverings and mask to minimise droplet dispersion and aerosolisation: A video case study. *Thorax*. 2020;75(11):1024–1025.

13. Hendrix MJ. Absence of apparent transmission of SARS-CoV-2 from two stylists after exposure at a hair salon with a universal face covering policy — Springfield, Missouri, May 2020. *MMWR Morbidity Mortality Weekly Report* [Internet]. 2020 [cited 2021 Apr 6];69. Available from: https://www.cdc.gov/mmwr/volumes/69/wr/mm6928e2.htm.

14. Wang Y, Tian H, Zhang L, Zhang M, Guo D, Wu W, *et al.* Reduction of secondary transmission of SARS-CoV-2 in households by face mask use, disinfection and social distancing: A cohort study in Beijing, China. *BMJ Global Health*. 2020;5(5):e002794.

15. Lyu W, Wehby GL. Community use of face masks and COVID-19: evidence from a natural experiment of state mandates in the US. *Health Affairs*. 2020;39(8):1419–1425.

16. Kai D, Goldstein G-P, Morgunov A, Nangalia V, Rotkirch A. Universal masking is urgent in the COVID-19 pandemic: SEIR and agent based models, empirical validation, policy recommendations. arXiv:200413553 [physics, q-bio] [Internet]. 2020 Apr 22 [cited 2021 Mar 11]; Available from: http://arxiv.org/abs/2004.13553.

17. Gandhi M, Beyrer C, Goosby E. masks do more than protect others during COVID-19: Reducing the inoculum of SARS-CoV-2 to protect the wearer. *Journal of General Internal Medicine*. 2020;35(10):3063–3066.

18. Reiner RC, Barber RM, Collins JK, Zheng P, Adolph C, Albright J, *et al.* Modeling COVID-19 scenarios for the United States. *Nature Medicine*. 2021;27(1):94–105.

19. Liang M, Gao L, Cheng C, Zhou Q, Uy JP, Heiner K, *et al.* Efficacy of face mask in preventing respiratory virus transmission: A systematic review and meta-analysis. *Travel Medicine and Infectious Disease*. 2020;36:101751.

20. Mantzari E, Rubin GJ, Marteau TM. Is risk compensation threatening public health in the covid-19 pandemic? *BMJ*. 2020 Jul 26;370:m2913.
21. Doung-ngern P, Suphanchaimat R, Panjangampatthana A, Janekrongtham C, Ruampoom D, Daochaeng N, *et al*. Case-control study of use of personal protective measures and risk for SARS-CoV 2 Infection, Thailand — Volume 26, Number 11—November 2020 — Emerging Infectious Diseases journal — CDC. *EID Journal* [Internet]. 2020 Nov [cited 2021 Apr 6];26. Available from: https://wwwnc.cdc.gov/eid/article/26/11/20-3003_article.
22. Ejemot RI, Ehiri JE, Meremikwu MM, Critchley JA. Hand washing for preventing diarrhoea. *Cochrane Database of Systematic Reviews*. 2008;(1):CD004265.
23. Rabie T, Curtis V. Handwashing and risk of respiratory infections: A quantitative systematic review. *Tropical Medicine and International Health*. 2006;11(3):258–267.
24. Zhang D, Liu W, Yang P, Zhang Y, Li X, Germ KE, *et al*. Factors associated with household transmission of pandemic (H1N1) 2009 among self-quarantined patients in Beijing, China. *PLoS One* [Internet]. 2013 Oct 18 [cited 2021 Apr 6];8(10). Available from: https://www.ncbi.nlm.nih.gov/pmc/articles/PMC3799752/.
25. Aiello AE, Coulborn RM, Perez V, Larson EL. Effect of hand hygiene on infectious disease risk in the community setting: A meta-analysis. *American Journal of Public Health*. 2008;98(8):1372–1381.
26. Kratzel A, Todt D, V'kovski P, Steiner S, Gultom M, Thao TTN, *et al*. Inactivation of severe acute respiratory syndrome Coronavirus 2 by WHO-recommended hand rub formulations and alcohols — CDC. *EID Journal* [Internet]. 2020 Jul [cited 2021 Mar 11];26(7). Available from: https://wwwnc.cdc.gov/eid/article/26/7/20-0915_article.
27. Alzyood M, Jackson D, Aveyard H, Brooke J. COVID-19 reinforces the importance of handwashing. *Journal of Clinical Nursing* [Internet]. 2020 May 14 [cited 2021 Apr 18]. Available from: https://www.ncbi.nlm.nih.gov/pmc/articles/PMC7267118/.
28. BCCDC. Hand Washing [Internet]. 2021 [cited 2021 Feb 20]. Available from: http://www.bccdc.ca/health-info/diseases-conditions/covid-19/prevention-risks/hand-washing.
29. Government of Canada HC. Hand sanitizers and children's safety: What you need to know [Internet]. 2020 [cited 2021 Mar 11]. Available from: https://healthycanadians.gc.ca/recall-alert-rappel-avis/hc-sc/2020/73883a-eng.php.
30. CDC. Community, Work, and School [Internet]. Centers for Disease Control and Prevention, 2020 [cited 2021 Mar 12]. Available from: https://www.cdc.

gov/coronavirus/2019-ncov/community/schools-childcare/clean-disinfect-hygiene.html.

31. Canada H. Hard-surface disinfectants and hand sanitizers (COVID-19): List of disinfectants with evidence for use against COVID-19 [Internet]. aem. 2020 [cited 2021 Mar 11]. Available from: https://www.canada.ca/en/health-canada/services/drugs-health-products/disinfectants/covid-19/list.html#tbl1.

32. CDC. Coronavirus Disease 2019 (COVID-19) [Internet]. Centers for Disease Control and Prevention. 2020 [cited 2020 Mar 15]. Available from: https://www.cdc.gov/coronavirus/2019-ncov/prepare/managing-stress-anxiety.html.

33. Noakes C. Transmission of SARS-CoV-2 and Mitigating Measures. United States: Scientific Advisory Group on Emergencies; 2020 Jun, p. 26.

34. Chu DK, Akl EA, Duda S, Solo K, Yaacoub S, Schünemann HJ, *et al.* Physical distancing, face masks, and eye protection to prevent person-to-person transmission of SARS-CoV-2 and COVID-19: A systematic review and meta-analysis. *The Lancet*. 2020;395(10242):1973–1987.

35. Islam N, Sharp SJ, Chowell G, Shabnam S, Kawachi I, Lacey B, *et al.* Physical distancing interventions and incidence of coronavirus disease 2019: Natural experiment in 149 countries. *BMJ*. 2020;370:m2743.

36. Anderson RM, Heesterbeek H, Klinkenberg D, Hollingsworth TD. How will country-based mitigation measures influence the course of the COVID-19 epidemic? *The Lancet*. 2020;395(10228):931–934.

37. Jones NR, Qureshi ZU, Temple RJ, Larwood JPJ, Greenhalgh T, Bourouiba L. Two metres or one: What is the evidence for physical distancing in covid-19? *BMJ*. 2020;370:m3223.

38. Giallonardo V, Sampogna G, Del Vecchio V, Luciano M, Albert U, Carmassi C, *et al.* The impact of quarantine and physical distancing following COVID-19 on mental health: Study protocol of a multicentric Italian population trial. *Frontiers in Psychiatry* [Internet]. 2020 Jun 5 [cited 2021 Mar 12];11. Available from: https://www.ncbi.nlm.nih.gov/pmc/articles/PMC7290062/.

39. Kennedy DM, Zambrano GJ, Wang Y, Neto OP. Modeling the effects of intervention strategies on COVID-19 transmission dynamics. *Journal of Clinical Virology*. 2020;128:104440.

Part 5

Interventions in Healthcare

Chapter 10

Hospital Infection Control

Andrea Simmonds[*,†] and Titus Wong[‡,§]

[*]*School of Population and Public Health, University of British Columbia, Vancouver, Canada*

[†]*BC Children's Hospital, Vancouver, Canada*

[‡]*Vancouver General Hospital, Jim Pattison Pavilion, Vancouver, Canada*

[§]*Department of Pathology and Laboratory Medicine, Vancouver, Canada*

Key Message

- Hospital prevention and control methods to manage the SARS-CoV-2 crisis have evolved since the pandemic began. IPC measures can be characterised using the established hierarchy of controls, as described by the United States Center for Disease Control.
- Elimination of the hazard is the most effective approach to minimise the risk of infection. This is accomplished through screening of patients, isolation of suspected or confirmed SARS-CoV-2 patients, minimising non-essential patient visits, limiting of visitors, encouraging non-essential personnel to work from home, and keeping personnel at home when ill.
- Engineering and environmental control measures such as physical separation and spatial barriers, ventilation, cleaning and disinfection, and waste management help reduce virus transmission.

- Administrative controls change the way people work within a hospital to help stop the spread of infection. This includes surge capacity, staffing modifications, training HCWS to function in a pandemic setting, vaccination of HCWs, enhanced communication with staff, adaptive surgery, obstetrics, and critical care protocols; and management of dead bodies.
- PPE classically falls to the bottom of the IPC hierarchy, but there has been an increasing focus on the importance of this measure in preventing transmission of SARS-CoV-2 in a healthcare setting. The major risks for transmission in HCWs are failure to appropriately identify and isolate affected patients, inadequate PPE availability, and improper use of PPE. Appropriate PPE varies based on risk level to the healthcare worker.

1. Introduction

With the WHO declaration of a global SARS-CoV-2 pandemic on March 11, 2020, hospital administrators were faced with an unprecedented outbreak scenario. Infection prevention and control (IPC) measures and protocols have long been established at most institutions, but the novelty, urgency, and magnitude of the COVID-19 pandemic required a coordinated and rapidly-evolving approach to management. In fact, in the first six weeks after declaration of the outbreak, the world saw a higher number of SARS-CoV-2 infections and higher mortality from the novel virus than the entire SARS-CoV outbreak of 2003.[1,2]

The response at the hospital level has evolved along with our understanding of the virus, the burden of disease, access to equipment and resources, and governmental support, guidance, and regulation. Variation exists in the type and breadth of change required of an institution, which is dependent on the type and capacity of the hospital, the local control measures and case numbers, and the individual characteristics of the institution.

Hospital prevention and control methods can be characterised using the established hierarchy of controls, as described by the United States Center for Disease Control (CDC).[3] This framework provides a basis for organisation of response to SARS-CoV-2 at an institutional level

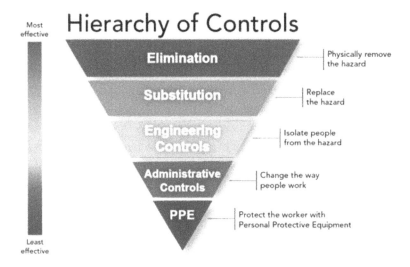

Figure 1: CDC representation of the hierarchy of controls. The control methods at the top of graphic are considered more effective and protective than those at the bottom.[3]

(Figure 1). The goal of employing this organisational structure is to implement a combination of interventions that will minimise transmission at an occupational and community-wide level, and reduce the burden of disease.

2. Elimination and Substitution

Elimination of the hazard (SARS-CoV-2 infection or exposure) is the most effective approach to minimise the risk of infection. Coronaviruses have been detected in sputum, nasal and nasopharyngeal secretions, endotracheal aspirate, bronchoalveolar lavage, urine, feces, tears, conjunctival secretions, and blood and lung tissues.[4] Several strategies have been used to reduce introduction of the virus into the hospital, and to prevent nosocomial transmission.

2.1 *Screening of patients*

Anyone entering a healthcare facility (patients, visitors, and HCWs) should be screened at the point of entry. Ideally, this should be done through active screening, in the form of checking for fever or SARS-CoV-2 symptoms, and asking about possible exposures or recent travel. Any patient who screens positively should be given a mask and directed to triage for further evaluation. As per the US CDC, a healthcare worker who screens positive should be sent home for self-quarantine. If possible, separate entrances for HCWs and patients/visitors should be established to decrease risk of cross-infection and improve flow through the entrances.[5]

Signage should be placed in every entrance instructing visitors not to enter if they have any symptoms of SARS-CoV-2. Hospitals must adopt policies regarding patient supports and visitors.[6] These protocols have evolved over the course of the pandemic, and are dependent on the type of hospital, caseload in the local area, and by the specifics related to the patient, on a case-by-case basis.

Additional screening is recommended for patients presenting to the hospital for scheduled visits such as clinic appointments, diagnostics, and procedures. Before presenting to the healthcare facility, patients are typically asked to complete a screening survey for symptoms of SARS-CoV-2. This may be done through telephone calls, questionnaires, or on-line forms. Upon arrival, screening is completed again. Depending on the reason for their visit, some facilities may require point of care testing as well. Mitra *et al.* found that the sensitivity of screening patients with temperature checks was 19% for detection of a positive SARS-CoV-2 diagnosis, and thus determined that this practice has negligible value for control of SARS-CoV-2.[7]

Patients presenting to the emergency room who have any symptoms suggestive of SARS-CoV-2 infection should be placed in segregated areas of the emergency room, where healthcare workers use full PPE including respirators. If a case of COVID-19 is confirmed, activity mapping and contact tracing should be carried out to determine whether any patients or staff may have been exposed without adequate protection.[8]

Paediatric patients represent a unique challenge with screening due to the increased likelihood of having minimal symptoms or no symptoms of COVID-19 and the close nature of relationships with household contacts and caregivers. Therefore, screening of children should include assessment of caregiver and household members for symptoms of SARS-CoV-2.[9]

A detailed description of screening measures for SARS-CoV-2 can be found in the Chapter 7.

2.2 *Isolation of suspected or confirmed SARS-CoV-2 patients*

Early diagnosis and rapid isolation of COVID-19 patients is essential to reduce exposure to SARS-CoV-2 in a healthcare setting. These patients should be placed in private rooms if available. Due to shortages of isolation rooms in response to the large number of infected patients, most international guidelines were updated to allow cohorting of COVID-positive patients into larger, shared rooms.[4]

Shared bathroom use should be minimised when possible. Toilet flushing may generate contaminated bioaerosols, which may remain in the air for over 30 minutes after flushing, suggesting the possibility of faecal droplet transmission.[10] Shared toilets should be cleaned and disinfected at least three times a day and private patient toilets should be cleaned at least twice daily by staff wearing appropriate PPE.[6]

2.3 *Minimising non-essential patient visits*

Outside of necessary or emergent care, patients should be encouraged to stay out of the hospital to reduce exposure to both HCWs and patients.[5] The WHO recommends using telehealth whenever possible to provide outpatient consults during the pandemic in lieu of face-to-face visits.[6]

If patients must be seen in person, every effort must be made to minimise foot traffic and crowding within the healthcare facility. Ideally, patients attending appointments should be directed immediately to an examination room. If one is not available, an alternate strategy should be employed to avoid patients congregating in a common waiting room. More common options include a well-ventilated space allowing appropriate distancing between patients and access to hand hygiene, or having patients wait outside the facility or in their car until notified by phone or text that their appointment is ready.[11]

2.4 *Limitation of visitors*

Site-specific guidelines on patient support people and visitors vary widely. The US CDC recommends limiting visitors to only those deemed essential for the patient's physical or emotional well-being and encouraging the use of alternate means of communication such as video or phone calls. All visitors should be educated on the facility's policies on hand hygiene, PPE use, and movement within the hospital.[11]

In cases where a patient is positive for SARS-CoV-2, additional measures should be undertaken. The facility should evaluate the appropriateness of the presence of the visitor or care-giver on a case-by-case basis. Visitors should be instructed to visit only the patient's room and avoid other areas within the hospital. PPE should be provided and used as per the institutional policies. Visitors should not be present during any aerosol generating procedures (AGPs).[11]

2.5 *Encouraging non-essential personnel to work from home*

Personnel who are not considered essential workers, or those not directly involved in patient care, such as research staff, administrators, vendors, and some office assistants, should be encouraged to work from home whenever possible. Conducting virtual meetings, and implementing mechanisms for telework and telehealth minimises foot traffic and risk of exposure in the hospital setting.[5]

2.6 *Keeping personnel at home when ill*

WHO recommends encouraging workers to stay at home if unwell, and developing flexible sick leave policies that do not lead to loss of income for unwell staff in order to facilitate this directive. Furthermore, HCWs should be encouraged to report any occupational or non-occupational exposures to SARS-CoV-2 without adequate protection. These exposures should be investigated on a case-by-case basis, and recommendations should be made for return to work according to protocol.[6]

3. Engineering and Environmental Controls

Engineering and environmental control measures aim to reduce transmission of SARS-CoV-2 in a hospital setting by removing or minimising hazardous conditions that could encourage the spread of disease.

3.1 *Physical separation and spatial barriers*

The CDC recommends approximately 2 metres/6 feet of distance between patients, while WHO suggests that 1 metre is sufficient. This can be accomplished with physical barriers such as plastic or glass windows, tables, or through geographic distancing using benches, chairs, or caution tape.[6]

The CDC and WHO agree that waiting areas, hospital entrances, and patient check-in areas should have hand hygiene stations, masks, tissues, and a no-touch waste bin available to patients and visitors at all times. Basic education on hand hygiene, limiting surfaces touched, and use of PPE should be provided for visitors. This is commonly in the form of posters and signs in strategic places.[6,11]

The distancing guidelines and enforcement should also apply to spaces such as staff offices, common areas, and elevators. Signage should be clearly posted in these areas with the maximum number of people allowed within the space.

3.2 *Ventilation*

Ensuring that a hospital maximises the ability to care for SARS-CoV-2 patients requires in-depth knowledge of the air-exchange capabilities of every area within the institution and coordination with a facilities maintenance team. The CDC suggests consulting with facility engineers to improve indoor air quality in all shared spaces within a healthcare facility. Specifically, air-handling systems should be optimised by ensuring appropriate directionality, filtration, exchange rate, proper installation, and up to date maintenance. Portable HEPA filtration systems can improve air quality in areas where a more permanent system is not achievable.[11]

Additional ventilation engineering is necessary wherever AGPs are performed. As per the US CDC, airborne infection isolation rooms (AIIRs) should have a minimum of six, but ideally twelve air changes per hour, and the air should be either directly exhausted to the outdoors, or filtered through a HEPA filter before recirculation. Variations exist with regard to standards for recommended temperature, airflow patterns, relative humidity, pressurisation relative to surroundings, and filtration standards.[12] Facilities should regularly monitor the negative pressure of these rooms, and entry and exit to the room should be kept to a minimum with the doors always closed when not necessary for entry/exit.[11]

3.3 *Routine cleaning and disinfection*

Fomite elimination through frequent use of broad-spectrum disinfectants with proven anti-viral activity is paramount in a hospital setting. In the setting of the pandemic, disposable equipment should be used when possible. Viable SARS-CoV-2 has been detected at 72 hours post-application onto plastic and stainless-steel surfaces.[13] Multiple-use devices such as stethoscopes and thermometers should be disinfected thoroughly after each use.[6]

Organic and non-organic debris should be pre-cleaned before disinfection, particularly if the surface is visibly soiled. Following this, chemical disinfectants are used to break the outer lipid layer of coronaviruses.[14] Many countries have a publicly available list of disinfectants suitable for use against SARS-CoV-2. The Canadian government lists over 600 approved disinfectants.[15] Disinfectants should be used according to manufacturing instructions; each has a label contact time necessary for efficacy. Many of the EPA-approved products have a wet-contact time of 10 minutes, but have been shown to eliminate pathogens in time frames as short as one minute.[16]

No touch cleaning systems can be used to supplement cleaning and disinfection practices and increase the likelihood of thorough surface disinfection. This can be accomplished through ultraviolet light emitters or ultraviolet germicidal irradiation, which have been shown to reduce the virulence of microorganisms.[12] Similarly, hydrogen peroxide vapour has also been shown to exhibit virucidal activity against coronaviruses.[14]

Cadnum *et al.* found that after a minimal manual pre-cleaning, application of a dilute sodium hydrochlorite disinfectant using an electrostatic sprayer effectively and rapidly eliminated SARS-CoV-2 from the surfaces tested.[17] The combination of cleaning and disinfection with no touch systems can shorten the contact time to fully disinfect surfaces, and ensure adequate disinfection of hard-to-clean surfaces such as wheelchairs and portable equipment.

3.4 *Waste management*

The pandemic has dramatically increased waste production within a healthcare setting. Ilyas *et al.* outline best practices for disposal of this waste safely and effectively. The first step should be establishing clearly marked bins for COVID-waste, and ensuring the bins are placed in areas where they will be required. Before transporting the waste to temporary storage, the bins/bags should be disinfected and sealed in double-layer bags, which are usually yellow in colour. Ideally, the waste is then processed via incineration, alternative thermal techniques, or chemical techniques. In addition, a disinfectant containing 2 g/L chlorine should be sprayed four times daily in areas of COVID-waste.[18]

4. Administrative Controls

Measures that change the way people work within a hospital can help keep patients and workers safe, and limit the nosocomial spread of SARS-CoV-2.

4.1 *Surge capacity*

The SARS-CoV-2 pandemic placed an unparalleled strain on the resources and treatment capabilities of hospitals around the world, rapidly exceeding the surge capacity protocols previously employed by most institutions. A systematic review of the models employed by a diverse array of health authorities showed that a variety of models can be used to help predict the caseload projection and hospital capacity management of an institution. They vary based on their projected outputs: some are better for longer term planning, some incorporate age-stratification, and others are better for predicting patient pathways and detailed patient flow. With a collective, improved understanding of the complex response necessary to manage a pandemic of this magnitude, Klein *et al.* hope that these models can be refined to better prepare hospitals for response to a similar outbreak in the future.[19]

In order to accommodate increased clinical burdens during the pandemic, many hospitals have developed strategies to increase capacity and improve patient flow. Kumar *et al.* recommend encouraging and supporting SARS-CoV-2 patients with mild symptoms to stay home by leveraging remote care options. In addition, hospitals should increase bed capacity and prepare to efficiently discharge patients once appropriate as they recover. Options for increasing capacity include developing mobile hospital units, reactivating decommissioned beds, increasing bed capacity per room, modifying existing units or areas within an institution, and using non-healthcare facilities to treat patients.[20]

In particular, increasing ICU capacity to accommodate patients with severe disease has become an important consideration. Aziz *et al.* suggest allocating resources for one in five hospitalised COVID-19 patients to require ICU admission. In addition, they recommend planning for 70% of these ICU patients to need ventilatory support. Therefore, hospitals should increase the number of ventilators available, and to develop protocols for use of high flow oxygen and non-invasive ventilation to decrease need for intubation.[21]

4.2 *Staffing considerations*

The rapid spread of SARS-CoV-2 across the globe required hospitals to adapt quickly to the unprecedented and evolving and staffing needs. Kim *et al.* describe a framework for this issue with six guiding principles: (1) create an organisational structure, (2) define the need, (3) identify and optimise the pool of healthcare providers, (4) create surge teams, (5) prepare and deliver orientation materials, and (6) optimise working conditions for staff.[22]

They recommend using real-time, local data to predict the number of anticipated admissions, and deploy staff accordingly. Care should be taken to ensure adequate numbers of staff are available to meet the immediate demand, yet keep staff available for a surge in admissions.

When redeploying staff to care for COVID patients, consideration is given to their training, recognising that those with internal medicine backgrounds are likely to be more comfortable caring for these patients than those in surgical specialties. In addition, the furloughed group should be diverse in terms of race, gender, age, and experience, to ensure balance in those deployed. Pregnant HCWs, those aged over 65, or immunosuppressed staff were not asked to directly care for COVID patients.[22] The WHO also recommend that HCWs who are considered higher risk for development of severe illness from SARS-CoV-2 infection due to older age, pre-existing medical conditions, or pregnancy, should not be expected to carry out tasks or patient care with a high risk of exposure.[6]

Care teams should be created with a tiered structure; experienced physicians are in charge of the less experienced members, and the number of providers on a team is kept relatively small. Typically, two front line workers such as nurse practitioners or physician assistants are paired with one attending physician. Three to four of these teams are overseen by one supervising hospitalist. They are tasked with 10–12 patients per team.[22]

Finally, work schedules are created to mitigate burnout; 4-days on, 4-days off with 12-hour shifts is Kim *et al.*'s preferred model.[22] The WHO recommends five 8-hour shifts or four 10-hour shifts per week.[23]

WHO recognises the increased physical and emotional demands on healthcare workers during the SARS-CoV-2 crisis. Through the pandemic, HCWs have often been met with heavier workloads, insufficient time for rest, and higher levels of risk and stress in the workplace. These conditions can lead to physical and emotional fatigue, which may result in decreased alertness, coordination, and efficiency; increased reaction time; impaired cognition; and emotional blunting or mood changes.[6]

Pappa *et al.*'s systematic review on mental health of HCWs during the pandemic showed a pooled prevalence of depression to be 22.8%.[24] Khajuria *et al.* conducted the largest international cross-sectional study of mental health in healthcare workers through the SARS-CoV-2 pandemic. They found that workplace factors including availability of appropriate PPE, redeployment to areas such the ICU, and accessibility of mental health support were significantly associated with mental health during COVID-19.[25]

Strategies to mitigate the toll that the pandemic may have on HCWs' mental health include stockpiling PPE to ensure that frontline staff are appropriately protected, adequately training frontline and furloughed workers, providing flexible sick leave policies, and offering comprehensive and accessible mental health support.

4.3 *Training healthcare workers*

WHO recommends confirming documentation that all health workers have received training for IPC and COVID-19-related protocols and procedures, as it relates to their role. This includes IPC during healthcare for suspected and confirmed COVID-19, dead body management, and rational and extended use of personal protective equipment (PPE) and masks.[6]

Just-in-time training has been used globally to address the need for equip healthcare workers with new knowledge and skills in response to the SARS-CoV-2 pandemic. The main areas in which healthcare workers require additional training are IPC including public-health measures, and disaster medicine principles.[26]

Adequately training healthcare workers is also essential for preventing nosocomial spread of SARS-CoV-2 that can lead to outbreaks within a healthcare facility. Most HCWs infected with COVID-19 work outside of the high-acuity units that manage infected patients.[27–29] Chu *et al.* found that over 70% of nosocomial infections occurred in HCWs not assigned to front-line work.[29] Gagneux *et al.* hypothesise that ICU workers complete more intensive training compared to their peers in non-COVID-19 wards.[27]

Healthcare workers who do not receive adequate training through work may turn to other avenues to access information on SARS-CoV-2. Bhagavathula *et al.* found that 60% of healthcare workers used social media as a source of information on COVID-19. They showed that large knowledge gaps exist among HCWs, especially surrounding mode of transmission and incubation period of the virus.[30] Therefore, strategies to ensure consistent messaging and education are essential to healthcare worker training. A central source of information from a governing body should be used to guide training and education of HCWs.[31]

Due to the transmission dynamics of SARS-CoV-2, in-person training of healthcare workers is not always feasible or advisable. Many institutions have had success with video-based instruction, particularly for education on donning and doffing PPE. Christensen *et al.* found no significant difference in post-training donning and doffing scores between HCWs educated via instructor-led courses and video-based training.[32]

Simulation training for HCWs has also gained popularity during the pandemic. This educational modality allows for a review of clinical management of critically ill patients, workflow issues, as well as proper donning and doffing of PPE. Foong *et al.* found that in situ simulation early in the pandemic resulted in improvements in both timing for key events during resuscitation and in team competencies.[33]

4.4 *Vaccination of healthcare workers*

Healthcare workers were prioritised globally for SARS-CoV-2 vaccinations, once these vaccinations became available. This is supported by both WHO and the CDC. WHO recommends identifying priority groups of health workers for COVID-19 vaccination based on workplace risk assessment and medical conditions and organising immunisation campaigns and recording of vaccination status.[6] The CDC placed the estimated 24 million healthcare workers in the United States in phase 1a of their COVID-19 vaccination program, alongside long-term care residents.[34]

Vaccination of HCWs is important not only for protection of the workers, but also for decreasing transmission in a healthcare and community setting. Thompson *et al.* report that transmission risk in asymptomatic or pre-symptomatic individuals was lowered following vaccination, and acknowledged the importance of this finding for healthcare and frontline workers.[35] This sentiment was echoed by Shah *et al.*, who found that vaccination of healthcare workers was associated with a substantial reduction in transmission of infection to household contacts.[36]

4.5 *Communication*

Communication to frontline staff during the pandemic has been essential during the pandemic. Kuy *et al.* advocate for open lines of communication between staff and leadership, including a centralised COVID-19 response team (composed of supervisors from each clinical and administrative department), daily staff-wide dissemination of information, and virtual town halls at least twice per week.[5] Schaye *et al.* note that due to the immense volume of information requiring communication at a rapid pace to a large number of staff, multiple modes of communication are necessary. They found that a combination of intradepartmental operations calls, town halls, daily videoconferences, and regular emails worked best to meet this need.[37]

4.6 *Surgery protocols*

The management of emergent, urgent, and elective surgeries has been a complex and evolving challenge throughout the SARS-CoV-2 Pandemic. In response to the need for complex decision making and protocols to safely proceed with operations, a group of scientists and clinicians from around the world collaborated on a "Pandemic Surgery Guidance" report to help simplify the current understanding of safety during surgical care of patients.[38]

Surgeries were divided into emergency and planned categories, and recommendations were made for each type. The authors noted that decisions surrounding whether to proceed with non-emergency surgeries are dependent on the phase of urgency that the hospital is experiencing. The Australian and New Zealand Hepatic, Pancreatic, and Biliary Association (ANZHPBA) succinctly describes phases I through III in the COVID-19 response, ranging from the semi-urgent phase, to the urgent phase, and finally, to the "wartime" footing phase.[39] The COVIDSurg Collaborative — a group formed to aid with global guidance for surgical delivery during the pandemic — advocates for stratifying elective surgeries based on clinical urgency and resource availability.[40]

PPE recommendations are made based on a patient's risk stratification for SARS-CoV-2 infection. According to Brucher *et al.*, low risk PPE includes a surgical gown, double gloves, face shield ± goggles, head cover, and a N99 or N100 respirator. High risk PPE recommendations were that of low risk type, with the addition of overalls under the surgical gown, plastic poncho style gowns, and train dressing/undressing and observer.[38] In their systematic review, Jessop *et al.* also recommended respirator use in any high-risk areas where AGPs are performed, including operating theatres.[41] These recommendations are not universally accepted; a multi-disciplinary PPE taskforce from Stanford University created an algorithm for PPE use in the OR, recommending standard surgical attire for all patients who have negative PCR tests, or for those undergoing low-risk procedures and have a negative symptom screen.[42]

Patients requiring emergency surgery should be tested for SARS-CoV-2 and assessed for health risk prior to proceeding with surgery. Unless the patient is confirmed COVID-negative and considered low risk, high risk PPE should be worn for all emergency surgeries.[43] Additionally, pneumonia risk should be investigated through clinical exam and chest x-ray. Although controversial, many members of the ANZHPBA group advocated for chest CT scan as an early diagnostic and monitoring tool.[39]

Patients undergoing planned surgeries should also undergo health risk assessment and SAR-CoV-2 testing prior to surgery. The group recommends delaying planned surgeries if possible, and considering additional screening methods such as a walking or stair climbing test and blood gas analysis. To help determine whether a surgery should be deferred, the American College of Surgeons developed guidelines to triage procedures and decide which ones can be delayed or cancelled.[44] Low risk PPE can be worn for screened patients who are considered low risk of transmission.

Exposure risks associated with anaesthesia should be minimised. Avoidance of bag-mask ventilation and non-invasive ventilation in an OR setting can help limit exposure to HCWs. Both intubation and extubation should be performed in the OR due to potential aerosolisation of particles. Techniques to reduce patient coughing, especially during extubation should be used. Some centres have found success with increased physical barriers such as an "aerosol box" or vacuum shrouds for AGPs.[38,11]

Brindle *et al.* outline standard requirements for creation of a dedicated operating room for patients with confirmed SARS-CoV-2 or those considered high risk for the disease. This OR should be away from the high traffic areas within the surgical space. It should be completely emptied of all non-essential items, including equipment, stools, linens, disposable gloves, books, or signage. Ideally, a decontamination or anteroom should be present adjacent to the COVID OR, in which HCWs can don and doff PPE, and exchange equipment and medications as needed for the case. Instructional signage and necessary items for proper donning and doffing should be present in the anteroom.[45]

No unnecessary items should enter the designated COVID OR, including cell phones, pagers, bags, books, or pens. Any items brought into the OR should be disposed of after the case. HCWs should don disposable boot covers and caps, and discard these items immediately after exiting the OR into the anteroom.

Traffic should be minimised into and out of the room. Therefore, a team member should be designated as a runner. This person provides all equipment and materials required by the operating staff throughout the case and places it on a material exchange cart in the anteroom for the OR staff to collect as they need. Physicians are encouraged to choose surgical options that would minimise staff exposure and decrease operative time whenever possible.

In order to minimise transmission risk to those outside the room, the patient should be recovered in the operating room, and then transferred directly to an isolation or ICU room. This should be accomplished through the most direct route possible, with a team member travelling ahead of the patient to clear the path.[45]

4.7 *Obstetrics protocols*

Minimising exposure risk to patients and HCWs in the labour and delivery areas presents a unique challenge to the hospital during the SARS-CoV-2 pandemic. Many centres have adopted a protocol encouraging early epidural analgesia to reduce likelihood of requiring an emergency caesarean section under general anaesthesia. Furthermore, precipitous transfer of labouring patients between wards and units should be avoided to decrease the risk of nosocomial transmission.[46]

There has been debate throughout the pandemic regarding allowing a support person to accompany a labouring woman. Ultimately, hospitals must adopt protocols to reflect local risk, but there has certainly been a trend towards promoting a support person on the maternity ward who is compliant with hand washing and masking guidelines.[46]

4.8 *Critical care protocols*

An additional patient care complexity with respiratory viruses such as SARS-CoV-2 is the management of patients requiring supplemental cardiopulmonary support. These patients commonly require the use of AGPs as part of their care.

The WHO defines AGPs as: tracheal intubation, non-invasive ventilation (e.g. BiPAP and CPAP), tracheotomy, cardiopulmonary resuscitation, manual ventilation before intubation, bronchoscopy, sputum induction induced by using nebulised hypertonic saline, and autopsy procedures.[6]

The decision to intubate a COVID-19 patient evolved as the pandemic progressed. Initially, the clinical approach favoured by many institutions was early intubation and avoidance of high-flow nasal cannula oxygen supplementation and non-invasive ventilation.[47] However, as the number of critically ill patients increased around the globe, so too did international guidelines regarding intensive care. A trend towards using non-invasive respiratory support and delaying or avoiding endotracheal intubation was favoured in all those except the more critically ill patients displaying hypoxemia, tachypnea, increased work of breathing, and decreased gas exchange.[48]

In order to minimise risk to HCWs and maximise patient outcomes, many centres developed comprehensive airway policies to guide airway management. Only experienced operators who are part of a dedicated COVID-19 team perform endotracheal intubation, which is done in a negative pressure room using a rapid sequence induction and a video laryngoscope. Appropriate PPE for AGPs is used by all team members in the room, and the patient is then moved to an ICU bed by a multidisciplinary care team.[47]

Similarly, cardiac arrest policies were modified at many institutions to reflect the increased risk of exposure to HCWs during cardiopulmonary resuscitation. Mechanical compression devices were introduced to reduce the number of health workers responding to an arrest, and all members in attendance must don appropriate PPE for an AGP.[47]

4.9 *Deceased patients*

Current WHO guidelines recommend standard ICP precautions for handling of dead bodies, including hand hygiene and use of appropriate PPE (eye protection, medical mask, impermeable gown, closed footwear, and gloves). Leakage of bodily fluids should be avoided, movement or handling of the body should be minimised, and any area exposed to the deceased should be thoroughly disinfected. Standard burial and ritual measures should be respected. Immediate cremation of bodies is not required.[49]

While the WHO recommends using standard mortuary practice guidelines for body bag use, the Australian, Chinese, and United Kingdom guidelines suggest use of body bags in all patients. The Chinese guidelines advocate for placing gauze in the mouth, nose, ears, anus, and any open wound or tracheotomy site.[4]

Additional safety measures are required for deceased patients with suspected or confirmed COVID-19. Appropriate PPE must be used including a scrub suit, a long-sleeved fluid-resistant gown, gloves (either two pairs or one pair of autopsy gloves), a medical mask, eye protection (face shield or goggles), and boots/footwear protection. A respirator should be used for aerosol generating procedures such as washing of intestines or use of power saws. The autopsy should be performed in an adequately ventilated and well-lit room, ideally with negative pressure.[49]

5. Personal Protective Equipment (PPE)

In the hierarchy of infection control, PPE classically falls to the bottom of prevention and control methods. However, in the healthcare setting, there has been an increasing focus on the importance of this measure in preventing transmission of SARS-CoV-2. Agius *et al.* note that the scale of the pandemic did not allow time for adequate re-engineering of hospitals to meet the need for suitable ventilation, physical barriers, and adaptation of work practices. Therefore, they challenge the traditional view of PPE as the "last line of defense".[50]

In hospitals, the most common pathway of transmission of SARS has been the contact of the mucosae with infectious respiratory droplets or fomites.[51] Transmission may occur before, during, or after symptom onset, or even in the absence of symptoms. There has been much debate over the extent to which aerosol spread occurs in SAR-CoV-2, and thus the PPE recommendations for healthcare workers has varied across and within healthcare regions globally.

Shenoy *et al.* report that the major risks for SARS-CoV-2 transmission in healthcare workers are failure to appropriately identify and isolate affected patients, inadequate PPE availability, and improper use of PPE. They stress that the proper use of PPE plays a prominent role in the prevention of spread of COVID-19 within a healthcare setting.[52] A cross-sectional survey of HCWs during the beginning of the pandemic found that only one-third of the respondents were able to correctly identify the appropriate order to remove PPE equipment, potentially leading to HCW infections and nosocomial spread.[53]

Additionally, PPE recommendations have changed over the course of the pandemic. A global shortage of PPE and insufficient stockpiling of supplies at individual institutions required modification of guidelines, and these recommendations have evolved along with our understanding of the SARS-CoV-2 virus. The WHO, US CDC, and ECDC guidelines all recommend surgical masks (as opposed to N95 respirators) for healthcare workers who are not involved in AGPs, but there has been debate regarding the appropriateness of this recommendation. Many feel N95 respirators should be worn by all HCWs due to the potential for aerosolisation of the virus, the transmission dynamics of SARS-CoV-2, and the repeated exposure of HCWs due to lengthy periods in confined spaces.[4]

Nevertheless, appropriate PPE varies based on risk level to the healthcare worker. All HCWs should be trained on proper donning and doffing techniques, as well as proper disposal and disinfection of PPE. Up-to-date fit testing for N95 respirators is essential, and if powered air purifying respirators are to be used, education on use of these devices is required.[5]

Table 1: A guideline for PPE consistent with recommendations from the US CDC, WHO, and the PHAC.[6,11,54]

PPE type	Care of confirmed or suspected COVID + patients	Participation in aerosol generating procedures	Triage station	Care of COVID — or low risk patient	Area without direct patient contact/>2 metre distance maintained
Hand hygiene	WHO: Required CDC: Required PHAC: Required	WHO: Required CDC: Required PHAC: Required	WHO: Required CDC: Required PHAC: Required	WHO: Required CDC: Required PHAC: Required	WHO: Required CDC: Required PHAC: Required
Choice of mask type	WHO: Medical CDC: Medical PHAC: Medical, but N95 optional	WHO: N95 CDC: N95 PHAC: N95	WHO: N95 CDC: N95 PHAC: N95	WHO: Medical CDC: Medical PHAC: Medical	WHO: None CDC: Medical PHAC: Medical
Isolation gown or apron	WHO: Apron + Gown CDC: Gown PHAC: Gown	WHO: Required CDC: Required PHAC: Required	WHO: Required CDC: Required PHAC: Required	WHO: Recommended CDC: Not required PHAC: Not required	WHO: No CDC: No PHAC: No
Disposable gloves	WHO: Required CDC: Required PHAC: Required	WHO: Required CDC: Required PHAC: Required	WHO: Required CDC: Required PHAC: Required	WHO: Recommended CDC: Not required PHAC: Recommended	WHO: No CDC: No PHAC: No
Eye protection/ face shield	WHO: Required CDC: Required PHAC: Required	WHO: Required CDC: Required PHAC: Required	WHO: Required CDC: Required PHAC: Required	WHO: Recommended CDC: Required PHAC: Required	WHO: No CDC: No PHAC: No
Hair cover	WHO: Optional CDC: Optional PHAC: Optional	WHO: Optional CDC: Optional PHAC: Optional	WHO: Optional CDC: Optional PHAC: Optional	WHO: Not required CDC: Not required PHAC: Not required	WHO: No CDC: No PHAC: No

Table 1: Personal protective equipment (PPE) and control measure recommendations to prevent nosocomial transmission of SARS-CoV-2 in the hospital setting, based on exposure type. Guidelines are consistent with recommendations from the United States Center for Disease Control, World Health Organization, and the Public Health Agency of Canada. Adapted from Cheng *et al.*[55]

6. Conclusions

Hospital policies have changed rapidly since the onset of the pandemic, and will continue to evolve to meet the needs of the institution and the community that it serves. The ultimate goal remains providing patient care while reducing risk of exposure and transmission within the hospital walls.

References

1. World Health Organization. Novel Coronavirus (2019-nCoV): Situation Report, 3.
2. Cheng VC, Lau SK, Woo PC, Yuen KY. Severe acute respiratory syndrome coronavirus as an agent of emerging and reemerging infection. *Clinical Microbiology Reviews*. 2007;20(4):660–694.
3. Hierarchy of Controls. The National Institute for Occupational Safety and Health. [Internet]. 2015 Jan 13 [cited 12 Mar 2021] Available from: https://www.cdc.gov/niosh/topics/hierarchy/default.html.
4. Islam MS, Rahman KM, Sun Y, Qureshi MO, Abdi I, Chughtai AA, Seale H. Current knowledge of COVID-19 and infection prevention and control strategies in healthcare settings: A global analysis. *Infection Control & Hospital Epidemiology*. 2020;41(10):1196–1206.
5. Kuy S, Gupta R, Correa R, Tsai R, Vohra S. Best practices for a Covid-19 preparedness plan for health systems. *NEJM Catalyst Innovations in Care Delivery*. 2020;1(2).
6. World Health Organization. Infection prevention and control health-care facility response for COVID-19: A module from the suite of health service capacity assessments in the context of the COVID-19 pandemic: Interim guidance, 20 October 2020. World Health Organization; 2020.
7. Mitra B, Luckhoff C, Mitchell RD, O'Reilly GM, Smit DV, Cameron PA. Temperature screening has negligible value for control of COVID-19. *Emergency Medicine Australasia*. 2020;32(5):867–869.

8. Wee LE, Fua TP, Chua YY, Ho AF, Sim XY, Conceicao EP, Venkatachalam I, Tan KB, Tan BH. Containing COVID-19 in the emergency department: The role of improved case detection and segregation of suspect cases. *Academic Emergency Medicine*. 2020;27(5):379–387.

9. Infection Prevention and Control (IPC). Protocol for Pediatric Surgical Procedures During COVID-19: BC CDC.

10. Knowlton SD, Boles CL, Perencevich EN, Diekema DJ, Nonnenmann MW. Bioaerosol concentrations generated from toilet flushing in a hospital-based patient care setting. *Antimicrobial Resistance & Infection Control*. 2018; 7(1):1–8.

11. Interim Infection Prevention and Control Recommendations for Healthcare Personnel During the Coronavirus Disease 2019 (COVID-19) Pandemic [Internet]. 2021 Feb 23. Available from: https://www.cdc.gov/coronavirus/2019-ncov/hcp/infection-control-recommendations.html.

12. Saran S, Gurjar M, Baronia A, Sivapurapu V, Ghosh PS, Raju GM, Maurya I. Heating, ventilation and air conditioning (HVAC) in intensive care unit. *Critical Care*. 2020;24:1–1.

13. Van Doremalen N, Bushmaker T, Morris DH, Holbrook MG, Gamble A, Williamson BN, Tamin A, Harcourt JL, Thornburg NJ, Gerber SI, Lloyd-Smith JO. Aerosol and surface stability of SARS-CoV-2 as compared with SARS-CoV-1. *New England Journal of Medicine*. 2020;382(16): 1564–1567.

14. Choi H, Chatterjee P, Lichtfouse E, Martel JA, Hwang M, Jinadatha C, Sharma VK. Classical and alternative disinfection strategies to control the COVID-19 virus in healthcare facilities: A review. *Environmental Chemistry Letters*. 2021:1–7.

15. Hard-surface disinfectants and hand sanitizers (COVID-19): List of disinfectants with evidence for use against COVID-19. [Internet]. 2021 Apr 14. Available from: https://www.canada.ca/en/health-canada/services/drugs-health-products/disinfectants/covid-19/list.html.

16. Rutala WA, Weber DJ. Monitoring and improving the effectiveness of surface cleaning and disinfection. *American Journal of Infection Control*. 2016;44(5):e69–e76.

17. Cadnum JL, Jencson AL, Livingston SH, Li DF, Redmond SN, Pearlmutter B, Wilson BM, Donskey CJ. Evaluation of an electrostatic spray disinfectant technology for rapid decontamination of portable equipment and large open areas in the era of SARS-CoV-2. *American Journal of Infection Control*. 2020;48(8):951–954.

18. Ilyas S, Srivastava RR, Kim H. Disinfection technology and strategies for COVID-19 hospital and bio-medical waste management. *Science of the Total Environment.* 2020;749:141652.
19. Klein MG, Cheng CJ, Lii E, Mao K, Mesbahi H, Zhu T, Muckstadt JA, Hupert N. COVID-19 models for hospital surge capacity planning: A systematic review. *Disaster Medicine and Public Health Preparedness.* 2020:1–7.
20. Kumar P, Kattan O, Broome B, Singhal S. Reassessing Covid-19 needs: How providers can reexamine their surge capacity, supply availability, workforce readiness, and financial resiliency. *NEJM Catalyst Innovations in Care Delivery.* 2020;1(3).
21. Aziz S, Arabi YM, Alhazzani W, Evans L, Citerio G, Fischkoff K, Salluh J, Meyfroidt G, Alshamsi F, Oczkowski S, Azoulay E. Managing ICU surge during the COVID-19 crisis: Rapid guidelines. *Intensive Care Medicine.* 2020;46:1303–1325.
22. Kim MK, Rabinowitz LG, Nagula S, Dunn A, Chalil J, Xu T, Barna E, Raucher B, Thomas DC, Murphy B. A primer for clinician deployment to the medicine floors from an epicenter of Covid-19. *NEJM Catalyst Innovations in Care Delivery.* 2020;1(3).
23. World Health Organization. Coronavirus disease (COVID-19) outbreak: Rights, roles and responsibilities of health workers, including key considerations for occupational safety and health: Interim guidance, 19 March 2020. World Health Organization; 2020.
24. Pappa S, Ntella V, Giannakas T, Giannakoulis VG, Papoutsi E, Katsaounou P. Prevalence of depression, anxiety, and insomnia among healthcare workers during the COVID-19 pandemic: A systematic review and meta-analysis. *Brain, Behavior, and Immunity.* 2020.
25. Khajuria A, Tomaszewski W, Liu Z, Chen JH, Mehdian R, Fleming S, Vig S, Crawford MJ. Workplace factors associated with mental health of healthcare workers during the COVID-19 pandemic: An international cross-sectional study. *BMC Health Services Research.* 2021;21(1):1–1.
26. Ragazzoni L, Barco A, Echeverri L, Conti A, Linty M, Caviglia M, Merlo F, Martini D, Pirisi A, Weinstein E, Barone-Adesi F. Just-in-time training in a tertiary referral hospital during the COVID-19 pandemic in Italy. *Academic Medicine.* 2020 Jul 14.
27. Gagneux-Brunon A, Pelissier C, Gagnaire J, Pillet S, Pozzetto B, Botelho-Nevers E, Berthelot P. SARS-CoV-2 infection: Advocacy for training and social distancing in healthcare settings. *Journal of Hospital Infection.* 2020;106(3):610–612.

28. Sahu AK, Amrithanand VT, Mathew R, Aggarwal P, Nayer J, Bhoi S. COVID-19 in health care workers — A systematic review and meta-analysis. *The American Journal of Emergency Medicine*. 2020;38(9):1727–1731.

29. Chu J, Yang N, Wei Y, Yue H, Zhang F, Zhao J, He L, Sheng G, Chen P, Li G, Wu S. Clinical characteristics of 54 medical staff with COVID-19: A retrospective study in a single center in Wuhan, China. *Journal of Medical Virology*. 2020;92(7):807–813.

30. Bhagavathula AS, Aldhaleei WA, Rahmani J, Mahabadi MA, Bandari DK. Novel coronavirus (COVID-19) knowledge and perceptions: A survey on healthcare workers. *MedRxiv*. 2020 Jan 1.

31. Ali S, Noreen S, Farooq I, Bugshan A, Vohra F. Risk assessment of healthcare workers at the frontline against COVID-19. *Pakistan Journal of Medical Sciences*. 2020;36(COVID19-S4):S99.

32. Christensen L, Rasmussen CS, Benfield T, Franc JM. A randomized trial of instructor-led training versus video lesson in training health care providers in proper donning and doffing of personal protective equipment. *Disaster Medicine and Public Health Preparedness*. 2020;14(4):514–520.

33. Foong TW, Ng ES, Khoo CY, Ashokka B, Khoo D, Agrawal R. Rapid training of healthcare staff for protected cardiopulmonary resuscitation in the COVID-19 pandemic. *British Journal of Anaesthesia*. 2020 May 6.

34. Dooling K. The Advisory committee on immunization practices' updated interim recommendation for allocation of COVID-19 vaccine — United States, December 2020. MMWR. *Morbidity and Mortality Weekly Report*. 2021;69.

35. Thompson MG, Burgess JL, Naleway AL, Tyner HL, Yoon SK, Meece J, Olsho LE, Caban-Martinez AJ, Fowlkes A, Lutrick K, Kuntz JL. Interim estimates of vaccine effectiveness of BNT162b2 and mRNA-1273 COVID-19 vaccines in preventing SARS-CoV-2 infection among health care personnel, first responders, and other essential and frontline workers — eight US locations, December 2020–March 2021. *Morbidity and Mortality Weekly Report*. 2021;70(13):495.

36. Shah AS, Gribben C, Bishop J, Hanlon P, Caldwell D, Wood R, Reid M, McMenamin J, Goldberg D, Stockton D, Hutchinson S. Effect of vaccination on transmission of COVID-19: An observational study in healthcare workers and their households. *MedRxiv*. 2021 Jan 1.

37. Schaye VE, Reich JA, Bosworth BP, Stern DT, Volpicelli F, Shapiro NM, Hauck KD, Fagan IM, Villagomez SM, Uppal A, Sauthoff H. Collaborating across private, public, community, and federal hospital systems: Lessons learned from the Covid-19 pandemic response in NYC. *NEJM Catalyst Innovations in Care Delivery*. 2020 Oct 21;1(6).

38. Brücher BL, Nigri G, Tinelli A, Lapeña JF, Espin-Basany E, Macri P, Matevossian E, Ralon S, Perkins R, Lück R, Kube R. COVID-19: Pandemic surgery guidance. *4open*. 2020;3:1.

39. Australian and New Zealand Hepatic, Pancreatic and Biliary Association (ANZHPBA) (2020), Considerations for HPB Surgeons in a Complex Triage Scenario COVID-19. April 06, 2020. Available from https://www.anzhpba.com/covid-19-guidelines/ [Accessed 06 April 2020].

40. Collaborative C. Global guidance for surgical care during the COVID-19 pandemic. *The British Journal of Surgery*. 2020 Aug.

41. Jessop ZM, Dobbs TD, Ali SR, Combellack E, Clancy R, Ibrahim N, Jovic TH, Kaur AJ, Nijran A, O'Neill TB, Whitaker IS. Personal protective equipment for surgeons during. *British Journal of Surgery*. 2020;107(10):1262–1280.

42. Forrester JD, Nassar AK, Maggio PM, Hawn MT. Precautions for operating room team members during the COVID-19 pandemic. *Journal of the American College of Surgeons*. 2020;230(6):1098–1101.

43. Moletta L, Pierobon ES, Capovilla G, Costantini M, Salvador R, Merigliano S, Valmasoni M. International guidelines and recommendations for surgery during Covid-19 pandemic: A systematic review. *International Journal of Surgery*. 2020 May 23.

44. American College of Surgeons (ACS) (2020), COVID-19: Elective case triage guidelines for surgical care. March 24, 2020. Available from: https://www.facs.org/covid-19/clinical-guidance/elective-case [Accessed March 2020].

45. Brindle ME, Gawande A. Managing COVID-19 in surgical systems. *Annals of Surgery*. 2020 Mar 20.

46. Morau E, Bouvet L, Keita H, Vial F, Bonnet MP, Bonnin M, Le AG, Chassard D, Mercier FJ, Benhamou D. Anaesthesia and intensive care in obstetrics during the COVID-19 pandemic. *Anaesthesia, Critical Care & Pain Medicine*. 2020;39(3):345–349.

47. Griffin KM, Karas MG, Ivascu NS, Lief L. Hospital preparedness for COVID-19: A practical guide from a critical care perspective. *American Journal of Respiratory and Critical Care Medicine*. 2020;201(11): 1337–1344.

48. Tobin MJ. Basing Respiratory Management of COVID-19 on Physiological Principles. *American Journal of Respiratory and Critical Care Medicine*. 2020;201(11):1319–1320.

49. World Health Organization. Infection prevention and control for the safe management of a dead body in the context of COVID-19: Interim guidance, 4 September 2020. World Health Organization, 2020.

50. Agius RM, MacDermott N. Covid-19 and workers' protection: Lessons to learn, and lessons overlooked. *Occupational Medicine*. 2021 Mar 18.
51. Seto WH, Tsang D, Yung RW, Ching TY, Ng TK, Ho M, Ho LM, Peiris JS, Advisors of expert SARS group of Hospital Authority. Effectiveness of precautions against droplets and contact in prevention of nosocomial transmission of severe acute respiratory syndrome (SARS). *The Lancet*. 2003;361(9368):1519–1520.
52. Shenoy ES, Weber DJ. Lessons learned in infection prevention for Ebola virus disease and the coronavirus disease 2019 (COVID-19) pandemic — Principles underlying prevention. *Infection Control and Hospital Epidemiology*. 2021:1.
53. Piché-Renaud PP, Groves HE, Kitano T, Arnold C, Thomas A, Streitenberger L, Alexander L, Morris SK. Healthcare worker perception of a global outbreak of novel coronavirus (COVID-19) and personal protective equipment: Survey of a pediatric tertiary-care hospital. *Infection Control & Hospital Epidemiology*. 2020:1–7.
54. Infection prevention and control for COVID-19: Interim guidance for acute healthcare settings. [Internet]. 2021 Feb 12. Available from: https://www.canada.ca/en/public-health/services/diseases/2019-novel-coronavirus-infection/health-professionals/infection-prevention-control-covid-19-second-interim-guidance.html.
55. Cheng VC, Wong SC, Chen JH, Yip CC, Chuang VW, Tsang OT, Sridhar S, Chan JF, Ho PL, Yuen KY. Escalating infection control response to the rapidly evolving epidemiology of the coronavirus disease 2019 (COVID-19) due to SARS-CoV-2 in Hong Kong. *Infection Control & Hospital Epidemiology*. 2020;41(5):493–498.

Chapter 11

Long-Term Care Facilities

Sana Vahidy* and **Michael Schwandt***,†

School of Population and Public Health, University of British Columbia, Vancouver, Canada

†*Vancouver Coastal Health Authority, Vancouver, Canada*

Key Message

- Long-term care (LTC) facilities are regulated at a provincial level and can function on a for-profit or non-profit basis supported by governmental funding depending on the model.
- LTC facilities are particularly vulnerable to outbreaks due to the resident population being frail with multiple co-morbidities and poor structural design which can facilitate spread of infectious disease.
- An essential component of controlling these LTC outbreaks is supporting LTC staff who are also from vulnerable and sometimes marginalised populations, without job security necessitating part-time work at more than one LTC facility and lack of sick day leave which can facilitate spread of infectious disease.
- LTC facilities should adapt within structural limitations to ensure isolation rooms are allocated with adequate ventilation and sufficient personal protective supplies are provided to manage communicable disease outbreaks.

- The approach to this problem must reduce spread in both LTC residents and staff in order to manage outbreaks which requires time commitment and resources by local and provincial governments.
- There is a need to establish surveillance programs on a provincial level to monitor cases and outbreaks in for-profit and non-profit LTC facilities in Canada.

1. Introduction

In Canada and much of the Western hemisphere, it is estimated that up to 60–80% of COVID-19 deaths occurred in LTC homes.[1-4] However, one important limitation is the general paucity of scientifically rigorous studies evaluating morbidity and mortality in this vulnerable population over time in Canada and other countries. Fishman *et al.* (2020) evaluated LTC centers in Ontario, Canada compared to elderly living in the community from March to April 2020.[1] The COVID-19 mortality specific incidence rate ratios (IRR) of residents in LTC facilities compared to community dwelling residents 69 and older was 13.1 (95% CI, 9.9–17.3) which indicates those in LTC facilities are dying at a disproportionate rate compared to similarly aged persons in the community.[1] The authors also compared residents in LTC facilities to the entire provincial population which found the IRR was 90.4 (95% CI, 68.9–117.6).[1] These findings are alarming and suggest broader factors are at play contributing to this increased risk of death in residents of LTC facilities related to contracting COVID-19 infection.

1.1 *What are the important factors associated with increased risk in this population?*

This increased risk of morbidity and mortality in residents of LTC facilities is multi-faceted. First of all, these individuals are often frail and elderly with numerous co-morbidities posing increased risk of infection.[5-9] The second factor is the LTC staff can be from transient and marginalised communities working on a part-time basis.[9,10] This often necessitates working simultaneously at multiple facilities due to income and job insecurity with reluctance to take sick days and possibly lack of access to insured healthcare resources for themselves.[5,9,10] A strong predictor of death in these LTC facilities was poor identification of active infection in staff and unfortunately, resultant lag times, particularly, 2-day and 6-day lag times were associated with the highest risk of death in LTC residents.[1]

Estabrooks *et al.* (2020) highlight a simultaneous "workforce crisis" in LTC facilities which significantly impacts the health of residents in these LTC facilities and structural shortcomings in the design of these facilities.[14] Estabrooks *et al.* (2020) propose a 9-step method to mitigate this "workforce crisis" simultaneously occurring in LTC facilities as a call to action to federal and provincial governments.[14] In Canada, these LTC facilities are not regulated at a national level but frequently at a provincial level following different models of care.[5,11] There are variable funding supports depending on the province and some of these facilities may operate on a for-profit basis.[5,11] Some of these facilities may have multiple residents per room with inadequate spacing as a cost-saving measure.[5,11] There may be inadequate rooms allocated and poor ventilation systems for appropriate isolation of cases.[5,7,11] In addition, these LTC facilities are often old and outdated in design and represent a neglected part of the wider healthcare system.[9,11]

In a recent Canadian study, Stall *et al.* (2020) investigated LTC outbreaks in Ontario, Canada and whether these LTC facilities operated on a non-profit or for-profit basis.[11] Outbreaks were not more likely to occur in for-profit LTC homes but in the event of an active outbreak, for profit LTC homes were associated with greater extent and increased COVID-19 specific mortality in residents.[11] Municipally funded LTC homes were found to be associated with the least risk.[11] The higher risk associated with for-profit LTC homes was considered to be related to older design and infrastructure more commonly found in for-profit operation models.[11]

2. Reducing Transmission in Long-Term Care Facilities

British Columbia (BC) was the first province in Canada to identify a COVID-19 outbreak in a LTC facility.[4] Liu *et al.* (2020) compare the handling of LTC outbreaks in Ontario to British Columbia and highlight key deficiencies in LTC organisation in Ontario as being problematic and resulting in poor public health response.[5,7,12] Some of the successful measures used in BC include proactive and universal masking policies mandated early for all staff and visitors of LTC facilities.[5,12] Adequate supply of personal protective equipment (PPE) is essential with pre-planned alternate supply chains if stocks run low.[4] Another common measure was strict restrictions on visitors to LTC facilities and mandatory screening of visitors when visits were unavoidable.[5,9,12] A recently published mixed methods study surveyed key leaders in COVID-19 free LTC facilities in BC.[4] Overall, these leaders adhered to the BC Center for Disease Control (BCCDC) recommendations although some facilities had some design constraints not conducive to single room occupancy and private toilets.[4] However, these facilities overcame some barriers by allocating certain LTC staff to each room to reduce cross-contamination due to staff going from different residents' rooms during the shifts.[4] Also, communication between leadership and LTC staff was integral to maintain trust and avoid conflict.[4] Strategies employed by successful LTC leaders included engaging staff, residents and families through electronic messages and newsletters to avoid undue fear and anxiety.[4]

Another important point is the need for intensive surveillance and isolation of COVID-19 positive cases in residents or staff at these LTC facilities.[5,7,9,12] As mentioned before, contact tracing measures must be in place at LTC facilities to effectively reduce lag times in identifying the infected staff member and timely initiating of isolation to avoid spread to other staff and residents.[1] Some experts propose a lower threshold to declare outbreaks in LTC facilities (compared to other health facilities) by setting a lower number of required cases necessary to declare an outbreak.[5] Furthermore, it is critical to have a pre-planned and coordinated health teams that can be deployed in a timely manner to address and mitigate spread of outbreaks.[4,5,7,12]

2.1 *What other measures need to be continued in these facilities?*

Outbreaks at LTC facilities are often related to transmission and outbreaks in the local communities and health regions.[11] The LTC facilities must provide ongoing emphasis on hand hygiene and reasonable measures for enforcement such as auditing.[6,7] Adequate PPE must be provided with appropriate donning and doffing education and videos.[6,7,12] Surgical masks should be provided for routine care and then appropriate N95 and face shields for aerosol generating procedures.[12] Contingency plans must be in place for staffing and PPE shortages in the event of outbreaks.[6,7] For example, backup staffing support rosters should be established in the event of a large-scale exposure and/or outbreak.[1–3]

Each LTC needs to consider its own complexity of residents, human resource needs and limitations of their respective facilities (shared patient rooms, poor ventilation, and shared meal spaces) and limiting use of communal spaces to reduce transmission.[5–7,12] There needs to be an ongoing and unwavering commitment from LTC staff and residents to adhere to the above-mentioned strategies with ongoing reassessment at each site after outbreaks occur.[10,11] Some advocate for asymptomatic rapid screening of LTC staff on a weekly basis to identify cases in a pre-symptomatic phase.[9,12] Also, it is important that strict measures be applied to staff only areas such as break rooms to reduce transmission from staff to staff in these LTC facilities.[12]

3. Vaccination in the LTCF Population

The federal government procures the vaccine supply and distributes it to provincial and territorial jurisdictions appropriately.[15] Provinces and territories then distribute the supply to priority groups: LTC residents (potentially, their caregivers) and LTC staff.[15] As of February 2021, most provinces have confirmed that almost 100% of LTC residents have received the first dose of the vaccine.[15] In British Columbia, approximately 95% of LTC residents and 89% of LTC staff have received their first dose.[15]

A recently published Morbidity and Mortality Weekly Report examined the impact of partial vaccination in two nursing facilities in Connecticut experiencing COVID-19 outbreaks.[13] Partial vaccination referred to the status of residents of the facility having received the initial dose of the Pfizer vaccine more than 14 days ago and included residents who received the second dose within 7 days through vaccination clinics held at the site.[13] Partial vaccination was found to be approximately 63% effective in this population (95% confidence intervals of 33–79%).[13] This highlights the need for residents of LTC facilities and staff working at these sites be a COVID-19 vaccination priority to reduce the spread of COVID-19.[9,13]

4. Framework to Address Outcome Disparity

Andrew *et al.* (2020) construct an ecological framework to approach this disparity of COVID-19 specific mortality in residents of LTC facilities.[10] There are many elements that contribute to this disparity and disproportionate disadvantage to those living in LTC facilities from an individual level to families and caregivers, to institutions and health services/systems, communities and governmental policies.[10] On an individual, family and caregivers' level, frailty and isolation contribute directly and potentially, indirectly to morbidity and mortality.[10] LTC facilities are often designed as communal living spaces with shared rooms and dining spaces which have potential to enhance transmission.[10,12] On a community level, LTC staff are often part-time employees without benefits or job security so often work at multiple sites increasing risk of transmission.[4,10] These LTC staff may be less likely to take sick days and may live in crowded and marginalised communities themselves subject to higher COVID-19 positivity rates.[10,12] Government policies vary from region to region with different funding models and connection to local health services which can put LTC facilities at higher risk for outbreaks due to lack of supplies.[10,12]

We propose a framework below similar to the model by Andrew *et al.* (2020).[10] Figure 1 demonstrates the impact of vaccination on individual and staff risk in LTC facilities.

At the individual level, frailty and co-morbidities are important factors making residents of LTC facilities vulnerable.[1–8,12] At an administrative and staff level, many of the same principles are relevant such as LTC staff being a vulnerable population with minimal job and income security and likely a higher risk of acquiring COVID-19 themselves.[3–5,10–12] By LTC staff avoiding and delaying sick days, residents of LTC can

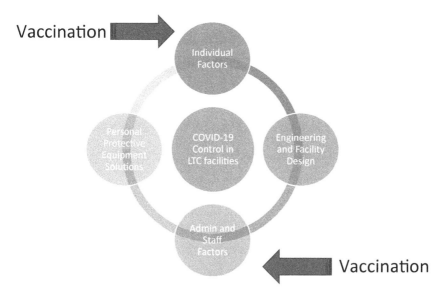

Figure 1: Framework of COVID-19 control in long-term care (LTC) facilities.

become infected which can spread easily to other residents resulting in an outbreak.[1,4,12] Due to limited funding often at these sites, the supply of PPE can be precarious and it may not be accompanied by appropriate education and training.[3–5,10–12] These deficiencies put LTC residents and staff at risk as well as the overarching community and health region.

Part of the ease of transmission at LTC facilities is related to poor engineering such as communal nature of these facilities and outdated buildings with lack of adequate ventilation.[1,4,10,12] Also, these LTC facilities are often designed as communities which can be detrimental in outbreaks and result in further spread of communicable disease.[4,7,10,12]

To overcome these deficiencies, a complex strategy must be implemented which focuses on modifiable factors to mitigate risk of transmission and reduce mortality. The most modifiable factors are likely providing assured income for sick days for infected LTC staff and a one-site work order.[4,12,14] Other modifiable factors are optimised use of existing LTC facilities and appropriate PPE supply with relevant education.[4,12,14] Optimised use of LTC facilities should utilise local expertise to designate appropriately ventilated and isolated resident rooms for infected LTC residents.[10,12,14] Each resident room should have a private toilet and handwashing station.[4,7] LTC facilities should limit use of communal spaces and provide virtual engagement to residents instead to avoid loneliness.[4,7,10,12]

5. Future Efforts and Pandemic Preparedness

The pandemic has unmasked underlying disparities and health inequities in LTC facilities and ultimately, there is no easy solution to this multi-faceted problem. Governments must commit time and resources to improve the function of these LTC facilities and preserve the health of the vulnerable population.[14] It is important to ensure LTC facilities are well designed and equipped with personal protective supplies to manage communicable disease outbreaks, whether respiratory or non-respiratory in etiology.[4,14]

There is a need to collect standardised data from LTC facilities to obtain accurate incident cases and associated COVID-19 specific mortality rates.[4,10] This data collection needs to be part of current provincial surveillance systems. In addition, a shift in focus must occur to further evaluate environmental, engineering and staffing deficiencies in LTC facilities which impact COVID-19 transmission and make LTC residents vulnerable to infection.[4]

References

1. Fisman DN, Bogoch I, Lapointe-Shaw L, McCready J, Tuite AR. Risk factors associated with mortality among residents with coronavirus disease 2019 (COVID-19) in long-term care facilities in Ontario, Canada. *JAMA Network Open*. 2020;3(7):e2015957.
2. Team EPHE, Danis K, Fonteneau L, Georges S, Daniau C, Bernard-Stoecklin S, *et al*. High impact of COVID-19 in long-term care facilities, suggestion for monitoring in the EU/EEA, May 2020. *Eurosurveillance*. 2020;25(22).
3. D'Adamo H, Yoshikawa T, Ouslander JG. Coronavirus disease 2019 in geriatrics and long-term care: The ABCDs of COVID-19. *Journal of American Geriatrics Society*. 2020;68(5):912–917.
4. Havaei F, MacPhee M, Keselman D, Staempfli S. Leading a long-term care facility through the COVID-19 crisis: Successes, barriers and lessons learned. *Healthcare Quaterly*. 2021;23(4):28–34.

5. Liu M, Maxwell CJ, Armstrong P, Schwandt M, Moser A, McGregor MJ, *et al.* COVID-19 in long-term care homes in Ontario and British Columbia. *CMAJ*. 2020;192(47):E1540–E6.

6. McMichael TM, Currie DW, Clark S, Pogosjans S, Kay M, Schwartz NG, *et al.* Epidemiology of Covid-19 in a long-term care facility in King County, Washington. *New England Journal of Medicine*. 2020;382(21):2005–2011.

7. Yen MY, Schwartz J, King CC, Lee CM, Hsueh PR, Society of Taiwan Long-term Care Infection P, *et al.* Recommendations for protecting against and mitigating the COVID-19 pandemic in long-term care facilities. *Journal of Microbiology Immunology and Infection*. 2020;53(3):447–453.

8. Du RH, Liang LR, Yang CQ, Wang W, Cao TZ, Li M, *et al.* Predictors of mortality for patients with COVID-19 pneumonia caused by SARS-CoV-2: A prospective cohort study. *European Respiratory Journal*. 2020.

9. Hashan MR, Smoll N, King C, Ockenden-Muldoon H, Walker J, Wattiaux A, *et al.* Epidemiology and clinical features of COVID-19 outbreaks in aged care facilities: A systematic review and meta-analysis. *EClinicalMedicine*. 2021;33:100771.

10. Andrew M, Searle SD, McElhaney JE, McNeil SA, Clarke B, Rockwood K, *et al.* COVID-19, frailty and long-term care: Implications for policy and practice. *Journal of Infection in Developing Countries*. 2020;14(5): 428–432.

11. Stall NM, Jones A, Brown KA, Rochon PA, Costa AP. For-profit long-term care homes and the risk of COVID-19 outbreaks and resident deaths. *CMAJ*. 2020;192(33):E946–E55.

12. Gosch M, Heppner HJ, Lim S, Singler K. Recommendations for the management of COVID-19 pandemic in long-term care facilities. *Journal of Gerontology Geriatrics*. 2021.

13. Britton A, Jacobs Slifka KM, Edens C, Nanduri SA, Bart SM, Shang N, *et al.* Effectiveness of the Pfizer-BioNTech COVID-19 vaccine among residents of two skilled nursing facilities experiencing COVID-19 Outbreaks — Connecticut, December 2020-February 2021. *MMWR Morbidity and Mortality Weekly Report*. 2021;70(11):396–401.

14. Estabrooks CA, Straus S, Flood, CM, Keefe J, Armstrong P, Donner G, Boscart V, Ducharme F, Silvius J, Wolfson M. Restoring trust: COVID-19 and the future of long-term care. *Royal Society of Canada*. 2020.

15. Sinha S, Feil C and Iciaszczyk N. The rollout of the COVID-19 vaccines in care homes in Canada as of 16th February 2021. Article in LTCcovid.org, International Long-Term Care Policy Network, CPEC-LSE.

Part 6

Therapeutics

Chapter 12

Therapeutics for COVID-19

Jorge Andres Delgado-Ron[*], Reza Hosseini[*],
Srinivas Murthy[*,†], and David Sweet[‡,§]

[*]*School of Population and Public Health, University of British Columbia,*
Vancouver, Canada

[†]*BC Children's Hospital, Vancouver, Canada*

[‡]*Department of Emergency Medicine, Faculty of Medicine,*
University of British Columbia, Diamond Health Care Centre
Vancouver, Canada

[§]*Division of Critical Care Medicine, Department of Medicine,*
Vancouver General Hospital Jim Pattison Pavilion,
Vancouver, Canada

Key Message

- The coronavirus disease 2019 pandemic provoked an unprecedented wave of research aimed at containing the spread of the SARS-CoV-2 virus and fighting its catastrophic impacts in the worldwide population. New experimental studies were launched daily and international experts teamed up to analyze the results almost in real time through live network meta-analyses.
- While useful, network meta-analyses lack the nuance that allow physicians to pinpoint the most appropriate treatment for specific patients given their clinical status: patients in late stages, for instance, do not benefit as much from drugs that target the SARS-CoV-2 virus.

- Given the complexity of the host–virus interaction, different treatments should be applied depending on the aim: prophylaxis, viral neutralisation, immunomodulation, or vital support. The evidence is current as of April 2021 and includes drugs with proven efficacy for specific subgroups.
- Polyclonal antibodies work to prevent infection. Colchicine, proxalutamide, and convalescent plasma seem to benefit non-severe patients. Remdesivir and other antiviral treatments likely benefit patients with more severe infection. Finally, corticosteroids, interleukin inhibitors, Janus kinase inhibitors, and interferons might help those in critical stages.

1. Introduction

COVID-19 caused by severe acute respiratory syndrome coronavirus 2 (SARS-CoV-2) infected people in 18 different countries within five weeks of the publication of its first whole-genome sequence.[1] It managed to spread and sicken in big numbers precisely because we were ill-prepared to counter its infectious and pathogenic mechanisms. While the pandemic response has been equally impressive — with 2,846 active randomised human trials studying the Coronavirus Disease 2019 (COVID-19) as of April 19, 2021[2] — we remain challenged in producing rapid innovation and drug development. Under normal circumstances, the flow through discovery, animal studies, clinical trials, and approval processes takes a median of 6.7 years.[3] However, in practice, some potential treatments lead the way due to a well-known record of safety from previous approval processes.[4]

"Repurposed" drugs offer the advantage of reducing both development time and overall costs (a new drug costs an average of US$2.8 billion), making it more attractive to potential investors.[2,5] However, there are also drawbacks: readily available drugs may be first tested in observational studies, inducing heavy investments based on likely biased estimates. Several heads of state touted hydroxychloroquine based on poorly designed observational studies during the pandemic's first months. As of April 4, 2021, this drug ranks first among COVID-19 trials for treatments with the highest number of exposed participants (with lackluster results).[2,6] While institutional, organisational, and governmental factors are not the focus of our analysis, we have touched upon them to make a point: while drug development is standardised, many factors influence deciding who is ahead in the innovation race. As such, we caution the readers not to equate a lack of findings with a lack of possible effectiveness when some drugs have just begun testing. Such is the case with *de novo* molecules identified through computational methods, some of which could progress into phase III trials.

2. Making Sense of the Overwhelming Evidence

Based on previous epidemics experience, the World Health Organization (WHO) quickly identified (and later refined) the target product profiles for COVID-19 therapeutics. They include a set of preferred and minimum recommended outcomes to measure a drug's efficacy and safety.[7] They are also helpful because we can correlate them with the clinical phases of the COVID-19 (Figure 1).

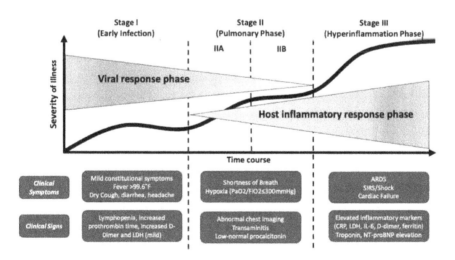

Figure 1: Cardinal clinical and laboratory features and phases of COVID-19 by Ibrahim Abaker Targio Hashem and colleagues under a CC-BY-ND 4.0 International license.
Source: https://doi.org/10.1101/2020.05.18.20105577.

The early infection starts with an asymptomatic period that precedes the fever, headache, dry cough, and other constitutional symptoms. Most patients spontaneously recover from this phase but still are highly contagious. The WHO conducted consultations regarding the role of therapeutics in prophylaxis but has yet to publish specific targets.[8] Hence, there are no specific options for asymptomatic patients, but useful drugs at this stage would need to measurably reduce the risk of probable or confirmed symptomatic infection.

Most infected people will become mild symptomatic cases. Drugs for these patients should, at minimum, reduce the duration of symptoms, measured by a standardised symptom scoring metric, or lessen the number of days to a negative polymerase chain reaction (PCR) test. An ideal treatment would also reduce the risk of disease progression.[7]

If the infection significantly compromises the lungs, the patients may develop clinical signs of pneumonia ("moderate to severe disease"). Here is where we see shortness of breath and other signs of respiratory distress. Meanwhile, the adaptive immune system actively counters the infection, therefore, reducing the viral load. An ideal treatment here should reduce mortality at 28 days. Other outcomes could be reduced risk of progression to critical disease or shorter duration of oxygen support.[7,9]

In some cases, patients require life-sustaining treatment due to acute respiratory distress syndrome, sepsis, or septic shock. Viral load may be declining, but symptoms worsen due to an over-active immune responses.[10] For both moderate-to-severe and critical care patients, 28 day survival remains a critical indicator. Length of hospital stay is also a valid indicator used in some trials. The need for, and duration of, mechanical ventilation are other key metrics.[7,9]

Well-established outcomes help researchers aggregate information from different studies to avoid type II errors. Network meta-analyses have the added advantage of calculating indirect effects between drugs that had never been tested against each other.[11,12] In the following sections, we thoroughly describe classes of therapies that, so far, have produced meaningful effects on the outcomes mentioned above in two living systematic reviews and network meta-analyses synthesising the extant evidence on COVID-19 preventive and treatment drugs.[2,13] Table 1 summarises the therapies recommended by at least one of WHO, United States National

Table 1: Summary of therapies recommended by at least one of WHO*, NIH*, or BCCTC* as effective for treating COVID-19 outside clinical trials. Not-recommended drugs are those that are agreed upon by all three agencies.[9,14,15]

	Pulmonary phase	Inflammatory phase	Other therapies

Recommended by at least one agency	• Remdesivir;
	• Polyclonal antibodies:
	  ○ Bamlanivimab-etesevimab
	  ○ Casirivimab-imdevimab
		• Corticosteroids;
		• IL-6* pathway inhibitors:
		  ○ Tocilizumab
		  ○ Sarilumab
		• Baricitinib (only in combination with remdesivir).
			• Antibacterial therapy (only when a bacterial infection is suspected);
			• Antithrombotic therapy (at prophylactic dose);
			• Prone ventilation;
			• ECMO.*

Raised in the literature but not currently recommended by any of three agencies	• Chloroquine; • Hydroxychloroquine; • Lopinavir/ritonavir; • Ivermectin; • hrsACE2.*	• IL-1 pathway inhibitors (anakinra); • Interferons; • Convalescent plasma; • Colchicine; • Proxalutamide.	

*WHO = *World Health Organization;* NIH = *[United States] National Institutes of Health;* BCCTC = *British Columbia COVID-19 Therapeutics Committee;* hrsACE2 = *Human Recombinant Soluble ACE2;* IL-6 = *Interleukin-6;* ECMO = *Extracorporeal Membrane Oxygenation.*

Institute of Health (NIH), or British Columbia COVID-19 Therapeutics Committee (BCCTC). We will also briefly review the evidence for supportive therapy for critical patients.

3. Pre-Exposure and Post-Exposure Prophylaxis

Asymptomatic individuals are the source of at least 50% of new COVID cases.[16] Moreover, people with symptoms do not seek medical care immediately, usually delaying their visit to a healthcare practitioner by a day or two. At this point, the number of viral copies has already started declining,[17] and most people would stop being infectious shortly after (Figure 2). From a public health perspective, virus-targeting approaches have the theoretical advantage of reducing transmission. However,

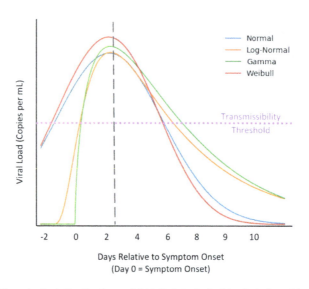

Figure 2:   Hypothetical distributions of SARS-CoV-2 viral load. A dotted horizontal line indicating the threshold of transmissibility (106 copies per mL). The intersection of the dotted line with the various curves would show when an individual becomes contagious. A vertical dashed line shows when an individual might seek medical consultation. Assuming patients do not seek medical care for 2.5 days, the light shaded region refers to the area where data is lacking, Image by Christina Savvides and Robert Siegel (2020)[19] under a CC-BY-ND 4.0 international license.

researchers have found it challenging to treat the early stages of infection.[18]

A systematic review looking at studies for prophylactic candidates against COVID-19 concluded a lack of evidence in clinical trials with results published up to December 13, 2020, all of them for hydroxy-chloroquine either as pre-exposure ($n = 1,615$) or post-exposure therapy ($n = 3,756$). However, there are still ongoing trials for antivirals, antibod-ies, antibiotics, vaccines for other microorganisms, several supplements, mouthwashes, and nasal sprays.[20–22] Among those, the most promising result comes from an interim analysis of 400 participants enrolled in a phase-III randomised clinical trial evaluating a mix of gamma immunoglobulins.[26]

3.1 *Polyclonal antibodies*

Initially approved by the United States Food and Drug Administration (US FDA) for intravenous use in outpatients with mild to moderate dis-ease who are at high risk for severe disease,[15,23–25] polyclonal antibodies (combination therapy of bamlanivimab-etesevimab and casirivimab-imdevimab) seem to be effective in preventing new infections when administered early on as a subcutaneous injection. These antibodies bind to epitopes of the spike protein of SARS-CoV-2. The interim analysis by Regeneron Pharmaceuticals on their antibody cocktail (casirivimab-imdevimab) showed that, on average, 20 patients would need to receive this therapy to prevent one new infection (RR: 0.52). However, the cock-tail prevented 100% of symptomatic infections (0/186), whereas 3.4% of patients in the placebo group (8/223) did develop symptoms and also had a higher peak viral load and more prolonged infections.[26] While these drugs are promising for tertiary prevention and reducing hospital work-load during peaks of the pandemic curve, they do not have an *ideal* pro-file as prophylactic agents or early treatment due to their formulation, storage requirements, and difficulty to scale up production in low-and-middle-income countries.[7] Some variants have evaded single (monoclo-nal) antibodies. Resistance to polyclonal (more than one) antibody cocktails might arise over time, although, as of April 2021, this is still a theoretical concern.[27]

4. Treatment of Non-Severe COVID-19 Patients

4.1 *Colchicine*

Colchicine is an old drug with analgesic and anti-inflammatory characteristics. An initial positive case series motivated a randomised clinical trial in 4,488 outpatients with death or hospitalisation as the primary outcomes.[28] Compared to those receiving placebo, patients with a confirmed PCR test who took 0.5 mg of colchicine daily (after taking a loading dose twice a day for three days) reduced their odds of both hospitalisation and death by 0.25 (95% CI: 0.01–0.57). Other trials in hospitalised patients also included moderate forms of the disease and were pooled in subsequent meta-analyses, showing positive results.[29] There is low certainty that colchicine also may reduce the risk of mechanical ventilation in outpatients with mild disease.[30]

4.2 *Proxalutamide*

Two clinical trials have studied the effects of this androgen receptor inhibitor. The theorised mechanism involves the downregulation of the transmembrane protease serine 2 (TMPRSS2), which modifies the SARS-CoV-2 spike protein to invade the type II pneumocytes. Proxalutamide (200 mg/day) accelerated viral clearance by real-time reverse transcription-PCR (cT > 40) from an average of 21.8 ± 13.0 days in the placebo arm to 4.2 ± 5.4 days. Clinical remission for all symptoms except the loss of taste or smell at seven days was also significantly different in the treatment arm (95.9%) compared to placebo (48.5%).[31] Another trial of mild ambulatory patients compared hospitalisation rates exclusively in men, finding significant differences between proxalutamide (0/114) and placebo (31/114). Other secondary outcomes were the need for mechanical ventilation (10/114) and death (2/114) versus 0 events of either in the treatment arm.[32]

4.3 *Convalescent plasma*

Most trials that used convalescent plasma have failed to find a positive effect on reducing mortality, hospitalisation, or clinical progression.

Even after pooling the results of the early trials, researchers were not able to find a benefit.[2] However, a retrospective analysis conducted on 3,082 patients who received a plasma transfusion found a dose-effect relationship between anti-SARS-CoV-2 antibody levels and the risk of death on those patients who were treated early (before mechanical ventilation). The use of high-titer antibodies reduced the risk of death by 34% (95% CI: 9–52%).[33] Following the publication of these results, a couple of studies experimented with high-titer plasma in the early stages of the disease. One trial in 160 senior adults with mild diseases showed a 48% reduction in the risk of progression to severe disease (95% CI: 6–71%).[34]

5. Viral-Based Treatment Options for the Pulmonary Phase

Therapeutics for the pulmonary phase mainly targeted the 3-chymotrypsin like protease (3CLpro), envelope, spike, ribonucleic acid (RNA) polymerase, and methyltransferase proteins.[35] So far, very few antivirals have significantly reduced mortality in well-designed trials[13] (Figure 3).

5.1 *Antiviral drugs*

Antiviral drugs can prevent the viral replication of SARS-CoV-2 through different mechanisms: inhibiting the virus from entering into human cells through angiotensin-converting enzyme 2 (ACE2) receptors, preventing the virus from fusion and endocytosis, or inhibiting the activity of its proteases or RNA polymerase.[37] These drugs are more effective during the viral response phase and should be used before the host inflammatory response phase.[38]

5.1.1 *Remdesivir*

Remdesivir is a nucleotide analog that binds to the RNA polymerase of the virus and terminates its RNA transcription prematurely, inhibiting the viral replication.[39,40] It was originally developed and tested for Ebola treatment.[14,39] Several clinical trials have investigated its effects among

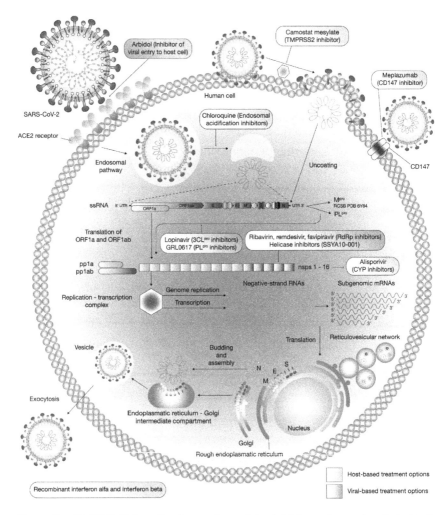

Figure 3: SARS-CoV-2 replication cycle and its inhibitors. Image by Ortiz-Prado and colleagues[36] under a CC-BY 4.0 international license. DOI: 10.20944/preprints 202004.0283.v1.

COVID patients.[41–45] Some of these studies demonstrated a beneficial effect on time to recovery, but they did not show an improvement in mortality, need for mechanical ventilation, or length of hospital stay.[14]

The Adaptive COVID-19 Treatment Trial (ACTT-1) is the most prominent study that suggests a benefit in administering remdesivir.[41]

It recruited 1,062 hospitalised COVID patients with lower respiratory tract infections from several countries. In their final report, the authors stated that remdesivir significantly reduced the median recovery time by five days. Their data also showed positive effects of remdesivir in lowering mortality by day 29, which did not reach statistical significance. Another supporting study is a randomised controlled trial by Spinner *et al.* on COVID patients with moderate severity that showed beneficial effects of remdesivir, compared to standard care, on clinical status after 11 days.[42]

On the other hand, the WHO Solidarity open-label trial ($n = 2,743$ and $n = 2,708$ in the remdesivir and control groups, respectively) is the leading study that found little or no effect from remdesivir on inpatients in terms of mortality, the need for ventilation, or length of hospital stay.[43] Additionally, in a controlled trial in China on 237 patients, the recovery time among remdesivir-treated patients, though faster than placebo, was not significantly better.[44] The same trial also reported higher percentages of early termination among patients receiving remdesivir, compared to placebo, due to adverse events.

Based on these trials and more, the US FDA came to the conclusion to approve remdesivir for the treatment of COVID-19.[46] Conversely, the WHO recommends against using remdesivir based on the same studies.[47] Moreover, studies suggest a 5-day course of remdesivir may be clinically preferable to a 10-day course,[42,45] a serendipitous discovery as remdesivir is an expensive drug with currently limited availability.

5.2 *Human recombinant soluble ACE-2*

To enter human cells, the SARS-CoV-2 binds with a membrane protein called ACE2. It is primarily found in the lung but is also present in the vascular system, heart, kidney, and intestine.[48] It has been shown *in vitro* that human recombinant soluble ACE2 (hrsACE2) can significantly block SARS-CoV-2 infections,[49] possibly by forcing the virus to bind to it instead of the host cell (Figure 4). Additionally, a case report on a COVID patient treated with hrsACE2 demonstrated successful treatment and rapid disappearance of the virus from the patient's serum.[50]

Phase I (NCT00886353) and phase II (NCT01597635) clinical trials have already been done on the hrsACE2 for acute respiratory distress

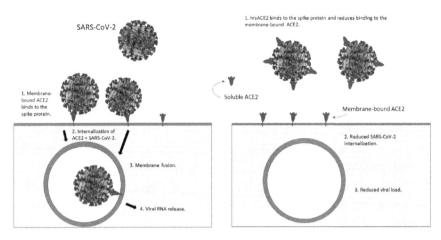

Figure 4:   Possible hrsACE2's mechanism of action in blocking SARS-CoV-2 infection. Graphic adapted from Vanessa Monteil and colleagues. DOI: 10.1016/j.cell.2020.04.004.

syndrome (ARDS), investigating its other probable effects on reducing inflammation, vasoconstriction, and vascular leak. Following them, a recent phase II trial (NCT04335136) assessing hrsACE2 as a treatment for patients with COVID-19 is yet to release its findings.

Another study on human organoids also suggested an additive effect of hrsACE2 on remdesivir in the treatment of COVID patients.[51] Further evidence is required to clarify the possible position of hrsACE2 in COVID treatment.

6. Host-Based Treatment Options for Pulmonary and Inflammatory Phases

Host-targeting approaches treat patients that, for the most, have low viral loads and are relatively well isolated.[19] From a public health perspective, these treatments are necessary because they reduce the risk of death and disease severity. By improving infected patients' clinical outcomes, healthcare systems can better support patients both related and unrelated to infectious outbreaks. These treatments aim to (a) interfere in the pathway from infection to disease and (b) modulate the hyperimmune response seen in COVID-19 patients.[35]

6.1 *Dexamethasone and other corticosteroids*

The anti-inflammatory effects of corticosteroids can be utilised to manage severely ill hospitalised COVID-19 patients prone to inflammation-mediated diffuse lung damage. Based on the current guidelines from WHO and NIH, corticosteroids are recommended for those patients who require supplemental oxygen (or more organ support).[15,47] NIH also recommends them as helpful in COVID patients with fluid-resistant septic shock,[15] although it rarely happens.

Among corticosteroids, the current evidence for the benefits of dexamethasone is the strongest. The most important study on using dexamethasone for COVID patients is the RECOVERY controlled trial in the United Kingdom. It recruited clinically-suspected or laboratory-confirmed patients to study the 28-day mortality as the primary outcome.[52] Of the recruited patients, 2,104 received dexamethasone (6 mg daily for up to 10 days) plus usual care and 4,321 received only usual care. Dexamethasone was able to significantly reduce mortality in patients in need of supplemental oxygen or mechanical ventilation. However, the result of dexamethasone use in patients who did not receive oxygen was towards a detrimental effect, though it did not reach statistical significance. A smaller controlled trial ($n = 299$) conducted in Brazil (the CoDEX trial) concluded that using dexamethasone at a higher dose (20 mg daily for five days, then 10 mg daily for another five days) can significantly increase the number of ventilator-free days for COVID patients.[53] However, it reported no benefit to all-cause 28-day mortality.

Current evidence for the use of other corticosteroids is limited. Studies evaluating hydrocortisone for COVID patients, including the REMAP-CAP[54] and the CAPE COVID[55] trials, though showing trends toward favourable effects in critically ill patients, did not reach statistical significance owing to early termination. Another study in Brazil, the Metcovid trial, on adjunct therapy with methylprednisolone for hospitalised COVID patients concluded that the mortality at 28 days was not lower for patients receiving methylprednisolone in the overall population but was lower for patients over 60 years old.[56]

Finally, a WHO working group conducted a meta-analysis on seven trials from 12 countries with a total of 1,703 severely ill COVID patients.[57]

In addition to data from four of the trials mentioned above, namely the RECOVERY, CoDEX, REMAP-CAP, and CAPE COVID trials, this meta-analysis also included the findings of three other trials that stopped early and did not publish their results. Six of these trials were assessed as having a low risk of bias. The authors concluded that the 28-day all-cause mortality is lower in critical patients that receive systemic corticosteroids. However, in subgroup analysis, the results were significant only for dexamethasone and not for hydrocortisone and methylprednisolone[57] Notwithstanding, other glucocorticoids, such as prednisone, methylprednisolone, or hydrocortisone, are recommended by different agencies when dexamethasone is not available.[14,15,58]

6.2 *Interleukin-6 pathway inhibitors*

As previously mentioned, controlling inflammation during dysregulated immune response in severe COVID-19 patients can be beneficial.[59] Examples of drug categories that can potentially inhibit immune dysregulation are interleukin (IL) 6 pathway inhibitors, IL-1 pathway inhibitors, and kinase inhibitors. The US FDA had previously approved two groups of IL-6 pathway inhibitors primarily for rheumatologic indications: anti-IL-6 receptor monoclonal antibodies, such as tocilizumab and sarilumab, and anti-IL-6 monoclonal antibodies, such as siltuximab. The current evidence for their usage in COVID treatment is most available for tocilizumab and sarilumab, respectively.

The two large, main trials on tocilizumab (and sarilumab with a smaller sample size) among severe COVID patients are the REMAP-CAP[60] and the RECOVERY[61] trials both of which reported improved survival with these drugs. However, tocilizumab failed to reduce mortality in smaller trials of COVACTA,[62] EMPACTA,[63] and BACC Bay,[64] although the EMPACTA trial showed a significant improvement in a composite measure of mechanical ventilation and death in patients receiving tocilizumab, compared to placebo. Finally, a recent Cochrane living review on COVID patients stated high confidence in the effect of tocilizumab on lowering the number of deaths but low confidence in sarilumab's results.[65]

Overall, according to the current recommendations from the NIH and United Kingdoms' National Health Service (NHS), tocilizumab can be used in combination with dexamethasone in hospitalised patients with severe respiratory decompensation outside clinical trials.[15,66]

6.3 *Janus kinase inhibitors*

Baricitinib is a Janus kinase (JAK) inhibitor that can suppress the immune response, similar to corticosteroids, and reduce the lung damage from inflammation.[67] It is also posited that baricitinib has antiviral activity by preventing the virus from entering human cells and infecting them.[68] Based on these characteristics and using artificial intelligence, baricitinib was suggested to be beneficial against COVID-19.[69] Subsequently, in a randomised controlled trial (ACTT-2) on 1,033 patients, its combination therapy with remdesivir improved patients' recovery time and clinical status, compared to remdesivir and placebo.[70] Although the improvement in median recovery time was statistically significant in this study, the difference was only one day (7 days for remdesivir+baricitinib, compared to 8 days for remdesivir+placebo). However, this difference increased to 8 days for those receiving non-invasive ventilation or high-flow oxygen.

An emergency use authorization (EUA) has been issued by US FDA for baricitinib to be used along with remdesivir in patients that require supplemental oxygen.[71] Owing to a lack of sufficient evidence, the current guidelines from the NIH only recommend the usage of baricitinib in combination with remdesivir in patients that cannot receive corticosteroids.[15]

6.4 *Other drugs under evaluation*

6.4.1 *Interleukin-1 pathway inhibitors*

Interleukin-1 (IL-1) pathway inhibitors can also potentially prevent the immune dysregulation caused by COVID-19. However, current evidence is not enough to warrant their usage. In a randomised controlled trial in France on mild to moderate COVID-19 pneumonia, anakinra, an IL-1 receptor antagonist, was not associated with an improvement in mortality or the need for mechanical ventilation.[72]

6.4.2 *Interferons*

Interferons have known immunomodulatory effects and have also been reported to inhibit SARS-CoV-2 replication *in vitro*.[73] Although a small trial ($n = 81$) earlier in the pandemic suggested interferons may reduce 28-mortality and increase discharge rate on day 14 among COVID patients,[74] more extensive studies later did not support those conclusions. As part of the WHO Solidarity trial, subcutaneous or intravenous interferon beta was compared with standard of care ($n = 2,050$ patients in each arm), and no significant change in 28-mortality happened.[43] As a result, the evidence for the clinical use of interferons is not conclusive yet.

7. Other Therapies

7.1 *Antibacterial therapy*

A living rapid review on 24 studies ($n = 3,338$ COVID patients) reported the prevalence of bacterial co-infection as 3.5% and secondary bacterial infection as 14.3%.[75] Antibiotics are recommended in patients with community-acquired or hospital-acquired pneumonia or sepsis only when infection with a bacterial agent is suspected.[15]

7.2 *Antithrombotic therapy*

COVID-19 can cause a hypercoagulable state.[76] The prevalence of venous thromboembolism (VTE) in patients admitted to intensive care units (ICU) has been reported up to 43% despite some of those patients receiving prophylactic-dose anticoagulation.[77] One small retrospective study that conducted complete duplex ultrasound as a standard of care on all inpatients even found an incidence of 69%.[78] Hospitalised non-ICU patients have a lower risk of VTE, but they are still hypercoagulable.

As of now, there is no concrete evidence on whether an approach apart from the pre-COVID era guidance on thromboprophylaxis for hospitalised patients is more appropriate.[79] The pre-print results of a multiplatform randomised clinical trial that combined the findings of three international adaptive platform trials, including REMAP-CAP (NCT02735707),

ACTIV-4 (NCT04505774 and NCT04359277), and ATTACC (NCT04372589), failed to show any benefit to hospital survival or organ support-free days among severe COVID patients receiving therapeutic-dose anticoagulation, compared to prophylactic doses.[80] Furthermore, there is no specific evidence on the preferred type of anticoagulation therapy to be used in these patients. Overall, the current recommendation by the WHO, NIH, BCCTC, and the American Society of Hematology states that hospitalised COVID-19 patients should receive prophylactic-dose anticoagulation.[9,14,15,81]

7.3 *Supportive care*

Conventional supportive measures are used to maintain hemodynamics and oxygenation in COVID patients. In particular, two recently-debated topics are presented below.

7.3.1 *Prone ventilation*

Prone positioning during ventilation was previously shown to improve oxygenation and mortality in a clinical trial on patients with ARDS.[82] Observational studies on COVID patients, with relatively small sample sizes, have reiterated that pronation is feasible to be maintained for several hours and can be beneficial on patients' respiratory rate and peripheral oxygen saturation.[83,84] However, it is yet to be confirmed if this maneuver can affect time to recovery, need for ventilation, or mortality among COVID patients. The WHO and NIH currently recommend prone ventilation for persistently hypoxemic awake COVID patients who increasingly need supplemental oxygen but do not have indication for endotracheal intubation.[9,15]

7.3.2 *ECMO*

When optimised mechanical ventilation and pronation fail to improve hypoxemia in critically ill patients, extracorporeal membrane oxygenation (ECMO) may be of benefit. Observational studies have suggested ECMO may be able to reduce mortality among these patients.[85] The WHO recommends ECMO for COVID patients with ARDS when there is access to expertise.[9] As implementing and using ECMO is resource-intensive, its implication in a pandemic is limited to highly selected patients in previously established facilities, and investing resources in other prevention and treatment areas is probably more cost-effective.[86]

References

1. World Health Organization. Novel Coronavirus (2019-nCoV): Situation report [Internet]. Geneva: World Health Organization; 2020. Available from: https://apps.who.int/iris/handle/10665/330760.
2. Boutron I, Chaimani A, Meerpohl JJ, Hróbjartsson A, Devane D, Rada G, *et al*. The COVID-NMA project: Building an evidence ecosystem for the COVID-19 pandemic. *Annals of Internal Medicine*. 2020;173:1015–1017.
3. DiMasi JA, Grabowski HG, Hansen RW. Innovation in the pharmaceutical industry: New estimates of R&D costs. *Journal of Health Economics*. 2016;47:20–33. Available from: https://www.sciencedirect.com/science/article/pii/S0167629616000291.
4. Pushpakom S, Iorio F, Eyers PA, Escott KJ, Hopper S, Wells A, *et al*. Drug repurposing: Progress, challenges and recommendations. *Nature Reviews Drug Discovery*. 2019;18(1):41–58. Available from: https://doi.org/10.1038/nrd.2018.168.
5. Martin JH, Bowden NA. Drug repurposing in the era of COVID-19: A call for leadership and government investment. *Medical Journal of Australia*. 2020;212(10):450–452.e1. Available from: https://doi.org/10.5694/mja2.50603.
6. Renoux C, Azoulay L, Suissa S. Biases in evaluating the safety and effectiveness of drugs for covid-19: Designing real-world evidence studies. *American Journal of Epidemiology*. 2021; Available from: https://doi.org/10.1093/aje/kwab028.
7. World Health Organization. COVID-19 Therapeutics Target Product Profile for Hospitalized Patients [Internet]. 2020. Available from: https://www.who.int/docs/default-source/coronaviruse/rd-blueprint-therapeutics-tpp-v20oct2020-final-(009).pdf?sfvrsn=d981c3cf_3&download=true [Accessed 5 April 2021].
8. WHO Working Group on Protocols for Therapeutics in COVID-19 PrEP and PEP. Informal consultation on the role of therapeutics in COVID-19 prophylaxis and post-exposure prophylaxis [Internet]. 2020. Available from: https://

www.who.int/docs/default-source/blue-print/covid-19-therapeutics-in-prep-pep-working-group-meeting-notes-2020-05-01.pdf?sfvrsn=fab1bbbf_1&download=true [Accessed 5 April 2021].

9. World Health Organization. COVID-19 Clinical management: Living guidance [Internet]. 2021. Available from: https://apps.who.int/iris/rest/bitstreams/1328457/retrieve [Accessed 5 April 2021].

10. van Kampen JJA, van de Vijver DAMC, Fraaij PLA, Haagmans BL, Lamers MM, Okba N, *et al.* Duration and key determinants of infectious virus shedding in hospitalized patients with coronavirus disease-2019 (COVID-19). *Nature Communication.* 2021;12(1):8–13.

11. Mills EJ, Thorlund K, Ioannidis JPA. Demystifying trial networks and network meta-analysis. *British Medical Journal.* 2013;346:f2914. Available from: http://www.bmj.com/content/346/bmj.f2914.abstract.

12. Salanti G, Del Giovane C, Chaimani A, Caldwell DM, Higgins JPT. Evaluating the quality of evidence from a network meta-analysis. *PLoS One.* 2014;9(7):e99682.

13. Siemieniuk RAC, Bartoszko JJ, Ge L, Zeraatkar D, Izcovich A, Kum E, *et al.* Drug treatments for COVID-19: Living systematic review and network meta-analysis. *BMJ.* 2020;370:m2980. Available from: http://www.bmj.com/content/370/bmj.m2980.abstract.

14. British Columbia COVID-19 Therapeutics Committee (CTC). Therapies for COVID-19 — BC Centre for Disease Control [Internet]. 2021. Available from: http://www.bccdc.ca/Health-Professionals-Site/Documents/Therapies_for_COVID-19.pdf [Accessed 7 April 2021].

15. National Institutes of Health. Coronavirus Disease 2019 (COVID-19) Treatment Guidelines [Internet]. Available from: https://covid19treatmentguidelines.nih.gov/ [Accessed 14 March 2021].

16. Johansson MA, Quandelacy TM, Kada S, Prasad PV, Steele M, Brooks JT, *et al.* SARS-CoV-2 transmission from people without COVID-19 symptoms. *JAMA Network Open.* 2021;4(1):e2035057–e2035057. Available from: https://doi.org/10.1001/jamanetworkopen.2020.35057.

17. He X, Lau EHY, Wu P, Deng X, Wang J, Hao X, *et al.* Temporal dynamics in viral shedding and transmissibility of COVID-19. *Nature Medicine.* 2020;26(5): 672–675. Available from: https://doi.org/10.1038/s41591-020-0869-5.

18. Kim PS, Read SW, Fauci AS. Therapy for Early COVID-19: A Critical Need. *JAMA.* 2020;324(21):2149–50. Available from: https://doi.org/10.1001/jama.2020.22813.

19. Savvides C, Siegel R. Asymptomatic and presymptomatic transmission of SARS-CoV-2: A systematic review. *medRxiv.* 2020;2020.06.11.20129072.

Available from: http://medrxiv.org/content/early/2020/06/17/2020.06.11.201 29072.abstract.

20. Burton MJ, Clarkson JE, Goulao B, Glenny A-M, McBain AJ, Schilder AGM, *et al*. Antimicrobial mouthwashes (gargling) and nasal sprays to protect healthcare workers when undertaking aerosol-generating procedures (AGPs) on patients without suspected or confirmed COVID-19 infection. *Cochrane Database of Systematic Reviews*. 2020;(9). Available from: https://doi.org//10.1002/14651858.CD013628.pub2.

21. Burton MJ, Clarkson JE, Goulao B, Glenny A-M, McBain AJ, Schilder AGM, *et al*. Antimicrobial mouthwashes (gargling) and nasal sprays administered to patients with suspected or confirmed COVID-19 infection to improve patient outcomes and to protect healthcare workers treating them. *Cochrane Database of Systematic Reviews*. 2020;(9). Available from: https://doi.org//10.1002/14651858.CD013627.pub2.

22. Smit M, Marinosci A, Agoritsas T, Calmy A. Prophylaxis for COVID-19: A systematic review. *Clinical Microbiology Infection*. 2021. Available from: https://doi.org/10.1016/j.cmi.2021.01.013.

23. U.S. Food and Drug Administration. Emergency Use Authorization (EUA) of Bamlanivimab [Internet]. Available from: https://www.fda.gov/media/143603/download [Accessed 14 March 2021].

24. U.S. Food and Drug Administration. Emergency Use Authorization (EUA) of Bamlanivimab and Etesevimab [Internet]. Available from: https://www.fda.gov/media/145802/download [Accessed 14 March 2021].

25. U.S. Food and Drug Administration. Emergency Use Authorization (EUA) of Casirivimab and Imdevimab [Internet]. Available from: https://www.fda.gov/media/143892/download [Accessed 14 March 2021].

26. Regeneron Pharmaceuticals Inc. Regeneron Reports Positive Interim Data with REGEN-COV™ Antibody Cocktail used as Passive Vaccine to Prevent COVID-19 [Internet]. 2021. Available from: https://investor.regeneron.com/news-releases/news-release-details/regeneron-reports-positive-interim-data-regen-covtm-antibody [Accessed 7 April 2021].

27. United States' Food and Drug Administration. FDA authorizes revisions to fact sheets to address SARS-CoV-2 variants for monoclonal antibody products under emergency use authorization [Internet]. 2021. Available from: https://www.fda.gov/drugs/drug-safety-and-availability/fda-authorizes-revisions-fact-sheets-address-sars-cov-2-variants-monoclonal-antibody-products-under [Accessed 7 April 2021].

28. Tardif J-C, Bouabdallaoui N, L'allier PL, Gaudet D, Shah B, Pillinger MH, *et al*. Efficacy of colchicine in non-hospitalized patients with COVID-19. *medRxiv*. 2021;2021.01.26.21250494.

29. Lopes MI, Bonjorno LP, Giannini MC, Amaral NB, Menezes PI, Dib SM, *et al*. Beneficial effects of colchicine for moderate to severe COVID-19: A randomised, double-blinded, placebo-controlled clinical trial. *RMD Open*. 2021;7(1).

30. Siemieniuk RAC, Bartoszko JJ, Ge L, Zeraatkar D, Izcovich A, Pardo-Hernandez H, *et al*. Drug treatments for covid-19: Living systematic review and network meta-Analysis. *The BMJ*. 2020;370.

31. Cadegiani FA, McCoy J, Gustavo Wambier C, Vaño-Galván S, Shapiro J, Tosti A, *et al*. Proxalutamide significantly accelerates viral clearance and reduces time to clinical remission in patients with mild to moderate COVID-19: Results from a randomized, double-blinded, placebo-controlled trial. *Cureus*. 2021;13(2).

32. Adsuara Cadegiani F, McCoy J, Gustavo Wambier C, Kovacevic M, Shapiro J, Sinclair R, *et al*. Proxalutamide (GT0918) reduces the rate of hospitalization and death in COVID-19 male patients: A randomized double-blinded placebo-controlled trial.

33. Joyner MJ, Carter RE, Senefeld JW, Klassen SA, Mills JR, Johnson PW, *et al*. Convalescent plasma antibody levels and the risk of death from COVID-19. *New England Journal of Medicine*. 2021;384(11):1015–1027.

34. Libster R, Pérez Marc G, Wappner D, Coviello S, Bianchi A, Braem V, *et al*. Early high-titer plasma therapy to prevent severe COVID-19 in older adults. *New England Journal of Medicine*. 2021;384(7):610–618.

35. Galindez G, Matschinske J, Rose TD, Sadegh S, Salgado-Albarrán M, Späth J, *et al*. Lessons from the COVID-19 pandemic for advancing computational drug repurposing strategies. *Nature Computational Science*. 2021;1(1):33–41. Available from: https://doi.org/10.1038/s43588-020-00007-6.

36. Ortiz-Prado E, Simbaña-Rivera K. Prevalence of retinopathy of prematurity: An institutional cross-sectional study of preterm infants in Ecuador View project Primary Care Capacity Building for Rural, Remote and Underserved Communities in Ecuador View project. *[Preprint]*. 2020.

37. Sanders JM, Monogue ML, Jodlowski TZ, Cutrell JB. Pharmacologic treatments for coronavirus disease 2019 (COVID-19): A review. *JAMA*. 2020;323(18):1824–1836.

38. Siddiqi HK, Mehra MR. COVID-19 illness in native and immunosuppressed states: A clinical-therapeutic staging proposal. *The Journal of Heart and Lung Transplantation*. 2020;39:405–407.

39. Warren TK, Jordan R, Lo MK, Ray AS, Mackman RL, Soloveva V, *et al*. Therapeutic efficacy of the small molecule GS-5734 against Ebola virus in rhesus monkeys. *Nature*. 2016;531(7594):381–385. Available from: https://doi.org/10.1038/nature17180.

40. Wang M, Cao R, Zhang L, Yang X, Liu J, Xu M, *et al*. Remdesivir and chloroquine effectively inhibit the recently emerged novel coronavirus (2019-nCoV) *in vitro*. *Cell Research*. 2020;30:269–271.

41. Beigel JH, Tomashek KM, Dodd LE, Mehta AK, Zingman BS, Kalil AC, *et al*. Remdesivir for the treatment of Covid-19 — final report. *N Engl J Med*. 2020;383(19):1813–1826.

42. Spinner CD, Gottlieb RL, Criner GJ, Arribas López JR, Cattelan AM, Soriano Viladomiu A, *et al*. Effect of Remdesivir vs standard care on clinical status at 11 days in patients with moderate COVID-19: A randomized clinical trial. *JAMA*. 2020;324(11):1048–1057.

43. Pan H, Peto R, Henao-Restrepo A-M, Preziosi M-P, Sathiyamoorthy V, Abdool Karim Q, *et al*. Repurposed antiviral drugs for Covid-19 — interim WHO solidarity trial results. *New England Journal of Medicine*. 2021; 384(6):497–511.

44. Wang Y, Zhang D, Du G, Du R, Zhao J, Jin Y, *et al*. Remdesivir in adults with severe COVID-19: A randomised, double-blind, placebo-controlled, multi-centre trial. *Lancet (London, England)*. 2020;395(10236):1569–1578.

45. Goldman JD, Lye DCB, Hui DS, Marks KM, Bruno R, Montejano R, *et al*. Remdesivir for 5 or 10 days in patients with severe Covid-19. *N Engl J Med*. 2020;383(19):1827–1837.

46. United States' Food and Drug Administration. VEKLURY® (remdesivir) [Internet]. 2020. Available from: https://www.accessdata.fda.gov/drugsatfda_docs/label/2020/214787Orig1s000lbl.pdf [Accessed 14 March 2021].

47. Siemieniuk R, Rochwerg B, Agoritsas T, Lamontagne F, Leo Y-S, Macdonald H, *et al*. A living WHO guideline on drugs for covid-19. *BMJ*. 2020;370:m3379.

48. Rodell CB. An ACE therapy for COVID-19. *Science Translational Medicine*. 2020;12(541):eabb5676. Available from: http://stm.sciencemag.org/content/12/541/eabb5676.abstract.

49. Monteil V, Kwon H, Prado P, Hagelkrüys A, Wimmer RA, Stahl M, *et al*. Inhibition of SARS-CoV-2 infections in engineered human tissues using clinical-grade soluble human ACE2. *Cell*. 2020;181(4):905–913.e7. Available from: https://doi.org/10.1016/j.cell.2020.04.004.

50. Zoufaly A, Poglitsch M, Aberle JH, Hoepler W, Seitz T, Traugott M, *et al*. Human recombinant soluble ACE2 in severe COVID-19. *Lancet Respiratory Medicine*. 2020;8(11):1154–1158. Available from: https://doi.org/10.1016/S2213-2600(20)30418-5.

51. Monteil V, Dyczynski M, Lauschke VM, Kwon H, Wirnsberger G, Youhanna S, *et al*. Human soluble ACE2 improves the effect of remdesivir in

SARS-CoV-2 infection. *EMBO Molecular Medicine*. 2021;13(1):e13426. Available from: https://doi.org/10.15252/emmm.202013426.

52. The RECOVERY Collaborative Group. Dexamethasone in hospitalized patients with Covid-19. *New England Journal of Medicine*. 2020;384(8):693–704. Available from: https://doi.org/10.1056/NEJMoa2021436.

53. Tomazini BM, Maia IS, Cavalcanti AB, Berwanger O, Rosa RG, Veiga VC, *et al*. Effect of dexamethasone on days alive and ventilator-free in patients with moderate or severe acute respiratory distress syndrome and COVID-19: The CoDEX randomized clinical trial. *JAMA*. 2020;324(13):1307–1316. Available from: https://doi.org/10.1001/jama.2020.17021.

54. Angus DC, Derde L, Al-Beidh F, Annane D, Arabi Y, Beane A, *et al*. Effect of hydrocortisone on mortality and organ support in patients with severe COVID-19: The REMAP-CAP COVID-19 corticosteroid domain randomized clinical trial. *JAMA*. 2020;324(13):1317–1329.

55. Dequin P-F, Heming N, Meziani F, Plantefève G, Voiriot G, Badié J, *et al*. Effect of hydrocortisone on 21-day mortality or respiratory support among critically ill patients with COVID-19: A randomized clinical trial. *JAMA*. 2020;324(13):1298–1306.

56. Jeronimo CMP, Farias MEL, Val FFA, Sampaio VS, Alexandre MAA, Melo GC, *et al*. Methylprednisolone as adjunctive therapy for patients hospitalized with COVID-19 (Metcovid): A randomised, double-blind, phase IIb, placebo-controlled trial. *Clinical Infectious Diseases*. 2020.

57. WHO Rapid Evidence Appraisal for COVID-19 Therapies (REACT) Working Group. Association between administration of systemic corticosteroids and mortality among critically ill patients with COVID-19: A meta-analysis. *JAMA*. 2020;324(13):1330–1341. Available from: https://doi.org/10.1001/jama.2020.17023.

58. World Health Organization. Corticosteroids for COVID-19: Living guidance, 2 September 2020 [Internet]. Geneva; 2020. Available from: https://apps.who.int/iris/handle/10665/334125.

59. Mehta P, McAuley DF, Brown M, Sanchez E, Tattersall RS, Manson JJ. COVID-19: Consider cytokine storm syndromes and immunosuppression. *Lancet (London, England)*. 2020;395:1033–1034.

60. Gordon AC, Mouncey PR, Al-Beidh F, Rowan KM, Nichol AD, Arabi YM, *et al*. Interleukin-6 receptor antagonists in critically ill patients with Covid-19. *New England Journal of Medicine*. 2021.

61. Horby PW, Pessoa-Amorim G, Peto L, Brightling CE, Sarkar R, Thomas K, *et al*. Tocilizumab in patients admitted to hospital with COVID-19

(RECOVERY): Preliminary results of a randomised, controlled, open-label, platform trial. *medRxiv*. 2021;2021.02.11.21249258. Available from: http://medrxiv.org/content/early/2021/02/11/2021.02.11.21249258.abstract.

62. Rosas IO, Bräu N, Waters M, Go RC, Hunter BD, Bhagani S, *et al*. Tocilizumab in hospitalized patients with severe COVID-19 pneumonia. *New England Journal of Medicine*. 2021. Available from: https://doi.org/10.1056/NEJMoa2028700.

63. Salama C, Han J, Yau L, Reiss WG, Kramer B, Neidhart JD, *et al*. Tocilizumab in patients hospitalized with COVID-19 pneumonia. *New England Journal of Medicine*. 2021;384(1):20–30.

64. Stone JH, Frigault MJ, Serling-Boyd NJ, Fernandes AD, Harvey L, Foulkes AS, *et al*. Efficacy of tocilizumab in patients hospitalized with COVID-19. *New England Journal of Medicine*. 2020;383(24):2333–2344.

65. Ghosn L, Chaimani A, Evrenoglou T, Davidson M, Graña C, Schmucker C, *et al*. Interleukin-6 blocking agents for treating COVID-19: A living systematic review. *Cochrane Database Systematic Review*. 2021;(3). Available from: https://doi.org//10.1002/14651858.CD013881.

66. United Kingdoms' National Health Service (NHS). Interim Clinical Commissioning Policy: Tocilizumab for hospitalised patients with COVID-19 pneumonia (adults) [Internet]. Available from: https://www.cas.mhra.gov.uk/ViewandAcknowledgment/ViewAttachment.aspx?Attachment_id=103773 [Accessed 14 March 2021].

67. Zhang W, Zhao Y, Zhang F, Wang Q, Li T, Liu Z, *et al*. The use of anti-inflammatory drugs in the treatment of people with severe coronavirus disease 2019 (COVID-19): The Perspectives of clinical immunologists from China. *Clinical Immunology*. 2020;214:108393.

68. Stebbing J, Phelan A, Griffin I, Tucker C, Oechsle O, Smith D, *et al*. COVID-19: Combining antiviral and anti-inflammatory treatments. *Lancet Infectious Diseases*. 2020;20(4):400–402.

69. Stebbing J, Krishnan V, de Bono S, Ottaviani S, Casalini G, Richardson PJ, *et al*. Mechanism of baricitinib supports artificial intelligence-predicted testing in COVID-19 patients. *EMBO Molecular Medicine*. 2020;12(8):e12697.

70. Kalil AC, Patterson TF, Mehta AK, Tomashek KM, Wolfe CR, Ghazaryan V, *et al*. Baricitinib plus Remdesivir for hospitalized adults with Covid-19. *New England Journal of Medicine*. 2021;384(9):795–807.

71. United States' Food and Drug Administration. Emergency Use Authorization (EUA) Of Baricitinib [Internet]. Available from: https://www.fda.gov/media/143823/download [Accessed 14 March 2021].

72. The CORIMUNO-19 Collaborative group. Effect of anakinra versus usual care in adults in hospital with COVID-19 and mild-to-moderate pneumonia (CORIMUNO-ANA-1): A randomised controlled trial. *Lancet Respiratory Medicine.* 2021;9(3):295–304.

73. Clementi N, Ferrarese R, Criscuolo E, Diotti RA, Castelli M, Scagnolari C, *et al.* Interferon-β-1a inhibition of severe acute respiratory syndrome-Coronavirus 2 *in vitro* when administered after virus infection. *Journal of Infectious Diseases.* 2020;222(5):722–725.

74. Davoudi-Monfared E, Rahmani H, Khalili H, Hajiabdolbaghi M, Salehi M, Abbasian L, *et al.* A randomized clinical trial of the efficacy and safety of interferon β-1a in treatment of severe COVID-19. *Antimicrobial Agents and Chemotherapy.* 2020;64(9):e01061-20. Available from: http://aac.asm.org/content/64/9/e01061-20.abstract.

75. Langford BJ, So M, Raybardhan S, Leung V, Westwood D, MacFadden DR, *et al.* Bacterial co-infection and secondary infection in patients with COVID-19: A living rapid review and meta-analysis. *Clinical Microbiology and Infection.* 2020;26(12):1622–1629. Available from: https://www.science direct.com/science/article/pii/S1198743X20304237.

76. Connors JM, Levy JH. COVID-19 and its implications for thrombosis and anticoagulation. *Blood.* 2020;135(23):2033–2040. Available from: https://doi.org/10.1182/blood.2020006000.

77. Helms J, Tacquard C, Severac F, Leonard-Lorant I, Ohana M, Delabranche X, *et al.* High risk of thrombosis in patients with severe SARS-CoV-2 infection: A multicenter prospective cohort study. *Intensive Care Medicine.* 2020;46(6):1089–1098. Available from: https://doi.org/10.1007/s00134-020-06062-x.

78. Llitjos J-F, Leclerc M, Chochois C, Monsallier J-M, Ramakers M, Auvray M, *et al.* High incidence of venous thromboembolic events in anticoagulated severe COVID-19 patients. *Journal of Thrombosis Haemostasis.* 2020;18(7): 1743–1746.

79. Maldonado E, Tao D, Mackey K. Antithrombotic therapies in COVID-19 disease: A systematic review. *Journal of General Internal Medicine.* 2020;35(9):2698–2706. Available from: https://doi.org/10.1007/s11606-020-05906-y.

80. The REMAP-CAP and ACTIV-4a and ATTACC Investigators. Therapeutic anticoagulation in critically ill patients with COVID-19 — preliminary report [Internet]. *medRxiv.* 2021 Mar. Available from: http://medrxiv.org/content/early/2021/03/12/2021.03.10.21252749.abstract.

81. Cuker A, Tseng EK, Nieuwlaat R, Angchaisuksiri P, Blair C, Dane K, *et al.* American Society of Hematology 2021 guidelines on the use of anticoagulation for thromboprophylaxis in patients with COVID-19. *Blood Advances.* 2021;5(3):872–888.

82. Guérin C, Reignier J, Richard J-C, Beuret P, Gacouin A, Boulain T, *et al.* Prone positioning in severe acute respiratory distress syndrome. *New England Journal of Medicine.* 2013;368(23):2159–2168. Available from: https://doi.org/10.1056/NEJMoa1214103.

83. Sartini C, Tresoldi M, Scarpellini P, Tettamanti A, Carcò F, Landoni G, *et al.* Respiratory parameters in patients with COVID-19 after using noninvasive ventilation in the prone position outside the intensive care unit. *JAMA.* 2020;323(22):2338–2340. Available from: https://doi.org/10.1001/jama.2020.7861.

84. Coppo A, Bellani G, Winterton D, Di Pierro M, Soria A, Faverio P, *et al.* Feasibility and physiological effects of prone positioning in non-intubated patients with acute respiratory failure due to COVID-19 (PRON-COVID): A prospective cohort study. *Lancet Respiratory Medicine.* 2020;8(8): 765–774. Available from: https://doi.org/10.1016/S2213-2600(20)30268-X.

85. Shaefi S, Brenner SK, Gupta S, O'Gara BP, Krajewski ML, Charytan DM, *et al.* Extracorporeal membrane oxygenation in patients with severe respiratory failure from COVID-19. *Intensive Care Medicine.* 2021;47(2):208–221. Available from: https://doi.org/10.1007/s00134-020-06331-9.

86. MacLaren G, Fisher D, Brodie D. Preparing for the most critically ill patients with COVID-19: The potential role of extracorporeal membrane oxygenation. *JAMA.* 2020;323(13):1245–1246. Available from: https://doi.org/10.1001/jama.2020.2342.

Part 7

Vaccines

Chapter 13

Overview of Vaccine Designs and Performance

Emma Ackermann[*] and **Manish Sadarangani**[†,‡]

[*]*School of Population and Public Health, University of British Columbia, Vancouver, Canada*

[†]*Department of Pediatrics, University of British Columbia, Vancouver, Canada*

[‡]*Vaccine Evaluation Center, BC Children's Hospital Research Institute, Vancouver, Canada*

Key Message

- Whole inactivated vaccines are made from manufactured whole virus that is then inactivated. The whole inactivated virus induces an immune response in the vaccine recipient.
- Protein subunit vaccines are made from manufactured pieces of the virus. The pieces of virus induce an immune response in the vaccine recipient.
- Non-replicating viral vector vaccines use a viral vector to transport DNA instructions for making a piece of virus into the nucleus of the vaccine recipient's cells. The vaccine recipient's cells then read the DNA and manufacture pieces of virus. Those pieces of virus induce an immune response.

251

- RNA vaccines use lipid nanoparticles to transport RNA instructions for making a piece of virus into the cytoplasm of the vaccine recipient's cells. The vaccine recipient's cells then read the RNA and manufacture pieces of virus. Those pieces of virus induce an immune response.

1. Introduction

The COVID-19 pandemic has seen the fastest vaccine development in history. While vaccine development normally takes over ten years, the first COVID-19 vaccine entered clinical trials on March 16, 2020, only 63 days after the SARS-CoV-2 genetic sequence was published.[1,2] By December 2, 2020, less than a year after the pandemic began, the first vaccine with published phase 3 trial data was approved for emergency use.[3]

Rapid vaccine development was due, in part, to global coordination and funding. As it cannot be known which vaccines will succeed and which will fail, funding a large diverse selection of vaccine candidates was the best move. The World Health Organization (WHO); Gavi, the Vaccine Alliance; and the Coalition for Epidemic Preparedness Innovations (CEPI) collaboratively created COVAX, a program with the aim of providing equitable access to COVID-19 vaccines.[4] COVAX helped fund a broad portfolio of vaccine candidates chosen by CEPI's experts.[5] The United States of America's Operation Warp Speed (OWS), the largest source of COVID-19 vaccine funding worldwide, set out to support two vaccines from each of four vaccine categories in order to maximise the probability of success.[6,7]

The WHO released target product profiles to guide vaccine evaluation.[8] A minimal efficacy point estimate was set at 50% with a goal of 70% efficacy.[8] Emphasis was also placed on stable vaccines with only mild and temporary side effects that could be administered to a broad population regardless of age or health concerns.[8] Unlike traditional frameworks for evaluating vaccines, no criteria of cost-effectiveness are present.[8,9] Given the extent and severity of the COVID-19 pandemic, there is no question that vaccines are necessary, regardless of cost or logistical challenges.

As of March 30, 2021 there are 84 COVID-19 vaccines in clinical development and a further 184 in pre-clinical development.[10] This chapter provides an overview of vaccines approved for use somewhere in the world prior to a cut-off point of February 18, 2021. Efficacy estimates from interim phase 3 trial results are presented for each vaccine where available. Vaccine efficacy is important as more effective vaccines will require fewer people to be vaccinated to achieve the herd immunity as dictated by the reproductive number R.

The vaccine efficacy estimates cannot be directly compared as the phase 3 trials are taking place in different parts of the world, at different times, with different SARS-CoV-2 variants present, and among participants with different inclusion/exclusion criteria. Additionally, the trials calculated efficacy based on inconsistent criteria. Both the number of days after vaccination used as the start of the efficacy measurement period as well as the definition of a case of COVID-19 varied significantly.

2. Whole Inactivated Virus Vaccines

This vaccine type is quite simple; whole active virus is manufactured, inactivated, and then used to vaccinate people.

As of February 18, 2021, ten inactivated virus vaccines candidates are in the clinical phase of development.[10] Four of these have been approved for use in at least one country: China's Sinovac, Sinopharm — Beijing Institute of Biological Products, and Sinopharm — Wuhan Institute of Biological Products plus India's Bharat Biotech.[10,11]

All four of these vaccines share a similar manufacturing process and mechanism of action.

The SARS-CoV-2 strain selected for use in the vaccine is inoculated onto Vero Cells and cultured (normally in a large bioreactor) for 36–72 hours.[12–15] Vero cells are a cell line originally isolated from the epithelial cells from an African green monkey kidney.[16] Vero cells have a mutation making them susceptible to a wide range of pathogens and so are commonly used in vaccine manufacturing.[16,17]

After culturing in Vero cells, the supernatant is mixed with β-propiolactone for 20–48 hours to inactivate the virus.[12–15] β-propiolactone modifies the nucleic acids of the virus, inactivating it without changing the physical structure significantly.[18] The inactivated virus no longer poses a risk to human health, but is still recognised by the immune system and induces an immune response.[19] β-propiolactone has been widely used to inactivate viruses for use in vaccines.[20]

Next, the inactivated SARS-CoV-2 is purified (normally using column chromatography).[12–15] After purification, virus inactivation must be confirmed. Confirming that the inactivation process worked is vital as, if inactivation fails, then whole, active virus could make it into the vaccine. Inactivation is confirmed by inoculating the inactivated virus onto Vero cells again and checking for evidence of cytopathic effect (CPE).[12–14,21] CPEs are physical changes in a cell caused by a virus. For the SARS-CoV-2 vaccine, the inactivated virus (and positive and negative controls) is cultured in Vero cells for four days (Passage 1).[12–14,21] Afterwards, a sample of the supernatant is removed and inoculated onto fresh Vero cells and cultured for another four days (Passage 2).[12–14,21] This procedure is repeated for a total of three passages. Throughout this process, investigators check cells for signs of CPE.[12–14,21] If no CPE appears in the samples, then the inactivation process success is confirmed and the inactivated virus is ready for use in vaccines.[12–14,21]

Finally, the inactivated virus is mixed with an adjuvant. Adjuvants help boost the immune system's response to a vaccine.[22] The adjuvant used in all four vaccines is aluminum hydroxide which has been widely used in vaccines for many years.[12–14,22,23] While the exact mechanism of action of aluminum hydroxide is not completely understood, it has been shown to bring immune cells to the injection site, increase phagocytosis of the antigen by dendritic cells, and may increase the immune response duration by keeping the antigen at the injection site.[22,24,25]

As whole inactivated virus vaccines are an established and well-studied, relatively large-scale manufacturing facilities existed prior to the COVID-19 pandemic.[17,26] However, as large amounts of active virus must be created before inactivation, these vaccines require high biosafety manufacturing facilities so scaling up manufacturing quickly can be difficult.[27] Although inactivation is confirmed with every batch of vaccine, there can be public concerns about the inactivation process not working and active virus making it into the vaccine. An advantage of this vaccine type is that it is stable and can be stored at regular fridge temperature which improves the logistics of vaccine delivery.[14,28–30] Another advantage of this vaccine is, as whole virus is used, a broader immune response can be created. Researchers do not have to select the most important parts of a virus to create an immune response against as the whole virus is included in the vaccine.

2.1 *Sinovac biotech (CoronaVac)*

This vaccine is based on SARS-CoV-2 strain CN02.[31] The two dose vaccine may be administered 14–28 days apart but the phase 3 trials all use a 14 day interval.[32–34] It is stored at 2–8°C.[28,35]

The end point for the phase 3 trials is efficacy against symptomatic COVID-19 at least 14 days after dose 2 (confirmed by PCR).[33–35] The reported interim efficacy estimates from these trials are 83.50%, 50.65%, and 65.30%, respectively.[32,36,37] However, full results have not yet been published and peer reviewed. Refer to Appendix A.1 for further phase 3 trial information.

2.2 *Sinopharm — Beijing Institute of Biological Products (BBIBP-CorV)*

This vaccine is based on SARS-CoV-2 strain 19nCoV-CDC-Tan-HB02 (HB02).[13] It is administered in 2 doses spaced 21 days apart and stored at 2–8°C.[29,38] The end point for the phase 3 trials is efficacy against symptomatic COVID-19 at least 14 days after dose 2.[38,39] No data has been published and peer reviewed from phase 3 trials but Sinopharm has stated that the interim efficacy against symptomatic COVID-19 is 79.34%.[29] The source of this efficacy estimate is unclear. Refer to Appendix A.2 for further phase 3 trial information.

2.3 *Sinopharm — Wuhan Institute of Biological Products*

This vaccine is based on SARS-CoV-2 strain WIV04 (GenBank: MN996528.1). It is administered in 2 doses spaced 21 days apart and stored at 2–8°C.[14,38] The end point for the phase 3 trials is efficacy against symptomatic COVID-19 at least 14 days after dose 2.[38,40] No data has been published and peer reviewed from phase 3 trials but Sinopharm has stated that the interim efficacy against symptomatic COVID-19 is 72.51%.[41] The source of this efficacy estimate is unclear. Refer to Appendix A.3 for further phase 3 trial information.

2.4 *Bharat Biotech (Covaxin or BBV152B)*

This vaccine is based on SARS-CoV-2 strain NIV-2020-770.[23] It is administered in 2 doses spaced 28 days apart and stored at 2–8°C.[30] Efficacy estimates are based on an endpoint of symptomatic COVID-19 (confirmed by PCR) at least 14 days after dose 2.[42] The reported efficacy based on interim Phase 3 trial data is 80.60%, however, results have not yet been published and peer reviewed.[42] Refer to Appendix A.4 for further phase 3 trial information.

3. Protein Subunit Vaccines

Protein subunit vaccines, similar to whole inactivated vaccines, involve creating the virus outside of humans. However, while in whole inactivated vaccines the entire active virus is manufactured and inactivated, in protein subunit vaccines only a small portion of the virus needed to create an immune response is made.

As of February 18, 2021, there are 27 protein subunit vaccines for SARS-CoV-2 in the clinical phase of development.[10] Only one of these vaccines, that of Russia's State Research Center of Virology and Biotechnology VECTOR (known as the Vector Institute), has been approved for use in at least one country.[11] However, as there is little published information about this vaccine, this section will focus on the vaccine by the United States of America's (USA's) Novavax. While the Novavax vaccine is not approved for use in any country, its phase 3 trial in the United Kingdom (UK) just finished and imminent approval is likely.[43]

With protein subunit vaccines, instead of manufacturing the whole virus, only the small part of the virus needed to induce the necessary immune response is created. Thus the whole, active virus is not present at any point in the manufacturing process. In the Novavax vaccine, the portion of the virus selected for vaccine use is the full-length SARS-CoV-2 spike protein.[44] The spike protein is found on the outside of SARS-CoV-2 and enables the virus to enter host cells.[45,46] Previous experience with the SARS-CoV and MERS-CoV spike proteins made the SARS-CoV-2 spike protein immediately of interest for vaccine researchers.[45,46] As the SARS-CoV-2 spike protein was found to be quite immunogenic and antibodies against it were able to neutralise the virus, it became the primary vaccine target.[45,46]

In the wild, the SARS-CoV-2 spike protein exists in a prefusion state and then changes conformation to a post-fusion state after encountering a host cell.[47] A vaccine should ideally induce the creation of antibodies against the spike protein in its prefusion state as this is the state that will be present on the outside of whole active SARS-CoV-2 when it enters the body. However, the SARS-CoV-2 spike protein on its own is unstable and may change conformation into the post-fusion conformation.[47] To fix this, the spike protein in the vaccine has been modified through a mutation at the S1/S2 furin cleavage site and adding two proline substitutions.[44] These modifications make the spike protein resistant to cleavage and keep the protein in its prefusion state.[44]

The gene for the modified spike protein is then inserted into a baculovirus transfer vector.[44,48] Baculovirus transfer vectors were developed from baculoviruses, a family of viruses that infect insects.[49] The baculovirus transfer vector containing the gene for the modified spike protein is then inoculated onto Sf9 cells (a cell line derived from fall armyworm moths).[44,48] The baculovirus transfer vector infects the Sf9 cells which then manufacture large amounts of the modified spike protein.[44,48] The baculovirus–Sf9 cell expression system has been widely used for manufacturing viral proteins for many years.[49]

The spike proteins are then purified from the Sf9 cells and mixed with polysorbate 80 (PS 80) to form nanoparticles.[48,50] Similar to soap, PS 80 has a hydrophilic head and hydrophobic tail.[50] In water, it forms micelles, small balls with the hydrophilic heads on the surface and the hydrophobic tails in the middle.[50] In the vaccine, the spike proteins attach to micelles like they would stick out of wild SARS-CoV-2.[50] The portion of the spike protein that would normally be embedded in the SARS-CoV-2 membrane instead embeds in the micelles, creating nanoparticles covered in spike protein.[50]

Viral nanoparticles are mixed with an adjuvant to improve the immune system's response. The Novavax vaccine uses the proprietary Novavax adjuvant called Matrix-M™.[51] While the specific components of Matrix-M™ are not published, the adjuvant is based on saponin from the soapbark tree along with phospholipid and cholesterol.[51] This adjuvant has been shown to boost the immune response after vaccination.[44,52]

As with whole inactivated virus vaccines, an advantage of protein subunit vaccines is that they are well established and researched. Protein subunits are also stable and can be stored at regular fridge temperature.[44,53] Another advantage of these vaccines is that, unlike whole inactivated virus vaccines, it is not necessary to make whole active virus during manufacturing. However, researchers must choose the proteins to include as targets in protein subunit vaccines. This requires knowledge of the virus's structure and function to select the correct proteins. Additionally, in comparison to other vaccine types, protein subunit vaccines can be complicated and expensive to produce so scaling up production can be difficult.[54]

3.1 *Novavax (NVX-CoV2373)*

This vaccine is administered in 2 doses spaced 21 days apart and is stored at 2–8°C.[44,55] The primary endpoint for the phase 3 trials is symptomatic COVID-19 (confirmed by PCR) at least 7 days after dose 2.[43] Results from phase 3 trials have not yet been published and peer reviewed. The reported efficacy based on the results of the phase 3 trial in the United Kingdom is 89.7% (95% Confidence Interval (CI) = 80.2, 94.6).[43] The reported efficacy based on the results of the phase 2b trial in South Africa is 48.6% (95% CI = 28.4, 63.1).[43] Refer to Appendix A.5 for further phase 3 and phase 2b trial information.

3.2 *Vector Institute (EpiVacCorona)*

Very little information has been published about this vaccine.[56] It administered in 2 doses spaced 14–21 days apart and is stored at 2–8°C.[53]

Instead of the full length SARS-CoV-2 spike protein, EpiVacCorona only consists of three synthesised spike protein peptides.[56] The peptides are covalently bound to a modified SARS-CoV-2 nucleocapsid protein that is used as a carrier.[56] The vaccine is adsorbed onto the adjuvant aluminum hydroxide.[56] No efficacy data has been released. Refer to Appendix A.6 for further phase 3 trial information.

4. Non-Replicating Viral Vector Vaccines

Unlike whole inactivated virus or protein subunit vaccines, viral vector vaccines do not require manufacturing any portion of the virus outside of the human body. Like protein subunit vaccines, viral vector vaccines use a vector to deliver the instructions for making a portion of the virus to cells. Protein subunit vaccines delivered the instructions for making this portion of the virus to cells in culture with the resulting proteins then used to vaccinate people. Instead, viral vector vaccines cut out the cell culture step and give the instructions for making the portion of the virus directly to the cells of the person receiving the vaccine.

As of February 18, 2021, there are 12 non-replicating viral vector vaccines in the clinical phase of study.[10] Four of these vaccines have already been approved for use in at least one country: Swedish-British Oxford-AstraZeneca, Belgium's Janssen Pharmaceuticals (owned by USA's Johnson & Johnson), Russia's Gameleya National Center of Epidemiology and Microbiology, and China's CanSino Biologics (CanSinoBIO).[10,11]

All four of the currently approved viral vector vaccines use an adenovirus vector to transport the DNA for some form of the SARS-CoV-2 spike protein.[57–60] Adenoviruses are naturally occurring and circulate in the general human population causing cold and flu-like symptoms.[61] The adenoviruses in these vaccines have been modified so they cannot replicate.[57–60] Once injected into a vaccine recipient, the adenovirus vector transports the SARS-CoV-2 spike protein DNA into the nucleus of the person's cells.[57–60] The receiving cells read the DNA instructions and manufacture the spike protein. The newly manufactured spike protein induces an immune response.

An issue with viral vector vaccines is that they can also induce an immune response to the carrier vector itself.[62,63] This may be a particular problem for vaccines that require two doses as the immune system of the vaccine recipient may fight off the vector before it has time to deliver the DNA into the person's cells. However, it is also an issue in single-dose vaccines, as adenoviruses circulate in the human population so people may have some pre-existing immunity to the vector.[64,65]

With viral vector vaccines, as the vaccine DNA is delivered into the nucleus of a person's cells, there is some concern that the DNA of the vaccine could integrate into the recipient's genome.[27] However, this rarely happens with Adenovirus vectors and so should not pose a problem for these vaccines.[27,66,67]

As with protein subunit vaccines, an advantage of viral vector vaccines is that no active SARS-CoV-2 virus needs to be manufactured at any point. These vaccines are also stable and can be stored at regular fridge temperature.[57,59,68,69] An advantage of viral vector vaccines is that they can create a large immune response without the need for an adjuvant.[27]

4.1 *Janssen Pharmaceuticals (Ad26.COV2.S)*

This vaccine uses human adenovirus 26 vector (Ad26) that has been modified so it cannot replicate.[58,70] The vector delivers the DNA instructions to make a SARS-CoV-2 spike protein that has been stabilised in its pre-fusion conformation with two proline substitutions and a furin cleavage site mutation.[70] It is administered as a single dose.[71] While it is normally stored at 2–8°C, it can be stored at 9–25°C for up to 12 hours.[68] As the Janssen vaccine is only one dose, there is no concern of the first dose inducing an immune response against the vector that may reduce the efficacy of a second dose. However, as Ad26 is a human adenovirus that natural circulates in the population, there may be existing immunity against the vector.[65]

The primary endpoint of the phase 3 trials is moderate symptomatic COVID-19 (confirmed by PCR) at least 14 days after vaccination in participants who were seronegative at baseline.[72,71] Results have not yet been published and peer reviewed but the reported efficacy is 66.90% (95% CI = 59.0, 73.4).[72] Refer to Appendix A.7 for further phase 3 trial information.

4.2 *CanSino Biologics Inc. (Convidecia™ or Ad5-nCoV)*

This vaccine created uses a human adenovirus type 5 (Ad5) to transport the DNA instructions for the full-length SARS-CoV-2 spike protein.[73] It is stored at 2–8°C.[69] The vaccine is administered as a single dose so there is no concern of the first dose inducing an immune response against the vector that may reduce second dose efficacy. However, as Ad5 is a human adenovirus that natural circulates in the population, there may be existing immunity against the vector.[65] The proportion of the population with existing immunity against Ad5 is higher than that of Ad26.[65]

No data has been published from the studies yet but a CanSino press release states that the vaccine efficacy against symptomatic COVID-19 (confirmed by PCR) at least 14 days after vaccination was 68.83%.[69] It is unclear what data these estimates are based on and no 95% confidence intervals were provided. Refer to Appendix A.8 for further phase 3 trial information.

4.3 *Oxford-AstraZeneca (AZD1222 or Covishield)*

This vaccine uses ChAdOx1, a chimpanzee adenovirus vector that has been modified so it cannot replicate to deliver the DNA to make an unmodified, full-length SARS-CoV-2 spike protein.[57,74] As this vector is based on a chimpanzee adenovirus, existing immunity among the human population should not be an issue.[57] However, as the vaccine is administered as two doses and the ChAdOx1 vector is used for both doses, the first dose may induce an immune response against the vector that could reduce the uptake of the second dose. Phase 1/2 trials found that, although neutralising antibodies against the vector were induced after the first dose, the amount of anti-vector antibodies at the time of the second dose was not correlated with the anti-spike protein response after the second dose.[75] This suggests that reduced efficacy due to an anti-vector immune response may not be a major issue for this vaccine.

The primary endpoint of the phase 3 trials is symptomatic COVID-19 at least 15 days after dose 2.[74,76] The efficacy based on the published, peer-reviewed results of phase 3 trials is 66.7% (95% CI = 57.4, 74.0).[74] The reported efficacy based on interim results of another phase 3 trial is 76%

(95% CI = 68, 82).[77] Refer to Appendix A.9 for further phase 3 trial information.

As this vaccine is now in use, real-world effectiveness is being estimated. The results of these observational studies have been released in preprints but have not yet been published or peer-reviewed. A study of all adults 70 and older in England found an effectiveness 14–20 days after a single dose to be 60% (95% CI = 41, 73) against symptomatic COVID-19, rising to 73% (95% CI = 27, 90) 35 or more days after a single dose.[78] A study of the population of Scotland found an effectiveness of 94% (95% CI = 73, 99) against hospitalisation from COVID-19 28–34 days after a single dose.[79]

4.4 *Gamaleya National Center of epidemiology and microbiology* (*Sputnik V or Gam-Covid-Vac*)

This vaccine is a two dose vaccine administered 21 days apart that uses a different vector for each dose.[59] The first dose uses a human adenovirus type 26 (like Janssen's single dose) and the second dose uses a human adenovirus type 5 (like CanSino's single dose).[59] This two-vector approach avoids the problem of the first dose inducing an immune response against the vector that may reduce second dose efficacy. The vectors deliver the DNA instructions to make a full length SARS-CoV-2 spike protein.[59] The liquid form of the vaccine is stored at −18°C while a freeze dried version can be stored at 2–8°C.[59]

The primary endpoint of the phase 3 trials is symptomatic COVID-19 (confirmed by PCR) from the day of dose 2 (21 days after dose 1).[59,80] The efficacy based on published, peer-reviewed interim results of the phase 3 trial is 91.6% (95% CI = 85.6, 95.2).[59] Refer to Appendix A.10 for further phase 3 trial information.

5. RNA Vaccines

Similar to viral vector vaccines, RNA vaccines do not require manufacturing of any portion of the virus outside the human body. However, viral vector vaccines use a viral vector to deliver DNA instructions to make the SARS-CoV-2 spike protein to the nuclei of the cells of the person receiving the vaccine. That DNA is read to RNA and exported from the nucleus to the cytoplasm before being used to manufacture spike protein. In contrast, RNA vaccines deliver RNA directly to the cytoplasm of the cells of the vaccine recipient.

As of February 18, 2021, there are ten RNA-based SARS-CoV-2 vaccine candidates in the clinical phase of development.[10] Two of them, those made by the USA-Germany's Pfizer-BioNTech and by the USA's Moderna, have been approved for use in at least one country.[10,11]

Both of the currently approved vaccines consist of messenger RNA (mRNA) instructions for the full length SARS-CoV-2 spike protein.[81,82] The spike protein in both vaccines is modified with the same two proline substitutions seen in the Novavax protein subunit vaccine.[83,84] This mutation keeps the spike protein in its pre-fusion conformation in order to better represent the spike proteins on an intact SARS-CoV-2 virus.[47]

RNA is highly unstable and degrades easily.[85] Ribonucleases (RNases), small molecules that destroy RNA, are produced by almost every living thing.[85] To combat this, the mRNA in both the Pfizer-BioNTech and the Moderna vaccines is encapsulated in lipid nanoparticles (LNPs).[81,82] LNPs are tiny balls of fat that help protect and stabilise the mRNA while also promoting uptake into the cytoplasm of the vaccine recipient's cells.[85] In the cytoplasm, the mRNA instructions are read by the cell which then manufactures the modified spike protein.[85]

Unlike viral vector vaccines, there is no risk of developing immunity to a vector so multiple doses of mRNA vaccines can be administered without a reduction in uptake.[85] Additionally, as the instructions for the spike protein are coded in RNA rather than DNA there is no risk of integration into the genome of the person receiving the vaccine.[85] As with protein subunit and viral vector vaccines, no whole active virus needs to be manufactured. An additional advantage of RNA vaccines is that they are relatively quick and easy to produce, meaning that production can, in theory, be scaled up quickly.[27,86] However, as no RNA vaccines had been approved prior to the COVID-19 pandemic, no large scale manufacturing facilities existed.[27,86] In addition, as RNA vaccines are a new technology, no long term research exists on their efficacy or safety. Due to the unstable nature of RNA, these vaccines also have to be kept very cold which can make the logistics of vaccine delivery challenging.[87,88]

5.1 *Pfizer-BioNTech (COMIRNATY® or BNT162b2)*

This vaccine is administered in 2 doses spaced 21 days apart.[81] The vaccine is normally stored at –80 to –60°C but can be stored at –25°C to –15°C for 2 weeks and returned to –80 once.[87] It can be thawed and stored at 2–8°C for 120 hours before use, but cannot be refrozen once thawed.[87]

The primary endpoint for phase 3 trials is symptomatic COVID-19 (confirmed by PCR) at least 7 days after dose 2.[89] The efficacy based on the published, peer-reviewed phase 3 trial results is 95.0 (95% CI = 90.3, 97.6).[81] The efficacy based on more recent, unpublished, non-peer-reviewed results of the same trial is 91.3% (95% CI = 89.0, 93.2).[90] Refer to Appendix A.11 for further phase 3 trial information.

As the vaccine is now in widespread use, real-world effectiveness estimates are also being released. The Israel Ministry of Health reported an effectiveness of 97% against symptomatic COVID-19 and 94% against asymptomatic COVID-19 based on widespread use of the vaccine in Israel.[91] A pre-print from the United Kingdom found effectiveness of 86% (95% CI = 76, 97) against any COVID-19 (including asymptomatic) seven days after dose 2 based on observational data from a cohort of around 40,000 healthcare workers.[92] The Centers for Disease Control and Prevention (CDC) is conducting a combined observational study of the Moderna and Pfizer-BioNTech vaccines in frontline and essential workers in the USA. Their published interim results found these two vaccines to be 91% (95% CI = 73, 97) effective at preventing any COVID-19 (including asymptomatic infections) 14 or more days after dose 2.[93]

5.2 *Moderna (mRNA-1273)*

This vaccine is administered in 2 doses, 28 days apart.[82] It is normally stored at –25°C to –15°C but can be thawed and stored at 2–8°C for up to 30 days.[88] Once thawed, the vaccine cannot be refrozen.[88]

The primary endpoint of the phase 3 trials is symptomatic COVID-19 (confirmed by PCR) at least 14 days after dose 2.[82,94] The efficacy based on the published, peer-reviewed phase 3 trial results is 94.1% (95% CI = 89.3, 96.8).[82] Refer to Appendix A.12 for further phase 3 trial information.

Summary Table

Vaccine type	Developer (vaccine name)	Peer-reviewed phase 3 trial data	No. of approved countries[11]	Dosing frequency	Storage temperature	COVID-19 end point		Efficacy in phase 3 trial (95% confidence interval)
Whole inactivated	Sinovac (CoronaVac)	No	19	2 doses, 14–28 days apart[32]	2–8°C[28]	Symptomatic, ≥14 days after dose 2[35]	Turkey	83.5%[36,35]
							Brazil	50.65%[32,33]
							Indonesia	65.3%[37,34]
	Sinopharm-Beijing (BBIBP-CorV)	No	28	2 doses, 21 days apart[38]	2–8°C[29]	Symptomatic, ≥14 days after dose 2[38]	79.34%[29]	
	Sinopharm-Wuhan	No	2	2 doses, 21 days apart[38]	2–8°C[14]	Symptomatic, ≥14 days after dose 2[38]	72.51%[41]	
	Bharat (Covaxin; BBV152B)	No	5	2 doses, 28 days apart[30]	2–8°C[30]	Symptomatic, ≥14 days after dose 2[42]	80.6%[42]	
Protein subunit	Novavax (NVX-CoV2373)	No	0	2 doses, 21 days apart[55]	2–8°C[44]	Symptomatic, ≥7 days After dose 2[55]	United Kingdom	89.7%[43] (80.2, 94.6)
							South Africa	48.6%[43] (28.4, 63.1)
	Vector Institute (EpiVacCorona)	No	2	2 doses, 14–21 days apart[53]	2–8°C[53]	—	—	

(Continued)

(Continued)

				Doses	Storage temperature	Endpoint	Efficacy
Non-replicating viral vector	Janssen (Ad26.COV2.S)	No	37	1 dose[71]	2–8°C (9–25°C for up to 12 hours)[68]	Symptomatic, ≥14 days after vaccine[72]	66.9% (59.0–73.4)[72]
	CanSino (Convidecia™; Ad5-nCoV)	No	4	1 dose[73]	2–8°C[69]	Symptomatic, ≥14 days after vaccine[69,95]	68.83%[69]
	Oxford-AstraZeneca (AZD1222; Covishield)	Yes	82	2 doses, 4–12 weeks apart[76,77,96]	2–8°C[57]	Symptomatic, ≥15 days after dose 2[74,76]	United Kingdom,[97,98] Brazil,[99] South Africa[100] 66.7%[74] (57.4, 74.0); USA, Chile, Peru 76%[77] (68, 82)
	Gamaleya (Sputnik V; Gam-Covid-Vac)	Yes	59	2 doses, 21 days apart[59]	Liquid form: −18°C[59] Freeze dried form: 2–8°C[59]	Symptomatic, ≥ the day of dose 2[59]	91.6%[59] (85.6, 95.2)
RNA	Pfizer-BioNTech (COMIRNATY®; BNT162b2)	Yes	80	2 doses, 21 days apart[81]	−80 to −60°C (−25 to −15°C for 2 weeks) (2–8°C for 120 hours, cannot refreeze)[87]	Symptomatic, ≥7 days after dose 2[81]	91.3%[90,89] (89.0, 93.2)
	Moderna (mRNA-1273)	Yes	42	2 doses, 28 days apart[82]	−25°C to −15°C (2–8°C for up to 30 days, cannot refreeze)[88]	Symptomatic, ≥14 days after dose 2[82]	94.1%[82,94] (89.3, 96.8)

As referenced in Section 5.1, a combined observational study of the Moderna and Pfizer-BioNTech vaccines in frontline and essential workers in the USA found the real-world effectiveness of these two vaccines to be 91% (95% CI = 73, 97) at preventing any COVID-19 (including asymptomatic infections) 14 or more days after dose 2.[93]

Appendix A. Phase 3 Trial Information

A.1 *Sinovac Biotech (CoronaVac)*

Phase 3 trials are underway in Turkey, Brazil, and Indonesia.[33–35] Notably, the Brazilian trial only included medical staff. Demographic information has not been released. Table 1 shows a summary of the phase 3 trials.

A.2 *Sinopharm — Beijing Institute of Biological Products (BBIBP-CorV)*

The main multicenter phase 3 trial is ongoing in Bahrain, Egypt, Jordan, and the United Arab Emirates.[38] The vaccine is being trialed alongside the vaccine produced by Sinopharm — Wuhan Institute of Biological Products.[38] Another phase 3 trial of only BBIBP-CorV is underway in Argentina.[39] Demographic information has not been released.

Table 1:   Sinovac Biotech phase 3 trial summary.

	Trial	Turkey[35,36]	Brazil[32,33]	Indonesia[34,37]
	Age range	18–59	18+	—
No. of people in efficacy analysis	Total	10,216	12,396	~1,600
	Vaccine	6,648	—	—
	Placebo	3,568	—	—
COVID-19 cases	Total	41	253	25
	Vaccine	32	—	—
	Placebo	9	—	—
Efficacy against:	Symptomatic COVID-19	83.50%	50.65%	65.30%
	Moderate COVID-19	—	83.70%	—
	Severe COVID-19	100%	100%	—

A.3 *Sinopharm — Wuhan Institute of Biological Products*

The main multicenter phase 3 trial is ongoing in Bahrain, Egypt, Jordan, and the United Arab Emirates.[38,101] The vaccine is being trialed along side the vaccine produced by Sinopharm (Beijing).[38] Other phase 3 trials are underway in Peru and Morocco.[40,102] Demographic information has not been released for these trials.

A.4 *Bharat Biotech (Covaxin or BBV152B)*

A phase 3 trial is underway in India.[103] The study currently includes 4,500 people with comorbidities as well as 2,433 people over 60 years old.[42] Table 2 shows a summary of the phase 3 trial.

A.5 *Novavax (NVX-CoV2373)*

Two phase 3 trials are underway, one in the United Kingdom and one in the USA and Mexico.[55,104] The efficacy estimates were calculated among people who were seronegative at baseline.[43]

In the UK Phase 3 trial, among the 27% of the participants over 65, there were 10 cases of symptomatic COVID-19, 9 in the vaccine group and 1 in the vaccine group.[43] The majority of the cases in the

Table 2:   Bharat Biotech phase 3 trial summary.

	Trial	India[42,103]
	Age range	18–98
No. of people in efficacy analysis	Total	25,800
	Vaccine	~12,900
	Placebo	~12,900
COVID-19 cases	Total	43
	Vaccine	7
	Placebo	36
Efficacy against:	Symptomatic COVID-19	80.60%

Table 3: Novavax phase 3 and phase 2b trial summary.

	Trial	United Kingdom[43,55,105] Total	Original strain	B.1.1.7/ 501Y.V1 variant	South Africa[43,106] Total	HIV negative only
	Age range	18–84			18–65	
No. of people in efficacy analysis	Total	14,040			2,770	
	Vaccine	7,020			1,408	
	Placebo	7,020			1,362	
COVID-19 cases	Total	106	5		147	
	Vaccine	10	0		51	
	Placebo	96	5		96	
Efficacy against:	Symptomatic COVID-19 (95% Confidence Interval (CI))	89.7% (80.2, 94.6)	96.4% (73.8, 99.5)	86.3% (71.3, 93.5)	48.6% (28.4, 63.1)	55.4% (35.9, 68.9)
	Severe COVID-19	100%			100%	

South African 2b trial were from the B.1.351/501Y.V2 variant which may explain the lower efficacy estimate.[43] This trial also approximately 245 participants who were HIV positive.[105,106] No further demographic information about these trials has been released. Table 3 shows a summary of the phase 3 and phase 2b trials.

A.6 *Vector Institute* (*EpiVacCorona*)

A phase 3 trial of about 3,000 participants over 18 years old is underway in Russia but no efficacy data has been released.[107] Demographic information has not been released for this trial.

A.7 *Janssen Pharmaceuticals* (*Ad26.COV2.S*)

A multicenter phase 3 trial investigating a single dose is ongoing in the USA, Mexico, Argentina, Brazil, Chile, Colombia, Peru, and South Africa.[71]

Of the 39,321 participants included in the primary efficacy analysis population, 44.5% were female.[72] 65.4% of participants were aged 18–59, with the remaining 34.6% being aged 60 or older.[72] The participants were 62.1% white, 17.2% black, 3.5% Asian, 8.3% American Indian/Alaska Native, 0.3% Native Hawaiian or other Pacific Islander, 5.4% multiracial, and 3.2% unknown or unreported.[72] 45.1% of the participants were Hispanic or Latino and 39.9% of participants had comorbidities.[72]

Another multicenter phase 3 trial investigating a two dose schedule is also underway in the USA, Belgium, Brazil, Colombia, France, Germany, the Philippines, South Africa, Spain, and the UK but no efficacy data has been released yet.[108] Table 4 shows a summary of the phase 3 trials.

A.8 CanSino Biologics Inc. (*Convidecia*™ or *Ad5-nCoV*)

Multicenter phase 3 trials are underway in Argentina, Chile, Mexico, Pakistan, and Russia (~40,000 total participants).[95] CanSino also stated that the vaccine is 95.47% against severe COVID-19 from 14 days after vaccination.[69] Demographic information has not been released for this trial.

Table 4:   Janssen phase 3 trial summary.

	Trial	USA, Mexico, Argentina, Brazil, Chile, Colombia, Peru, South Africa[71,72]
	Age range	18+
No. of people in efficacy analysis	Total	39,321
	Vaccine	19,630
	Placebo	19,691
COVID-19 cases (Severe Cases)	Total	464
	Vaccine	116 (14)
	Placebo	348 (60)
Efficacy against	Moderate symptomatic COVID-19 (95% CI)	66.90% (59.0, 73.4)
	Severe COVID-19 (95% CI)	76.70% (54.6, 89.1)

A.9 Oxford-AstraZeneca (*AZD1222 or Covishield*)

The results of four trials (a phase 1/2 and a phase 2/3 trial from the UK, a phase 3 trial from Brazil, and a phase 1/2 trial from South Africa) were analyzed and published together.[57,74] Another multicenter phase 3 trial is ongoing in the USA, Chile, and Peru and, while no results are yet published, interim efficacy estimates have been released.[76,77] The phase 2/3 trial in the UK also assessed efficacy against asymptomatic COVID-19 through weekly nose and throat swaps that participants self-administered.[74]

During the phase 2/3 study in the UK, participants enrolled at the beginning of the study (May 31 to June 10, 2020) received a low first dose that was about half the strength of the standard dose (2.2×10^{10} viral particles instead of the intended 5×10^{10} viral particles).[57] Two methods were used to assess the number of viral particles in vaccine batches: quantitative PCR and spectrophotometry.[57] Due to interference from an ingredient in the vaccine, the spectrophotometry measurement mistakenly found a higher concentration of viral particles, almost double that of the quantitative PCR.[57] In order to ensure that the dose was within a safe range, the researchers decided to base the dosage off of the spectrophotometry measurement.[57] The source of the interference was later found, revealing that initial participants received a lower dose than intended.[57] From then on, a group of tests were used to determine the vaccine concentration so the low-dose participants received standard second doses and the participants enrolled later in the study received two standard doses.[57]

Of the 17,178 participants included in the primary efficacy analysis of the published trial data, 83.9% were aged 18–55, 10.4% were aged 56–69, and 5.7% were 70 or older.[74] 56.4% were female and 62.8% were workers in health and social care settings.[74] The ethnicity of the participants was 75.5% white, 9.9% black, 4.4% other, and 10.2% multiracial. 11.9% of the participants had cardiovascular disease, 10.1% had respiratory disease, and 2.6% had diabetes. Table 5 shows a summary of the phase 3 trials.

A.10 Gamaleya National Center of Epidemiology and Microbiology (*Sputnik V or Gam-Covid-Vac*)

A phase 3 trial is underway in Russia.[80] Of the 19,866 participants included in the primary efficacy analysis, 38.8% were female.[59] 98.5% of

Table 5: Oxford-AstraZeneca phase 3 trial summary.

| Trial | United Kingdom,[97,98] Brazil,[99] South Africa[74,100] | | | | | | USA, Chile, Peru[76,77] |
	Total		Only SD/SD		Only LD/SD		
Age range	18+		18+		18+		18+
No. of people in efficacy analysis — Total	17,178	8,207	14,380	5,443	2,798	2,764	32,449
Vaccine	8,597	4,071	7,201	2,692	1,396	1,379	—
Placebo	8,581	4,136	7,179	2,751	1,402	1,385	—
COVID-19 cases — Total	332	130	271	83	61	47	190
Vaccine	84	57	74	41	10	16	0
Placebo	248	73	197	42	51	31	8
Efficacy against: Symptomatic COVID-19 (95% CI)	66.7% (57.4, 74.0)		63.1% (51.8, 71.7)		80.7% (62.1, 90.2)		76% (68, 82)
Asymptomatic COVID-19[75] (95% CI)		22.2% (−9.9, 45.0)		2.0% (−50.7, 36.2)		49.3% (7.4, 72.2)	100%

Table 6: Gamaleya phase 3 trial summary.

Trial		Russia[59,80]
	Age range	18–111
No. people in efficacy analysis	Total	19,866
	Vaccine	14,964
	Placebo	4,902
COVID-19 cases (severe cases)	Total	78 (20)
	Vaccine	16 (0)
	Placebo	62 (20)
Efficacy against:	Symptomatic COVID-19 (95% CI)	91.6% (85.6, 95.2)
	Severe COVID-19	100%

the participants were white, 1.4% were Asian, and 0.05% were other races.[59] 10.7% were aged 18–30, 25.7% were aged 31–40, 29.4% were aged 41–50, 23.4% were aged 51–60, and 10.8% were aged 60 or older.[59] 24.8% had comorbidities, 75.1% did not, and the status of 0.15% was unknown.[59] Table 6 shows a summary of the phase 3 trial.

A.11 *Pfizer-BioNTech (COMIRNATY® or BNT162b2)*

A multicenter phase 3 trial in the USA, Argentina, Brazil, Germany, South Africa, and Turkey to test the vaccine is ongoing.[89] Peer reviewed results of the trial with a median follow-up time of 2 months were published on December 10, 2020.[81] The primary efficacy estimate was calculated only among HIV negative participants without significant protocol violations who had no evidence of being infected with SARS-CoV-2 at baseline.[81] Updated results with more follow-up time were released by press release on April 1, 2021.[90] It is unclear if this more recent efficacy estimate population also excludes HIV positive participants. The phase 3 trials are now being expanded to test the vaccine in younger age groups.[90] Pfizer-BioNTech has released interim efficacy estimates for a trial in adolescents age 12–15.[90] Further testing is also underway in children 5–11 years old and 2–5 years old, and expansion to children 6 months–2 years old is planned.

Table 7:   Pfizer-BioNTech phase 3 trial summary.

Trial	USA, Argentina, Brazil, Germany, South Africa, and Turkey[89]					USA
Date results published	Dec. 10, 2020[81]		April 1, 2021[90]			March 31, 2021[90]
				Severe case definition		
				CDC	FDA	
Age range	16+	12+	16+			12–15
No. of people in efficacy analysis — Total	36,523	43,385	46,307			2,260
Vaccine	18,198	21,669	—			1,131
Placebo	18,325	21,686	—			1,129
COVID-19 cases — Total	170	5	927	32	22	18
Vaccine	8	1	77	0	1	0
Placebo	162	4	850	32	21	18
Efficacy against: Symptomatic COVID-19 (95% CI)	95.0 (90.3, 97.6)		91.3% (89.0, 93.2)			100%
Severe COVID-19 (95% CI)		75.0 (−152.6, 99.5)		100% (88.0, 100.0)	95.3% (71.0, 99.9)	

Demographic information about the population used in the efficacy estimates was not reported, however demographic information of the main safety subset population was provided (all participants who received at least one vaccination (including HIV+) and were enrolled by October 9, 2020).[81] Of the 37,706 participants in the main safety subset, 49.4% were female.[81] 57.8% of the participants were aged 16–55 and 42.2% were aged 56 or older.[81] The population was 82.9% white, 9.3% black, 4.3% Asian, 0.5% Native American or Alaska Native, 0.2% Native Hawaiian or other Pacific Islander, 2.3% multiracial, and 0.6% unreported.[81] 28.0% of the population were Hispanic or Latino.[81] 20.5% had comorbidities and 35.1% were obese.[81] Table 7 shows a summary of the phase 3 trials.

A.12 *Moderna (mRNA-1273)*

The vaccine is being tested in a phase 3 trial in the USA.[94] The efficacy was calculated among participants who received both doses without significant protocol violations who also had no signs of prior SARS-CoV-2 infection.[82]

Of the 28,207 participants included in the primary efficacy population, 47.4% were female.[82] 74.7% of the population was aged 18–64 and 25.3% was aged 65 and older.[82] The population was 79.5% white, 9.7% black, 4.6% Asian, 0.8% American Indian or Alaska Native, 0.2% Native

Table 8:   Moderna phase 3 trial summary.

		Trial	**USA**[82,94]
		Age range	18+
No. of people in efficacy analysis	Total		28,207
	Vaccine		14,073
	Placebo		14,134
COVID-19 cases (Severe cases)	Total		196 (30)
	Vaccine		11 (0)
	Placebo		185 (30)
Efficacy against:	Symptomatic COVID-19 (95% CI)		94.1% (89.3, 96.8)
	Severe COVID-19		100%

Hawaiian or Other Pacific Islander, 2.1% other, 2.1% multiracial, and 0.9% unknown or unreported.[82] 19.7% of the population was Hispanic or Latino.[82] 4.8% had chronic lung disease, 5.0% had significant cardiac disease, 6.7% had severe obesity (BMI ≤ 40), 9.6% had diabetes, 0.7% had liver disease, and 0.6% were HIV positive.[82] Table 8 shows a summary of the phase 3 trial.

References

1. Pronker ES, Weenen TC, Commandeur H, Claassen EH, Osterhaus AD. Risk in Vaccine Research and Development Quantified. *PLoS ONE* [Internet]. 2013 Mar 20 [cited 2021 Apr 4];8(3). Available from: https://journals.plos.org/plosone/article?id=10.1371/journal.pone.0057755 doi: 10.1371/journal.pone.0057755.

2. Moderna. Moderna's Work on our COVID-19 Vaccine [Internet]. [place unknown]: Moderna; 2021 [cited 2021 Apr 4]. Available from: https://www.modernatx.com/modernas-work-potential-vaccine-against-covid-19.

3. Medicines and Healthcare products Regulatory Agency. UK medicines regulator gives approval for first UK COVID-19 vaccine [Internet]. [place unknown]: Government of the United Kingdom; 2020 Dec 20 [cited 2021 Apr 4]. Available from: https://www.gov.uk/government/news/uk-medicines-regulator-gives-approval-for-first-uk-covid-19-vaccine.

4. Berkley S. COVAX explained [Internet]. [place unknown]: Gavi, the Vaccine Alliance; 2020 Sep 3 [cited 2021 Apr 4]. Available from: https://cepi.net/covax/#content-the-scale-of-the-problem.

5. The Coalition for Epidemic Preparedness Innovations (CEPI). COVAX: CEPI's response to COVID-19 [Internet]. [place unknown]: CEPI; 2020 [cited 2021 Apr 4]. Available from: https://cepi.net/covax/.

6. Slaoui M, Hepburn M. Developing Safe and Effective Covid Vaccines — Operation Warp Speed's Strategy and Approach. New England Journal of Medicine [Internet]. 2020 Oct 29 [cited 2021 Apr 4];383(18):1701–1703. Available from: https://pubmed.ncbi.nlm.nih.gov/32846056/ doi: 10.1056/NEJMp2027405.

7. Kim JH, Hotez P, Batista C, Ergonul O, Figueroa JP, Gilbert S. Operation Warp Speed: Implications for global vaccine security. *Lancet Global Health* [Internet]. 2021 Mar 26 [cited 2021 Apr 4]. Available from: https://doi.org/10.1016/S2214-109X(21)00140-6 doi: 10.1016/S2214-109X(21)00140-6.

8. World Health Organization. WHO Target Product Profiles for COVID-19 Vaccines [Internet]. [place unknown]: WHO; 2020 Apr 9 [cited 2021 Apr 4]. Available from: https://www.who.int/publications/m/item/who-target-product-profiles-for-covid-19-vaccines.

9. Erickson LJ, De Wals P, Farand L. An analytical framework for immunization programs in Canada. *Vaccine* [Internet]. 2005 Mar 31 [cited 2021 Apr 4];23(19):2470–2476. Available from: https://pubmed.ncbi.nlm.nih.gov/15752833/ doi: 10.1016/j.vaccine.2004.10.029.

10. World Health Organization. Draft landscape and tracker of COVID-19 candidate vaccines [Internet]. [place unknown]: WHO; 2021 Mar 30 [cited 2021 Mar 30]. Available from: https://www.who.int/publications/m/item/draft-landscape-of-covid-19-candidate-vaccines.

11. Basta NE, Moodie EEM. Trials & approved vaccines by country [Internet]. Montreal: McGill University COVID19 Vaccine Tracker; 2021 Apr 4 [cited 2021 Apr 4]. Available from: https://covid19.trackvaccines.org/trials-vaccines-by-country/.

12. Gao Q, Bao L, Mao H, Wang L, Xu K, Yang M, *et al.* Development of an inactivated vaccine candidate for SARS-CoV-2. *Science* [Internet]. 2020 Jul 3 [cited 2021 Apr 4];369(6499):77–81. Available from: https://pubmed.ncbi.nlm.nih.gov/32376603/ doi: 10.1126/science.abc1932.

13. Wang H, Zhang Y, Huang B, Deng W, Quan Y, Wang W, *et al.* Development of an inactivated vaccine candidate, BBIBP-CorV, with potent protection against SARS-CoV-2. *Cell* [Internet]. 2020 Aug 6 [cited 2021 Apr 4]; 182(3):713–721. Available from: https://doi.org/10.1016/j.cell.2020.06.008 doi: 10.1016/j.cell.2020.06.008.

14. Xia S, Duan K, Zhang Y, Zhao D, Zhang H, Xie Z, *et al.* Effect of an inactivated vaccine against SARS-CoV-2 on safety and immunogenicity outcomes: Interim analysis of 2 randomized clinical trials. *JAMA* [Internet]. 2020 Sep 8 [cited 2021 Apr 4];324(10):951–960. Available from: https://doi.org/10.1001/jama.2020.15543 doi: 10.1001/jama.2020.15543.

15. Yadav PD, Ella R, Kumar S, Patil DR, Mohandas S, Shete AM, *et al.* Immunogenicity and protective efficacy of inactivated SARS-CoV-2 vaccine candidate, BBV152 in rhesus macaques. *Nature Communication* [Internet]. 2021 Mar 2 [cited 2021 Apr 4];12(1):Article 1386. Available from: https://doi.org/10.1038/s41467-021-21639-w doi: 10.1038/s41467-021-21639-w.

16. Osada N, Kohara A, Yamaji T, Hirayama N, Kasai F, Sekizuka T, *et al.* The genome landscape of the African green monkey kidney-derived vero cell line. *DNA Research* [Internet]. 2014 Sep 28 [cited 2021 Apr 4];

21(6):673–683. Available from: https://doi.org/10.1093/dnares/dsu029 doi: 10.1093/dnares/dsu029.

17. Barrett PN, Mundt W, Kistner O, Howard MK. Vero cell platform in vaccine production: Moving towards cell culture-based viral vaccines. *Expert Review Vaccines* [Internet]. 2014 Jan 9 [cited 2021 Apr 4];8(5):607–618. Available from: https://doi.org/10.1586/erv.09.19 doi: 10.1586/erv.09.19.

18. Budimir N, Meijerhof T, Wilschut J, Huckriede A, de Haan A. The role of membrane fusion activity of a whole inactivated influenza virus vaccine in (re)activation of influenza-specific cytotoxic T lymphocytes. *Vaccine* [Internet]. 2010 Dec 6 [cited 2021 Apr 4];28(52):8280–8287. Available from: https://doi.org/10.1016/j.vaccine.2010.10.007 doi: 10.1016/j.vaccine.2010.10.007.

19. Hartman FW, LoGrippo GA. Betapropiolactone in sterilization of vaccines, tissue grafts, and plasma. *Journal of American Medical Association* [Internet]. 1957 May 18 [cited 2021 Apr 4];164(3):258–260. Available from: https://doi.org/10.1001/jama.1957.02980030034008 doi: 10.1001/jama.1957.02980030034008.

20. Fan C, Ye X, Ku Z, Kong L, Liu Q, Xu C, *et al.* Beta-propiolactone inactivation of coxsackievirus A16 induces structural alteration and surface modification of viral capsids. *Journal of Virology* [Internet]. 2017 Mar 29 [cited 2021 Apr 4];91(8):e00038-17. Available from: https://dx.doi.org/10.1128%2FJVI.00038-17 doi: 10.1128/JVI.00038-17.

21. Ganneru B, Jogdand H, Dharam VK, Molugu NR, Prasad SD, Vellimudu S, *et al.* Evaluation of safety and immunogenicity of an adjuvanted, TH-1 skewed, whole virion inactivated SARS-CoV-2 vaccine — BBV152. *BioRxiv* [Preprint]. 2020 Sep 12 [cited 2021 Apr 4]. Available from: 10.1101/2020.09.09.285445 doi: https://doi.org/10.1101/2020.09.09.285445.

22. Lindblad EB. Aluminium compounds for use in vaccines. *Immunology and Cell Biology* [Internet]. 2004 Oct 1 [cited 2021 Apr 4];82(5):497–505. Available from: https://doi.org/10.1111/j.0818-9641.2004.01286.x doi: 10.1111/j.0818-9641.2004.01286.x.

23. Ella R, Reddy S, Jogdand H, Sarangi V, Ganneru B, Prasad S, *et al.* Safety and immunogenicity of an inactivated SARS-CoV-2 vaccine, BBV152: Interim results from a double-blind, randomised, multicentre, phase 2 trial, and 3-month follow-up of a double-blind, randomised phase 1 trial. *Lancet Infectious Diseases* [Internet]. 2021 Mar 8 [cited 2021 Apr 4];S1473-3099(21):00070-0. Available from: https://doi.org/10.1016/s1473-3099(21)00070-0 doi: 10.1016/S1473-3099(21)00070-0.

24. HogenEsch H, O'Hagan DT, Fox CB. Optimizing the utilization of aluminum adjuvants in vaccines: You might just get what you want. *NPJ Vaccines* [Internet]. 2018 Oct 10 [cited 2021 Apr 4];3(51). Available from: https://doi.org/10.1038/s41541-018-0089-x doi: 10.1038/s41541-018-0089-x.

25. Hogenesch H. Mechanism of immunopotentiation and safety of aluminum adjuvants. *Frontiers in Immunology* [Internet]. 2013 Jan 10 [cited 2021 Apr 4];3:Article 406. Available from: https://doi.org/10.3389/fimmu.2012.00406 doi: 10.3389/fimmu.2012.00406.

26. Nunnally BK, Turula VE, Sitrin RD. Inactivated Viral Vaccines. Vaccine Analysis: Strategies, Principles, and Control [Internet]. 2014 Nov 28 [cited 2021 Apr 4]:45–80. Available from: https://dx.doi.org/10.1007%2F978-3-662-45024-6_2 doi: 10.1007/978-3-662-45024-6_2.

27. Rauch S, Jasny E, Schmidt KE, Petsch B. New vaccine technologies to combat outbreak situations. *Frontiers in Immunology* [Internet]. 2018 Sep 19 [cited 2021 Apr 4];9:Article 1963. Available from: https://doi.org/10.3389/fimmu.2018.01963 doi: 10.3389/fimmu.2018.01963.

28. Palacios R, Patiño EG, de Oliveira Piorelli R, Conde MTRP, Batista AP, Zeng G, *et al.* Double-blind, randomized, placebo-controlled phase III clinical trial to evaluate the efficacy and safety of treating healthcare professionals with the adsorbed COVID-19 (inactivated) vaccine manufactured by Sinovac. Trials [Internet]. 2020 Oct 15 [cited 2021 Apr 4];21(1):Article 853. Available from: https://doi.org/10.1186/s13063-020-04775-4 doi: 10.1186/s13063-020-04775-4.

29. Sinopharm. 【中共中央纪律检查委员会】探访北京新冠疫苗生产现场 [Internet]. [place unknown]: Sinopharm; 2020 Dec 30 [cited 2021 Apr 4]. Available from: http://www.sinopharm.com/s/1223-4126-38871.html.

30. Bharat Biotech. COVAXIN® — India's First Indigenous COVID-19 Vaccine [Internet]. [place unknown]: Bharat Biotech; 2021 [cited 2021 Apr 4]. Available from: https://www.bharatbiotech.com/covaxin.html.

31. Zhang Y, Zeng G, Pan H, Li C, Hu Y, Chu K, *et al.* Safety, tolerability, and immunogenicity of an inactivated SARS-CoV-2 vaccine in healthy adults aged 18–59 years: A randomised, double-blind, placebo-controlled, phase 1/2 clinical trial. *Lancet Infectious Diseases* [Internet]. 2020 Nov 17 [cited 2021 Apr 4];21(2):181–192. Available from: https://doi.org/10.1016/S1473-3099(20)30843-4 doi: 10.1016/S1473-3099(20)30843-4.

32. Sinovac. 北京科兴中维生物技术有限公司新冠灭活疫苗克尔来福®获批附条件上市 [Internet]. [place unknown]: Sinovac; 2021 Feb 6 [cited 2021 Apr 4]. Available from: http://www.sinovac.com.cn/?optionid=468&auto_id=1872.

33. Clinical Trial of Efficacy and Safety of Sinovac's Adsorbed COVID-19 (Inactivated) Vaccine in Healthcare Professionals (PROFISCOV). 2020 Jul 2 [cited 2021 Apr 4]. In: ClinicalTrials.gov [Internet]. Bethesda (MD): National Library of Medicine (US). 2000 Feb 29 - . Available from: https://clinicaltrials.gov/ct2/show/NCT04456595?term=vaccine&cond=covid-19&draw=2 ClinicalTrials.gov Identifier: NCT04456595.

34. Efficacy, Safety and Immunogenicity Study of SARS-CoV-2 Inactivated Vaccine (COVID-19). 2020 Aug 11 [cited 2021 Apr 4]. In: ClinicalTrials.gov [Internet]. Bethesda (MD): National Library of Medicine (US). 2000 Feb 29 - . Available from: https://clinicaltrials.gov/ct2/show/NCT04508075 ClinicalTrials.gov Identifier: NCT04508075.

35. Clinical Trial For SARS-CoV-2 Vaccine (COVID-19). 2020 Oct 9 [cited 2021 Apr 4]. In: ClinicalTrials.gov [Internet]. Bethesda (MD): National Library of Medicine. 2000 Feb 29 - . Available from: https://clinicaltrials.gov/ct2/show/NCT04582344 ClinicalTrials.gov Identifier: NCT04582344.

36. Reuters Staff. Turkish study revises down Sinovac COVID-19 vaccine efficacy to 83.5% [Internet]. Istanbul: Reuters; 2021 Mar 3 [cited 2021 Apr 4]. Available from: https://www.reuters.com/article/idUSL5N2L12O7.

37. Mallapaty S. China COVID vaccine reports mixed results — what does that mean for the pandemic? [Internet]. [place unknown]: *Nature*. 2021 Jan 15 [cited 2021 Apr 4]. Available from: https://www.nature.com/articles/d41586-021-00094-z.

38. A Study to Evaluate The efficacy, safety and immunogenicity of inactivated SARS-CoV-2 vaccines (Vero Cell) in healthy population aged 18 years old and above (COVID-19). 2020 Aug 12 [cited 2021 Apr 4]. In: ClinicalTrials.gov [Internet]. Bethesda (MD): National Library of Medicine (US). 2000 Feb 29 - . Available from: https://clinicaltrials.gov/ct2/show/NCT04510207 ClinicalTrials.gov Identifier: NCT04510207.

39. Clinical trial to evaluate the efficacy, immunogenicity and safety of the inactivated SARS-CoV-2 Vaccine (COVID-19). 2020 Sep 23 [cited 2021 Apr 4]. In: ClinicalTrials.gov [Internet]. Bethesda (MD): National Library of Medicine (US). 2000 Feb 29 - . Available from: https://clinicaltrials.gov/ct2/show/NCT04560881?term=vaccine&cond=covid-19&draw=2 ClinicalTrials.gov Identifier: NCT04560881.

40. Efficacy, safety and immunogenicity of inactivated SARS-CoV-2 vaccines (Vero Cell) in healthy adult population in Peru (Cov-Peru). 2020 Nov 3 [cited 2021 Apr 4]. In: ClinicalTrials.gov [Internet]. Bethesda (MD): National Library of Medicine (US). 2000 Feb 29 - . Available from:

https://clinicaltrials.gov/ct2/show/NCT04612972 ClinicalTrials.gov Identifier: NCT04612972.

41. Wuhan Institute of Biological Products. 国药集团中国生物武汉生物制品研究所新冠灭活疫苗III期临床试验期中分析数据发布 [Internet]. [place unknown]: Sinopharm; 2021 Feb 24 [cited 2021 Apr 4]. Available from: http://www.wibp.com.cn/Chs/Detail.aspx?Id=14669.

42. Bharat Biotech. Bharat Biotech Announces Phase 3 Results of COVAXIN®: India's First COVID-19 Vaccine Demonstrates Interim Clinical [Internet]. Hyderabad: Bharat Biotech; 2021 Mar 3 [cited 2021 Apr 4]. Available from: https://www.bharatbiotech.com/images/press/covaxin-phase3-efficacy-results.pdf.

43. Novavax, Inc. Novavax confirms high levels of efficacy against original and variant COVID-19 strains in United Kingdom and South Africa trials [Internet]. [place unknown]: Novavax; 2021 Mar 11 [cited 2021 Apr 4]. Available from: https://ir.novavax.com/news-releases/news-release-details/novavax-confirms-high-levels-efficacy-against-original-and-0.

44. Keech C, Albert G, Cho I, Robertson A, Reed P, Neal S, *et al*. Phase 1–2 trial of a SARS-CoV-2 recombinant spike protein nanoparticle vaccine. *New England Journal of Medicine* [Internet]. 2020 Dec 20 [cited 2021 Apr 4];383(24):2320–2332. Available from: https://www.nejm.org/doi/full/10.1056/NEJMoa2026920 doi: 10.1056/NEJMoa2026920.

45. Salvatori G, Luberto L, Maffei M, Aurisicchio L, Roscilli G, Palombo F, *et al*. SARS-CoV-2 SPIKE PROTEIN: An optimal immunological target for vaccines. *Journal of Translational Medicine* [Internet]. 2020 Jun 3 [cited 2021 Apr 4];18:Article 222. Available from: https://doi.org/10.1186/s12967-020-02392-y doi: 10.1186/s12967-020-02392-y.

46. Dai L, Gao GF. Viral targets for vaccines against COVID-19. *Nature Review Immunology* [Internet]. 2021 Feb [cited 2021 Apr 4];21(2):73–82. Available from: https://doi.org/10.1038/s41577-020-00480-0 doi: 10.1038/s41577-020-00480-0.

47. Wrapp D, Wang N, Corbett KS, Goldsmith JA, Hsieh CL, Abiona O, *et al*. Cryo-EM structure of the 2019-nCoV spike in the prefusion conformation. *Science* [Internet]. 2020 Mar 13 [cited 2021 Apr 4];367(6483):1260-1263. Available from: https://doi.org/10.1126/science.abb2507 doi: 10.1126/science.abb2507.

48. Tian JH, Patel N, Haupt R, Zhou H, Weston S, Hammond H, *et al*. SARS-CoV-2 spike glycoprotein vaccine candidate NVX-CoV2373 immunogenicity in baboons and protection in mice. *Nature Communication* [Internet].

2021 Jan 14 [cited 2021 Apr 4];12:Article 372. Available from: https://www.nature.com/articles/s41467-020-20653-8 doi: 10.1038/s41467-020-20653-8.

49. Kost TA, Condreay JP, Jarvis DL. Baculovirus as versatile vectors for protein expression in insect and mammalian cells. *Nature Biotechnology* [Internet]. 2005 May 5 [cited 2021 Apr 4];23(5):567–575. Available from: https://doi.org/10.1038/nbt1095 doi: 10.1038/nbt1095.

50. Bangaru S, Ozorowski G, Turner HL, Antanasijevic A, Huang D, Wang X, *et al*. Structural analysis of full-length SARS-CoV-2 spike protein from an advanced vaccine candidate. Science [Internet]. 2020 Nov 27 [cited 2021 Apr 4];370(6520):1089-1094. Available from: https://science.sciencemag.org/content/370/6520/1089 doi: 10.1126/science.abe1502.

51. Novavax. Matrix-M™ adjuvant technology [Internet]. [place unknown]: Novavax; [cited 2021 Apr 4]. Available from: https://www.novavax.com/our-unique-technology#matrix-m-adjuvant-technology.

52. Bengtsson KL, Song H, Stertman L, Liu Y, Flyer DC, Massare MJ, *et al*. Matrix-M adjuvant enhances antibody, cellular and protective immune responses of a Zaire Ebola/Makona virus glycoprotein (GP) nanoparticle vaccine in mice. *Vaccine* [Internet]. 2016 Apr 7 [cited 2021 Apr 4]; 34(16):1927–1935. Available from: https://doi.org/10.1016/j.vaccine.2016.02.033 doi: 10.1016/j.vaccine.2016.02.033.

53. Rospotrebnadzor. ТОП-20 вопросов о вакцине ФБУН ГНЦ ВБ «Вектор» [Internet]. [place unknown]: Rospotrebnadzor; 2021 Mar 5 [cited 2021 Apr 4]. Available from: https://www.rospotrebnadzor.ru/about/info/news/news_details.php?ELEMENT_ID=15649&sphrase_id=3178707.

54. Chakraborty S, Mallajosyula V, Tato CM, Tan GS, Wang TT. SARS-CoV-2 vaccines in advanced clinical trials: Where do we stand? *Advance Drug Delivery Reviews* [Internet]. 2021 Jan 20 [cited 2021 Apr 4];172:314–338. Available from: https://doi.org/10.1016/j.addr.2021.01.014 doi: 10.1016/j.addr.2021.01.014.

55. A study looking at the effectiveness, immune response, and safety of a COVID-19 vaccine in adults in the United Kingdom. 2020 Oct 12 [cited 2021 Apr 4]. In: ClinicalTrials.gov [Internet]. Bethesda (MD): National Library of Medicine (US). 2000 Feb 29 - . Available from: https://clinicaltrials.gov/ct2/show/NCT04583995 ClinicalTrials.gov Identifier: NCT04583995.

56. Ryzhikov AB, Ryzhikov EA, Bogryantseva MP, Usova SV, Danilenko ED, Nechaeva EA, *et al*. A simple, blind, placebo-controlled, randomized study

of the safety, reactogenicity and immunogenicity of the "EpiVacCorona" vaccine for the prevention of COVID-19 in volunteers aged 18–60 years (phase I-II). *Russian Journal of Infection and Immunity* [Internet]. 2021 [cited 2021 Apr 4];11(2):283–296. Available from: https://doi.org/10. 15789/2220-7619-ASB-1699 doi: 10.15789/2220-7619-ASB-1699.

57. Voysey M, Clemens SAC, Madhi SA, Weckx LY, Folegatti PM, Aley PK, *et al.* Safety and efficacy of the ChAdOx1 nCoV-19 vaccine (AZD1222) against SARS-CoV-2: An interim analysis of four randomised controlled trials in Brazil, South Africa, and the UK. *Lancet* [Internet]. 2021 Jan 9 [cited 2021 Apr 4];397(10269):99–111. Available from: https://doi.org/10. 1016/S0140-6736(20)32661-1 doi: 10.1016/S0140-6736(20)32661-1.

58. Sadoff J, Le Gars M, Shukarev G, Heerwegh D, Truyers C, de Groot AM, *et al.* Interim results of a phase 1–2a trial of Ad26.COV2.S Covid-19 vaccine. *New England Journal of Medicine* [Internet]. 2021 Jan 13 [cited 2021 Apr 4]:NEJMoa2034201. Available from: https://doi.org/10.1056/ nejmoa2034201 doi: 10.1056/NEJMoa2034201.

59. Logunov DY, Dolzhikova IV, Shcheblyakov DV, Tukhvatulin AI, Zubkova OV, Dzharullaeva AS, *et al.* Safety and efficacy of an rAd26 and rAd5 vector-based heterologous prime-boost COVID-19 vaccine: An interim analysis of a randomised controlled phase 3 trial in Russia. *Lancet* [Internet]. 2021 Feb 20 [cited 2021 Apr 4];397(10275):671–681. Available from: https://doi.org/10.1016/s0140-6736(21)00234-8 doi: 10.1016/ S0140-6736(21)00234-8.

60. Zhu FC, Guan XH, Li YH, Huang JY, Jiang T, Hou LH, *et al.* Immunogenicity and safety of a recombinant adenovirus type-5-vectored COVID-19 vaccine in healthy adults aged 18 years or older: A randomised, double-blind, placebo-controlled, phase 2 trial. *Lancet* [Internet]. 2020 Aug 15 [cited 2021 Apr 4];396(10249):479–488. Available from: https://doi.org/10.1016/ s0140-6736(20)31605-6 doi: 10.1016/S0140-6736(20)31605-6.

61. Centers for Disease Control and Prevention. Adenoviruses [Internet]. [place unknown]: CDC; 2019 Aug 28 [cited 2021 Apr 4]. Available from: https:// www.cdc.gov/adenovirus/index.html#:~:text=Adenoviruses%20are%20 common%20viruses%20that,adenovirus%20infection%20at%20any%20 age.

62. Gregory SM, Nazir SA, Metcalf JP. Implications of the innate immune response to adenovirus and adenoviral vectors. *Future Virology* [Internet]. 2011 Mar 31 [cited 2021 Apr 4];6(3):357–374. Available from: https://doi. org/10.2217/fvl.11.6 doi: 10.2217/fvl.11.6.

63. Ahi YS, Bangari DS, Mittal SK. Adenoviral vector immunity: Its implications and circumvention strategies. *Current Gene Therapy* [Internet]. 2011 Aug [cited 2021 Apr 4];11(4):307–320. Available from: https://doi.org/10.2174/156652311796150372 doi: 10.2174/156652311796150372.

64. Thacker EE, Timares L, Matthews QL. Strategies to overcome host immunity to adenovirus vectors in vaccine development. *Expert Review Vaccines* [Internet]. 2009 Jun [cited 2021 Apr 4];8(6):761–777. Available from: https://doi.org/10.1586/erv.09.29 doi: 10.1586/erv.09.29.

65. Barouch DH, Kik SV, Weverling GJ, Dilan R, King SL, Maxfield LF, *et al*. International seroepidemiology of Adenovirus serotypes 5, 26, 35, and 48 in pediatric and adult populations. *Vaccine* [Internet]. 2011 Jul 18 [cited 2021 Apr 4];29(32):5203–5209. Available from: https://doi-org.ezproxy.library.ubc.ca/10.1016/j.vaccine.2011.05.025 doi: 10.1016/j.vaccine.2011.05.025.

66. Stephen SL, Montini E, Sivanandam VG, Al-Dhalimy M, Kestler HA, Finegold M, *et al*. Chromosomal Integration of Adenoviral Vector DNA In Vivo. *Journal of Virology* [Internet]. 2010 Oct [cited 2021 Apr 4]; 84(19):9987–9994. Available from: https://doi.org/10.1128/jvi.00751-10 doi: 10.1128/JVI.00751-10.

67. Hillgenberg M, Tönnies H, Strauss M. Chromosomal Integration pattern of a helper-dependent minimal adenovirus vector with a selectable marker inserted into a 27.4-kilobase genomic stuffer. *Journal of Virology* [Internet]. 2001 Oct 15 [cited 2021 Apr 4];75(20):9896–9908. Available from: https://doi.org/10.1128/JVI.75.20.9896-9908.2001 doi: 10.1128/JVI.75.20.9896–9908.2001.

68. Janssen Therapeutics. Storage, Dosage and Administration [Internet]. [place unknown]: Janssen Therapeutics, Division of Janssen Products, LP; 2021 Feb 27 [cited 2021 Apr 4]. Available from: https://www.janssencovid19vaccine.com/hcp/storage-dosing-administration.html.

69. CanSinoBIO. 康希诺生物新冠疫苗克威莎TM附条件上市申请获得国家药品监督管理局受理 [Internet]. Tianjin: CanSinoBIO; 2021 Feb 24 [cited 2021 Apr 4]. Available from: http://www.cansinotech.com.cn/html/1/179/180/806.html.

70. Bos R, Rutten L, van der Lubbe JEM, Bakkers MJG, Hardenberg G, Wegmann F, *et al*. Ad26 vector-based COVID-19 vaccine encoding a prefusion-stabilized SARS-CoV-2 Spike immunogen induces potent humoral and cellular immune responses. *NPJ Vaccines* [Internet]. 2020 Sep 28 [cited 2021 Apr 4];5:Article 91. Available from: https://doi.org/10.1038/s41541-020-00243-x doi: 10.1038/s41541-020-00243-x.

71. A Study of Ad26.COV2.S for the Prevention of SARS-CoV-2-Mediated COVID-19 in Adult Participants (ENSEMBLE). 2020 Aug 10 [cited 2021 Apr 4]. In: ClinicalTrials.gov [Internet]. Bethesda (MD): National Library of Medicine (US). 2000 Feb 29 - . Available from: https://clinicaltrials.gov/ct2/show/study/NCT04505722 ClinicalTrials.gov Identifier: NCT04505722.

72. Janssen Therapeutics. Clinical Trial Data for the Janssen COVID-19 Vaccine [Internet]. [place unknown]: Janssen Therapeutics, Division of Janssen Products, LP; 2021 [cited 2021 Apr 4]. Available from: https://www.janssencovid19vaccine.com/hcp/clinical-trial-data.html.

73. Zhu FC, Li YH, Guan XH, Hou LH, Wang WJ, Li JX, *et al.* Safety, tolerability, and immunogenicity of a recombinant adenovirus type-5 vectored COVID-19 vaccine: A dose-escalation, open-label, non-randomised, first-in-human trial. *Lancet* [Internet]. 2020 Jun 13 [cited 2021 Apr 4]; 395(10240):1845–1854. Available from: https://doi.org/10.1016/s0140-6736(20)31208-3 doi: 10.1016/S0140-6736(20)31208-3.

74. Voysey M, Clemens SAC, Madhi SA, Weckx LY, Folegatti PM, Aley PK, *et al.* Single-dose administration and the influence of the timing of the booster dose on immunogenicity and efficacy of ChAdOx1 nCoV-19 (AZD1222) vaccine: A pooled analysis of four randomised trials. *Lancet* [Internet]. 2021 Mar 6 [cited 2021 Apr 4];397(10277):881–891. Available from: https://doi.org/10.1016/s0140-6736(21)00432-3 doi: 10.1016/S0140-6736(21)00432-3.

75. Barrett JR, Belij-Rammerstorfer S, Dold C, Ewer KJ, Folegatti PM, Gilbride C, *et al.* Phase 1/2 trial of SARS-CoV-2 vaccine ChAdOx1 nCoV-19 with a booster dose induces multifunctional antibody responses. *Nature Medicines* [Internet]. 2021 Feb [cited 2021 Apr 4];27(2):279–288. Available from: https://doi.org/10.1038/s41591-020-01179-4 doi:10.1038/s41591-020-01179-4.

76. Phase III Double-blind, Placebo-controlled Study of AZD1222 for the Prevention of COVID-19 in Adults. 2020 Aug 18 [cited 2021 Apr 4]. In: ClinicalTrials.gov [Internet]. Bethesda (MD): National Library of Medicine (US). 2000 Feb 29 - . Available from: https://clinicaltrials.gov/ct2/show/NCT04516746?term=astrazeneca&cond=covid-19&draw=2 ClinicalTrials.gov Identifier: NCT04516746.

77. Kemp A. AZD1222 US Phase III primary analysis confirms safety and efficacy [Internet]. [place unknown]: AstraZeneca; 2021 Mar 25 [cited 2021 Apr 4]. Available from: https://www.astrazeneca.com/media-centre/press-releases/2021/azd1222-us-phase-iii-primary-analysis-confirms-safety-and-efficacy.html.

78. Bernal JL, Andrews N, Gower C, Stowe J, Robertson C, Tessier E, *et al*. Early effectiveness of COVID-19 vaccination with BNT162b2 mRNA vaccine and ChAdOx1 adenovirus vector vaccine on symptomatic disease, hospitalisations and mortality in older adults in England. *medRxiv* [Preprint]. 2021 Mar 2 [cited 2021 Apr 17]. Available from: https://www. medrxiv.org/content/10.1101/2021.03.01.21252652v1 doi: 10.1101/2021. 03.01.21252652.

79. Vasileiou E, Simpson CR, Robertson C, Shi T, Kerr S, Agrawal U, *et al*. Effectiveness of first dose of COVID-19 vaccines against hospital admissions in Scotland: National prospective cohort study of 5.4 million people. *SSRN* [Preprint]. 2021 Feb 19 [cited 2021 Apr 17]. Available from: https:// ssrn.com/abstract=3789264 doi: 10.2139/ssrn.3789264.

80. Clinical Trial of Efficacy, Safety, and Immunogenicity of Gam-COVID-Vac Vaccine Against COVID-19 (RESIST). 2020 Aug 28 [cited 2021 Apr 4]. In: ClinicalTrials.gov [Internet]. Bethesda (MD): National Library of Medicine (US). 2000 Feb 29 - . Available from: https://clinicaltrials.gov/ct2/show/ NCT04530396 ClinicalTrials.gov Identifier: NCT04530396.

81. Polack FP, Thomas SJ, Kitchin N, Absalon J, Gurtman A, Lockhart S, *et al*. Safety and Efficacy of the BNT162b2 mRNA Covid-19 Vaccine. *New England J Journal of Medicine* [Internet]. 2020 Dec 31 [cited 2021 Apr 4]; 383(27):2603–2615. Available from: https://doi.org/10.1056/nejmoa 2034577 doi: 10.1056/NEJMoa2034577.

82. Baden LR, El Sahly HM, Essink B, Kotloff K, Frey S, Novak R, *et al*. Efficacy and Safety of the mRNA-1273 SARS-CoV-2 Vaccine. *New England J Journal of Medicine* [Internet]. 2021 Feb 4 [cited 2021 Apr 4];384(5):403–416. Available from: https://doi.org/10.1056/nejmoa2035389 doi: 10.1056/NEJMoa2035389.

83. Corbett KS, Edwards DK, Leist SR, Abiona OM, Boyoglu-Barnum S, Gillespie RA, *et al*. SARS-CoV-2 mRNA vaccine design enabled by prototype pathogen preparedness. *Nature* [Internet]. 2020 Oct 22 [cited 2021 Apr 4];586(7830):567–571. Available from: https://doi.org/10.1038/ s41586-020-2622-0 doi: 10.1038/s41586-020-2622-0.

84. Walsh EE, Frenck Jr RW, Falsey AR, Kitchin N, Absalon J, Gurtman A, *et al*. Safety and Immunogenicity of Two RNA-Based COVID-19 Vaccine Candidates. *New England J Journal of Medicine* [Internet]. 2020 Dec 17 [cited 2021 Apr 4];383(25):2439-2450. Available from: https://doi. org/10.1056/nejmoa2027906 doi: 10.1056/NEJMoa2027906.

85. Pardi N, Tuyishime S, Muramatsu H, Kariko K, Mui BL, Tam YK, *et al*. Expression kinetics of nucleoside-modified mRNA delivered in lipid

nanoparticles to mice by various routes. *Journal of Control Release* [Internet]. 2015 Nov 10 [cited 2021 Apr 4];217:345–351. Available from: https://doi.org/10.1016/j.jconrel.2015.08.007 doi: 10.1016/j.jconrel. 2015.08.007.

86. Jackson NAC, Kester KE, Casimiro D, Gurunathan S, DeRosa F. The promise of mRNA vaccines: A biotech and industrial perspective. *NPJ Vaccines* [Internet]. 2020 Feb 4 [cited 2021 Apr 4];5:Article 11. Available from: https://doi.org/10.1038/s41541-020-0159-8 doi: 10.1038/s41541-020-0159-8.

87. Pfizer Canada ULC. Pfizer-BioNTech COVID-19 Vaccine [COVID-19 mRNA Vaccine] Product Monograph [Internet]. Kirkland (QC): Health Canada; 2021 Mar 3 [cited 2021 Apr 4]. Available from: https://covid-vaccine.canada.ca/info/pdf/pfizer-biontech-covid-19-vaccine-pm1-en.pdf.

88. Moderna US, Inc. Fact sheet for healthcare providers administering vaccine (vaccination providers) [Internet]. Cambridge (MA): ModernaTX, Inc.; 2021 Mar 31 [cited 2021 Apr 4]. Available from: https://www.modernatx. com/covid19vaccine-eua/eua-fact-sheet-providers.pdf.

89. Study to Describe the Safety, Tolerability, Immunogenicity, and Efficacy of RNA Vaccine Candidates Against COVID-19 in Healthy Individuals. 2020 Apr 30 [cited 2021 Apr 4]. In: ClinicalTrials.gov [Internet]. Bethesda (MD): National Library of Medicine (US). 2000 Feb 29 - . Available from: https://clinicaltrials.gov/ct2/show/study/NCT04368728 ClinicalTrials.gov Identifier: NCT04368728.

90. Pfizer Inc., BioNTech SE. Pfizer and BioNTech confirm high efficacy and no serious safety concerns through up to six months following second dose in updated topline analysis of landmark COVID-19 vaccine study [Internet]. New York (NY): Business Wire; 2021 Apr 1 [cited 2021 Apr 4]. Available from: https://www.businesswire.com/news/home/2021040100 5365/en/.

91. Pfizer-BioNTech, The Israel Ministry of Health. Real-world evidence confirms high effectiveness of Pfizer-Biontech COVID-19 vaccine and profound public health impact of vaccination one year after pandemic declared [Internet]. Jerusalem: Pfizer Inc.; 2021 Mar 11 [cited 2021 Apr 17]. Available from: https://www.businesswire.com/news/home/2021031100 5482/en/.

92. Hall V, Foulkes S, Saei A, Andrews N, Oguti B, Charlett A, *et al.* Effectiveness of BNT162b2 mRNA vaccine against infection and COVID-19 vaccine coverage in healthcare workers in England, multicentre prospective cohort study (the SIREN Study). *SSRN* [Preprint]. 2021 Feb 22

[cited 2021 Apr 17]. Available from: https://ssrn.com/abstract=3790399 doi: 10.2139/ssrn.3790399.

93. Thompson MG, Burgess JL, Naleway AL, Tyner HL, Yoon SK, Meece J, *et al.* Interim estimates of vaccine effectiveness of BNT162b2 and mRNA-1273 COVID-19 vaccines in preventing SARS-CoV-2 infection among health care personnel, first responders, and other essential and frontline workers — eight U.S. locations. MMWR Morbidity and Mortality Weekly Report [Internet]. 2021 Apr 2 [cited 2021 Apr 17];70(13):495–500. Available from: https://www.cdc.gov/mmwr/volumes/70/wr/mm7013e3.htm?s_cid=mm7013e3_w#T2_down doi: 10.15585/mmwr.mm7013e3.

94. A study to evaluate efficacy, safety, and immunogenicity of mRNA-1273 vaccine in adults aged 18 years and older to prevent COVID-19. 2020 Jul 14 [cited 2021 Apr 4]. In: ClinicalTrials.gov [Internet]. Bethesda (MD): National Library of Medicine (US). 2000 Feb 29 - . Available from: https://clinicaltrials.gov/ct2/show/NCT04470427 ClinicalTrials.gov Identifier: NCT04470427.

95. Phase III trial of a COVID-19 vaccine of adenovirus vector in adults 18 years old and above. 2020 Aug 26 [cited 2021 Apr 4]. In: ClinicalTrials.gov [Internet]. Bethesda (MD): National Library of Medicine (US). 2000 Feb 29 - . Available from: https://clinicaltrials.gov/ct2/show/NCT04526990?term=vaccine&cond=covid-19&draw=6 ClinicalTrials.gov Identifier: NCT04526990.

96. AstraZeneca Canada Inc. AstraZeneca COVID-19 Vaccine Product Monograph [Internet]. Mississauga (ON): Health Canada; 2021 Mar 24 [cited 2021 Apr 4]. Available from: https://covid-vaccine.canada.ca/info/pdf/astrazeneca-covid-19-vaccine-pm-en.pdf.

97. A study of a candidate COVID-19 vaccine (COV001). 2020 Mar 27 [cited 2021 Apr 4]. In: ClinicalTrials.gov [Internet]. Bethesda (MD): National Library of Medicine (US). 2000 Feb 29 - . Available from: https://clinical-trials.gov/ct2/show/NCT04324606 ClinicalTrials.gov Identifier: NCT04324606.

98. Investigating a vaccine against COVID-19. 2020 May 26 [cited 2021 Apr 4]. In: ClinicalTrials.gov [Internet]. Bethesda (MD): National Library of Medicine (US). 2000 Feb 29 - . Available from: https://clinicaltrials.gov/ct2/show/NCT04400838 ClinicalTrials.gov Identifier: NCT04400838.

99. A phase III study to investigate a vaccine against COVID-19. 2020 Jun 11 [cited 2021 Apr 4]. In: *ISRCTN registry* [Internet]. London: BMC. [date unknown] - . Available from: https://www.isrctn.com/ISRCTN89951424 ISRCTN Identifier: ISRCTN89951424.

100. COVID-19 vaccine (ChAdOx1 nCoV-19) trial in south african adults with and without hiv-infection. 2020 Jun 23 [cited 2021 Apr 4]. In: ClinicalTrials.gov [Internet]. Bethesda (MD): National Library of Medicine (US). 2000 Feb 29 - . Available from: https://clinicaltrials.gov/ct2/show/NCT04444674 ClinicalTrials.gov Identifier: NCT04444674.

101. Phase III clinical trial for inactivated novel coronavirus pneumonia (COVID-19) vaccine (Vero cells). 2020 Jul 18 [cited 2021 Apr 4]. In: *Chinese Clinical Trial Register* [Internet]. Chengdu (Sichuan): Ministry of Health (China). 2007 Jun 27 - . Available from: http://www.chictr.org.cn/showprojen.aspx?proj=56651 ClinicalTrials.gov Identifier: ChiCTR2000 034780.

102. A Phase III clinical trial for inactivated novel coronavirus pneumonia (COVID-19) vaccine (Vero cells). 2020 Oct 13 [cited 2021 Apr 4]. In: *Chinese Clinical Trial Register* [Internet]. Chengdu (Sichuan): Ministry of Health (China). 2007 Jun 27 - . Available from: http://www.chictr.org.cn/showprojen.aspx?proj=62581 ChiCTR Identifier: ChiCTR200003 9000.

103. An efficacy and safety clinical trial of an investigational COVID-19 vaccine (BBV152) in adult volunteers. 2020 Nov 23 [cited 2021 Apr 4]. In: ClinicalTrials.gov [Internet]. Bethesda (MD): National Library of Medicine (US). 2000 Feb 29 - . Available from: https://clinicaltrials.gov/ct2/show/NCT04641481 ClinicalTrials.gov Identifier: NCT04641481.

104. A study looking at the efficacy, immune response, and safety of a COVID-19 vaccine in adults at risk for SARS-CoV-2. 2020 Nov 2 [cited 2021 Apr 4]. In: ClinicalTrials.gov [Internet]. Bethesda (MD): National Library of Medicine (US). 2000 Feb 29 - . Available from: https://clinicaltrials.gov/ct2/show/NCT04611802?term=NCT04611802&draw=2&rank=1 ClinicalTrials.gov Identifier: NCT04611802.

105. Novavax, Inc. Novavax confirms high levels of NVX-CoV2373 vaccine efficacy against original and variant COVID-19 strains in United Kingdom and South Africa trials [Internet]. [place unknown]: Novavax; 2021 Mar 11 [cited 2021 Apr 4]. Available from: https://cdn.filestackcontent.com/ElibilscTt6AxPbxRugu.

106. A study looking at the effectiveness and safety of a COVID-19 vaccine in South African adults. 2020 Aug 31 [cited 2021 Apr 4]. In: ClinicalTrials.gov [Internet]. Bethesda (MD): National Library of Medicine (US). 2000 Feb 29 - . Available from: https://clinicaltrials.gov/ct2/show/NCT04533399?term=vaccine&cond=covid-19&draw=7 ClinicalTrials.gov Identifier: NCT04533399.

107. Study of the tolerability, safety, immunogenicity and preventive efficacy of the EpiVacCorona vaccine for the prevention of COVID-19. 2021 Mar 3 [cited 2021 Apr 4]. In: ClinicalTrials.gov [Internet]. Bethesda (MD): National Library of Medicine (US). 2000 Feb 29 - . Available from: https:// clinicaltrials.gov/ct2/show/NCT04780035 ClinicalTrials.gov Identifier: NCT04780035.

108. A study of Ad26.COV2.S for the prevention of SARS-CoV-2-mediated COVID-19 in adults (ENSEMBLE 2). 2020 Nov 4 [cited 2021 Apr 4]. In: ClinicalTrials.gov [Internet]. Bethesda (MD): National Library of Medicine (US). 2000 Feb 29 - . Available from: https://clinicaltrials.gov/ct2/show/ NCT04614948 ClinicalTrials.gov Identifier: NCT04614948.

Chapter 14

Vaccine Allocation and Prioritisation

Mara Balvers* and **Monika Naus**[*,†]

*School of Population and Public Health, University of British Columbia,
Vancouver, Canada*

†*Communicable Diseases & Immunization Service,
BC Centre for Disease Control, Vancouver, Canada*

Key Message

- COVID-19 vaccine allocation is a complex and dynamic process: complex due to limited vaccine supply and the differential impact of COVID-19 on certain populations, and dynamic since the virus and environment are constantly evolving.
- Vaccine nationalism directly opposes global vaccine equity: ineffective COVID-19 vaccine allocation due to vaccine nationalism results in preventable deaths, most pre-dominantly in low- and middle-income countries (LMICs). COVAX is a global initiative aimed at promoting global vaccine equity and combating vaccine nationalism, through subsidised allocation of vaccine to LMICs.
- Vaccine allocation frameworks, such as the WHO framework for allocation and prioritisation of COVID-19 vaccination, have helped guide vaccine prioritisation decisions. Other strategies such as

mathematical modelling and epidemiological research have further been used to identify risk factors of severe outcomes and predict mortality-minimising allocation strategies.

- Logistical challenges of vaccine distribution, rising levels of transmission and variants of concern (VOC), and vaccine hesitancy are just a few examples of the barriers to achieving widespread coverage of COVID-19 vaccination.

- Critical analysis of different vaccine allocation strategies and vaccine rollouts of varying success within and between countries is important for informing future allocation decisions as the COVID-19 pandemic continues.

1. Introduction

Who should be prioritised for vaccination? How are priority decisions made? These questions are important in the context of the COVID-19 pandemic because vaccine supply is limited. It has been estimated that around 11 billion doses will be required to vaccinate 70% of the world's population, given that two doses are needed per person.[1] This is the estimated proportion of people that must be vaccinated in order to achieve herd immunity for COVID-19. Although manufacturers estimate that 12 billion doses could be produced by the end of 2021, widespread allocation may not be actualised until the end of 2022 due to breakdowns in the supply chain and export restrictions.[1] Ineffective COVID-19 vaccine allocation could result in preventable deaths, due to lower risk individuals in some countries receiving vaccine before vulnerable people in other countries.[2]

2. Global Allocation of COVID-19 Vaccines

Allocation of COVID-19 vaccines is reminiscent of the "vaccine nationalism" which occurred during the 2009 H1N1 influenza pandemic: most of the global vaccine supply was purchased by high-income countries, which resulted in a scarcity of vaccines available for low- and middle-income countries (LMICs).[3] In the current pandemic, over eight billion doses of COVID-19 vaccines developed by Western manufacturers have been pre-ordered by high-income countries.[4] The United States (US) and European Union (EU) led in pre-orders, followed by the United Kingdom (UK) and Japan. The US, UK, Russia, China, and some EU countries have produced vaccines that have been widely approved and utilised.[5] Other high-income countries *without* the capacity to produce vaccines, such as Canada, depend entirely on investing in vaccine candidates. On the other hand, LMICs that cannot afford to invest in vaccine candidates have been reliant on the COVID-19 Vaccine Global Access Facility (COVAX), an initiative that was created to help promote equitable distribution of COVID-19 vaccines.[3,6]

2.1 *COVAX*

COVAX is led by the Coalition for Epidemic Preparedness Innovations (CEPI), Gavi, the Vaccine Alliance, and the World Health Organization (WHO).[6] To promote equitable global allocation, COVAX aims to provide participating countries with the resources to vaccinate 20% of their population, after which the WHO framework for COVID-19 vaccine allocation will be used to guide allocation based on priority.[3] As of August 2020, nine vaccine candidates had been confirmed for COVAX use and 172 countries had signed up, including high-income countries which used COVAX as an insurance policy against their pre-ordered vaccines. This, and AstraZeneca's pledge to keep vaccine prices low for LMICs for the duration of the pandemic, enabled funding to distribute vaccines to LMICs at around $1.6–$2 USD per dose.[3,7] As of April 1, 2021, COVAX had shipped over 33 million COVID-19 vaccines to 74 participating countries.[8]

2.2 *Cost of vaccine nationalism*

The direct opponent of vaccine equity is vaccine nationalism. Unequal vaccine allocation could result in a global loss of $1.23 trillion per year in gross domestic product (GDP) in the scenario whereby only vaccine nations[a] have access.[2] As long as the virus is not under control in *all*

---

[a] EU-27, US, China, UK, India, Russia.

regions of the world, the global economy will continue to suffer. Further, ineffective COVID-19 vaccine allocation could increase preventable deaths.[2] It is likely that many LMICs will only achieve widespread coverage by 2023, a year or more behind high-income countries.[9] In light of these realities, equity considerations are paramount in vaccine allocation strategies.

3. Vaccine Allocation Frameworks

3.1 *Integration of a new immunisation program*

To help improve equity of vaccination programs, Erickson *et al.* (2005) developed a generalised conceptual model for the integration of new vaccines using the following guiding concepts[10]:

- **Burden of disease** is a control program needed given the burden of disease?
- **Vaccine characteristics** are the vaccines effective and safe?
- **Immunisation strategy** is there an immunisation strategy that will allow for control goals to be attained?
- **Cost-effectiveness** is there sufficient funding?
- **Acceptability of vaccine program** does a high level of demand and acceptability exist for the program?
- **Feasibility of program** is implementation feasible given the available resources?
- **Ability to evaluate programs** can the program be evaluated?
- **Research questions** have research questions affecting implementation been addressed?
- **Other considerations** (equity, ethical, legal, political, conformity) have various other considerations been adequately addressed?

However, in the context of a global pandemic, this model is insufficient. The burden of the disease for COVID-19 is extremely high, resulting in the cost-effectiveness and ability to evaluate the vaccination program becoming less relevant. In contrast, the high burden of disease increases the importance of vaccine efficacy, feasibility of the program, and equitable access.

3.2 *COVID-19 vaccine allocation and prioritisation*

The WHO developed a framework specific to COVID-19 to be used by policy makers, advisors, and stakeholders making prioritisation decisions regarding vaccination allocation.[11] The core principles and objectives are summarised in Table 1.

This framework takes into account generalised vaccine prioritisation principles while incorporating principles specific to a global pandemic. We know that certain groups and countries are at higher risk than others,[12,13] and that frontline healthcare workers, police, educators and other essential workers[14] continue to incur additional risks in order to protect the wellbeing of others. For these reasons, we must consider COVID-19 vaccine allocation and prioritisation through this framework.

Table 1:   WHO Framework for allocation and prioritisation of COVID-19 vaccination.

Core principle	Key objectives
Human well-being	Reduce deaths and disease burden
	Reduce societal and economic disruption
	Protect continuing function of essential services
Equal respect	Treat interests of all individuals/groups with equal moral consideration as allocation decisions made
	Offer meaningful vaccination opportunity to all qualifying groups/individuals
Global equity	Ensure special risks taken into account (especially with regard to low- and middle-income countries)
	Ensure countries commit to meeting needs of other countries that cannot secure vaccine on their own
National equity	Ensure vaccine prioritisation within countries considers elevated risk due to societal, geographic or biomedical factors
	Take action to ensure equal access to all qualifying priority groups (delivery systems and infrastructure)
Reciprocity	Protect those with additional risks due to helping protect welfare of others (e.g. essential workers)
	Transparency of criteria used for allocation decisions
Legitimacy	Use best available evidence and expertise
	Ensure evidence used for prioritisation decisions is unbiased and transparent

4. Strategies for Informing Priority Decisions

4.1 *Modeling prioritisation strategies*

Mathematical models have been used to compare prioritisation strategies for COVID-19 vaccine allocation. Generally speaking, there are two main prioritisation approaches[15]:

1. Direct vaccination of the most vulnerable (highest risk for severe outcomes) populations.
2. Indirect protection of the most vulnerable via vaccination of populations with highest levels of transmission.

Bubar *et al.* (2021) compared age-stratified prioritisation strategies by outcomes of interest: cumulative incidence, mortality, and years of life lost (YLL). An age-stratified SEIR model (susceptible, exposed, infectious, recovered) was employed. Under scenarios of high transmission ($R_0 = 1.5$), prioritisation of adults 60+ years was the mortality-minimising strategy for all countries included in the model. However, for scenarios of lower transmission ($R_0 = 1.15$), prioritising adults 20–49 years was the mortality-minimising strategy for most of the countries included (Poland, China, Spain, US, Belgium). Prioritising adults 20–49 years of age also minimised cumulative incidence of COVID-19. Impact of prioritisation on deaths, hospitalisations, and ICU admissions from COVID-19 in the UK has been modelled by Cook and Roberts.[16] Priority groups were identified as per government recommendations (see Table 2).

Three scenarios were modelled: groups vaccinated by age only, groups vaccinated by age adjusted for healthcare and social care workers, and groups vaccinated by age adjusting for healthcare and social care workers, extremely clinically vulnerable, and those at high risk. Overall, it was found that the latter model predicted better outcomes relative to the first two. As indicated in Figure 1, when half of the adult population has been vaccinated, hospitalisations are predicted to be reduced by 80% and deaths by 95%.[16] At this point, it may be prudent to re-evaluate prioritisation.

Table 2: UK Priority groups for COVID-19 vaccine allocation. Adapted from Ref. 16.

Priority group	Characteristics of individuals (ages in years)
1	Care home residents
	Care home workers
2	Age 80+
	Healthcare workers
	Social care workers
3	Age 75–79
4	Age 70–74
	Clinically extremely vulnerable age <70
5	Age 65–69
6	At risk age <65
7	Age 60–64
8	Age 55–59
9	Age 50–54
10	Age 18–50

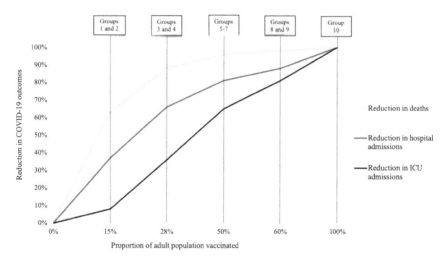

Figure 1: Cumulative impact of vaccination by priority group. Adapted from Ref. 16.

4.2 Evidence-based recommendations

Generally, vaccine allocation and prioritisation recommendations are made at the national level, and then each state or province or territory develops its own prioritisation plan. In Canada, the National Advisory Committee on Immunization (NACI) synthesises knowledge through epidemiological research of newly approved vaccines in order to make evidence-informed recommendations on national vaccine strategies.[17] In the US, the analogous organisation is the Centers for Disease Control and Prevention (CDC).[18] Provinces/territories and states are then at liberty to adjust their vaccine rollout as deemed fit, taking into account population demographics and equity considerations.[19]

4.2.1 Example: Epidemiological research (NACI)

Many risk factors that increase probability of hospitalisation and mortality from COVID-19 in Canada have been identified via a rapid review done by NACI on June 15, 2020.[17] Large associations were found between sociodemographic factors and hospitalisation, including homelessness, low socioeconomic status (income ≤25th versus >50th or 75th percentile), race (Black), and sex (male). Obesity, heart failure, diabetes, chronic kidney disease and Alzheimer's disease were identified as risk factors for hospitalisation, while liver disease predicted mortality. Older age was robustly associated with both hospitalisation and mortality (see Table 3).

4.3 Vaccine prioritisation in practice

4.3.1 Example: Vaccine rollout in British Columbia

The British Columbia (BC) immunisation plan is informed by NACI and aligns with the opinions of experts and individuals in the general Canadian population. High-risk populations are immunised first, with the general population following. This strategy is aimed to reduce the burden on the healthcare system and protect the most vulnerable.[20]

The first two phases are aimed at protecting the people who are most vulnerable to severe illness. Phase 1 focused on residents and staff of long-term care facilities, hospital workers providing care for COVID-19

Table 3:   Risk factors for severe COVID-19 outcomes.

Risk factor	Outcome	Magnitude of risk (confidence level)*
>80 versus ≤45 years	Hospitalisation	+++ (low)
	Mortality	+++ (low)
>70 versus ≤45 years	Hospitalisation	+++ (moderate)
	Mortality	+++ (moderate)
>60 versus ≤45 years	Hospitalisation	++/+++ (moderate/low)
	Mortality	++/+++ (moderate/low)
50–64 versus ≤45 years	Hospitalisation	++ (moderate)
	Mortality	++ (moderate)
45–54 versus ≤45 years	Hospitalisation	++ (moderate)
	Mortality	++ (low)

Magnitude of association was reported as ++ or +++, indicating a large associa-tion (OR or RR ≥2.00) or a very large association (OR or RR ≥5.00). Confidence in the association was reported as either low (possible association) or moderate (probable association).

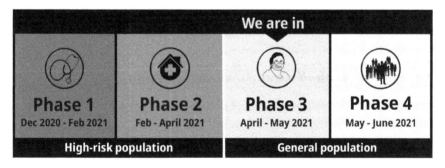

Figure 2:   BCCDC infographic for immunisation.
Source: Government of BC website.

patients in Intensive Care Units and emergency departments, and remote Indigenous communities (Figure 2). Phase 2 aimed to immunise seniors aged 80+ years in addition to Indigenous people aged 65+ years and con-tinued to immunise priority groups (e.g. hospital staff and vulnerable populations). Approximately 400,000 people were immunised during this phase with Pfizer or Moderna vaccines.[20]

Immunisations have continued to occur by descending age groups in five-year increments. In Phase 3, people aged 79 to 60 will be immunised, alongside people aged 69 to 16 who are "clinically extremely vulnerable". By Phase 4, people aged 59 to 18 in the Canadian general population can be immunised. The BC government also notes that front-line workers and essential workers outside of the eligible age groups may be immunised in Phase 3 pending approval of additional vaccines. Many people eligible for vaccination in Phase 3 have received the AstraZeneca vaccine; however, BC suspended the use of AstraZeneca vaccine for people under 55 years of age and frontline healthcare workers pending further investigation, and then allowed its use again for those over 30 with appropriate informed consent (see the "Vaccine Safety" section for more information).[20]

5. Further Considerations

In practice, there are many additional challenges and concerns for vaccine prioritisation and allocation. Logistical challenges may hinder the ability to efficiently immunise remote populations and countries without the infrastructure to distribute vaccines. High levels of transmission, low vaccine supply, timing of second dose administration, and vaccine hesitancy are all considerations that must be addressed.

5.1 *Logistical challenges of vaccine distribution*

The logistics of COVID-19 vaccine distribution can be broken down into three areas:[21]

- Cold chain capacity
- Storage requirements
- Last-mile delivery

"Cold chain" refers to the infrastructure used to transport temperature-sensitive vaccines from where they are produced to where they will be consumed. This is required for mRNA vaccines (e.g. Moderna and Pfizer BioNTech COVID-19 vaccines) since they become unviable if they are not transported at appropriately low temperatures.[21] Similarly, different vaccine types have different storage requirements, often requiring a lower temperature than typical refrigerators are capable of maintaining. LMICs generally do not have ultra-cold and cold chain capacity, meaning they will have to rely mostly on vaccines that can be stored with standard refrigeration, such as the AstraZeneca vaccine,[3] and distribution support from COVAX.[22] Recently, medical drones have allowed for transportation to harder-to-reach areas, addressing geographical barriers to equity.[23]

"Last-mile delivery" refers to the logistical challenges of vaccine distribution due to administrative issues and communication of prioritisation plans.[24] To improve efficiency of last-mile delivery, Israel, Italy, the UK, and Germany have converted stadiums, arenas, skating rinks, town squares, and museums into mass-vaccination sites.[25] These mass-vaccination sites have been a critical innovation for ensuring vaccines are used once delivered. Many countries, including the US and Canada, have distributed vaccines to pharmacies, where vaccination can occur by appointment.[26] Pharmacies will be particularly useful in vaccine rollout for vaccines which do not require cold storage.

5.2 *Rising levels of transmission and variants of concern*

With the rising levels of variants of concern (VOC) globally, a transmission control approach should be considered. Early on, this approach was only taken by Indonesia, which focused on vaccinating people aged 18 to 59 years, beginning with frontline workers.[27] However, Canadian public health modelling from late March 2021 indicate that cases are highest among young adults (aged 20–39 years), as they are more likely to be essential workers.[28] As of April 2021, Canada's approach has shifted away from a simple descending age prioritisation in order to account for essential workers that were left out in earlier phases, including daycare providers, bus drivers, and workers at meat packing plants.[29] This is in alignment with the Reciprocity principle outlined in the WHO framework for COVID-19 vaccine allocation. In light of the increasing prevalence of variants in Canada, high-risk regions, or "hotspots" are also being targeted to reduce transmission, including Whistler, BC[20] and York and Peel regions in Toronto, Ontario.[28]

5.3 *"Breadth versus depth" of doses*

Recommendations for dose intervals vary, both by vaccine product and jurisdiction. The WHO, European Medicines Agency, and US Centers for Disease Control recommend or support maximum deferral of a second dose up to six weeks, the UK government supports deferral up to twelve weeks, and NACI supports deferral up to sixteen weeks.[30] Under ideal circumstances, administration of dose two would occur between the minimum and authorised intervals; however, given the shortage of vaccines, many countries are prioritising "breadth" over "depth" of coverage. As of March 3, 2021, the official statement from the BC Centre for Disease Control was that partial immunity in more (vulnerable) people will lower cases and hospitalisations and save more lives.[30]

5.4 *Vaccine hesitancy*

Levels of mistrust in COVID-19 vaccines are high, based on studies of attitudes toward COVID-19 vaccination in the UK and US. In the UK study, 16% of respondents indicated high levels of mistrust, and 14% reported they did not intent to receive a COVID-19 vaccine.[31] Distrust of the vaccine was correlated to being part of an ethnic minority group, lower levels of education, lower income levels, and lower knowledge of COVID-19.[31] In a large US-based survey, it was found that only 36% of people willing to receive a vaccine identified as Black.[32] Mistrust of health systems by people of colour (POC) has been a long-lasting repercussion of systematic racism in healthcare and is a barrier against equitable COVID-19 vaccine allocation.[13] Research on COVID-19 vaccine hesitancy further highlights the need for rebuilding trust in public health institutions to increase vaccine equity.

6. Lessons from Israel's Vaccine Rollout

Israel is currently the forerunner in vaccination per capita.[33] Aside from its small population size and political incentivisation (i.e. Israel's 2021 election), there are several other key factors that influenced Israel's successful vaccine rollout:[34-36]

- Mobilisation of government funding for vaccine purchase and distribution (willingness to "overpay").
- Quick initial investment into large amount of vaccines.
- Use of clear prioritisation criteria in early phases of vaccine distribution.
- Comprehensive immunisation registry (pre-existing).
- Division of immunisation responsibility by priority group: people aged 60+ years and/or with pre-existing conditions were linked to non-profit health plans, nursing home residents were linked to a national emergency services organisation, and health workers were linked to their employer organisations.
- Innovative solutions to cold chain requirements of Pfizer-BioNTech COVID-19 vaccine.
- Strong efforts to minimise vaccine hesitancy and encourage prompt vaccination scheduling and turn-out.

Synergy of these factors within a coordinated, national response, has allowed Israel to surpass the US and UK in their vaccine rollouts.

7. Conclusion: No "One Size Fits All" Approach

There is no generalised solution for COVID-19 vaccine allocation, because different countries and regions have different environmental and social factors that lend to different priorities. While most countries are in agreement that healthcare works should be vaccinated first, there is less agreement for who comes next. This can depend on demographics, economic factors, and healthcare capacities, among other factors such as transmission rates and prevalence of VOC.[37] Ultimately, the goal of a COVID-19 immunisation program is to provide coverage to as many people as possible as quickly as possible, considering the principles of human wellbeing, equal respect of persons and groups, global and national equity, reciprocity and legitimacy.[11] A deeper analysis of different vaccine rollout strategies and outcomes will provide insight into how to best actualise these key principles throughout the current pandemic and in the future.

References

1. Irwin A. What it will take to vaccinate the world against COVID-19. *Nature.* 2021 Mar 25;d41586-021-00727-3.
2. RAND Corporation. COVID-19 and the cost of vaccine nationalism [Internet]. 2021 Jan 25 [cited 2021 Apr 5]. Available from: https://www.rand. org/randeurope/research/projects/cost-of-covid19-vaccine-nationalism.html.
3. Wouters OJ, Shadlen KC, Salcher-Konrad M, Pollard AJ, Larson HJ, Teerawattananon Y, *et al.* Challenges in ensuring global access to COVID-19 vaccines: Production, affordability, allocation, and deployment. *The Lancet.* 2021;397(10278):1023–1034.
4. Kim JH, Marks F, Clemens JD. Looking beyond COVID-19 vaccine phase 3 trials. *Nature Medicine.* 2021;27(2):205–211.
5. BBC News. Covax: How will Covid vaccines be shared around the world? [Internet]. 2021 Feb 24 [cited 2021 Mar 11]. Available from: https://www. bbc.com/news/world-55795297.
6. Gavi, The Vaccine Alliance. COVAX Explained [Internet]. 2021 [updates 2021 Feb 3; cited 2021 Feb 21]. Available from: https://www.gavi.org/ vaccineswork/covax-explained.
7. Burki T. Equitable distribution of COVID-19 vaccines. *The Lancet Infectious Diseases.* 2021;21(1):33–34.
8. Gavi, The Vaccine Alliance. COVAX vaccine roll-out: Country updates [Internet]. 2021 [updated 2021 Apr 1; cited 2021 Apr 5]. Available from: https://www.gavi.org/covax-vaccine-roll-out
9. Vaccine nationalism means that poor countries will be left behind. *The Economist* [Internet]. 2021 Jan 28 [cited 2021 Apr 10]; Available from: https://www.economist.com/graphic-detail/2021/01/28/vaccine-nationalism-means-that-poor-countries-will-be-left-behind.
10. Erickson LJ, De Wals P, Farand L. An analytical framework for immunization programs in Canada. *Vaccine.* 2005;23(19):2470–2476.
11. World Health Organization. WHO SAGE values framework for the allocation and prioritization of COVID-19 vaccination [Internet]. 2020 Sep 14 [cited 2021 Feb 21]. Available from: https://apps.who.int/iris/bitstream/ handle/10665/334299/WHO-2019-nCoV-SAGE_Framework-Allocation_ and_prioritization-2020.1-eng.pdf.
12. Nelson C. The Case for Equitable Vaccine Distribution [Internet]. [cited 2021 Apr 10]. Available from: https://www.ifc.org/wps/wcm/connect/NEWS_ EXT_CONTENT/IFC_External_Corporate_Site/News+and+Events/News/ Insights/Equitable-Vaccine-Distribution.

13. KFF. Latest data on COVID-19 vaccinations race/ethnicity [Internet]. 2021 Mar 31 [cited 2021 Apr 5]. Available from: https://www.kff.org/coronavirus-covid-19/issue-brief/latest-data-on-covid-19-vaccinations-race-ethnicity/.

14. Categories of Essential Workers: COVID-19 Vaccination | CDC [Internet]. 2021 [cited 2021 Apr 19]. Available from: https://www.cdc.gov/vaccines/covid-19/categories-essential-workers.html.

15. Bubar KM, Reinholt K, Kissler SM, Lipsitch M, Cobey S, Grad YH, *et al.* Model-informed COVID-19 vaccine prioritization strategies by age and serostatus. *Science.* 2021;371(6532):916–921.

16. Cook TM, Roberts JV. Impact of vaccination by priority group on UK deaths, hospital admissions and intensive care admissions from COVID-19. *Anaesthesia.* 2021;76(5):608–616.

17. Government of Canada. National Advisory Committee on Immunization (NACI): Statements and publications [Internet]. 2021 [updated 2021 Mar 3; cited 2021 Mar 11]. Available from: https://www.canada.ca/en/public-health/services/immunization/national-advisory-committee-on-immunization-naci.html.

18. Assistant Secretary for Public Affairs (ASPA). COVID-19 Vaccine Distribution: The Process [Internet]. HHS.gov. 2020 [cited 2021 Apr 19]. Available from: https://www.hhs.gov/coronavirus/covid-19-vaccines/distribution/index.html.

19. Kahn B, Brown L, Foege W, Gayle H. Framework for Equitable Allocation of COVID-19 Vaccine [Internet]. National Academies Press (US); 2020 [cited 2021 Apr 10]. Available from: https://www.ncbi.nlm.nih.gov/books/NBK564086/.

20. BC Centre for Disease Control. BC's COVID-19 Immunization Plan [Internet]. 2021 [updated 2021 Mar 1; cited 2021 Mar 11]. Available from: http://www.bccdc.ca/health-info/diseases-conditions/covid-19/covid-19-vaccine/bcs-plan-for-vaccine-distribution.

21. World Economic Forum. UNICEF calls on supply chain and transport industry to take COVID-19 vaccinations to the world [Internet]. 2021 Feb 5 [cited 2021 Apr 5]. Available from: https://www.weforum.org/agenda/2021/02/supply-chains-and-transport-industry-are-critical-in-getting-covid-19-vaccines-out-to-the-world/.

22. UNICEF. UNICEF outlining plans to transport up to 850 tonnes of COVID-19 vaccines per month on behalf of COVAX, in 'mammoth and historic' logistics [Internet]. 2020 Dec 18 [cited 2021 Apr 5]. Available from: https://www.unicef.org/press-releases/unicef-outlining-plans-transport-850-tonnes-covid-19-vaccines-month-behalf-covax.

23. Prabhu M. COVAX vaccines take to the air by drone [Internet]. 2021 Feb 26 [cited 2021 Apr 5]. Available from: https://www.gavi.org/vaccineswork/covax-vaccines-take-air-drone.

24. Lee TH, Chen AH. Last-Mile Logistics of Covid Vaccination — The Role of Health Care Organizations. *New England Journal of Medicine*. 2021; 384(8):685–687.

25. Goralnick E, Kaufmann C, Gawande AA. Mass-vaccination sites — An essential innovation to curb the COVID-19 pandemic. *New England Journal of Medicine*. 2021;NEJMp2102535.

26. Kominers SD, Tabarrok A. America's pharmacies can do a lot more vaccinations [Internet]. 2021 Feb 17 [cited 2021 Apr 5]. Available from: https://www.bloomberg.com/opinion/articles/2021-02-17/pharmacies-are-crucial-to-covid-19-vaccination-success.

27. Aditya A, Ho Y. Younger people get vaccines first in Indonesia's unusual rollout [Internet]. 2021 Dec 15 [cited 2021 Apr 6]. Available from: https://www.bloomberg.com/news/articles/2020-12-15/younger-people-get-vaccines-first-in-indonesia-s-unusual-rollout.

28. Want to get ahead of COVID-19 variants? Vaccinate young people, experts say [Internet]. Global News. [cited 2021 Apr 15]. Available from: https://globalnews.ca/news/7738013/coronavirus-vaccinating-young-people/.

29. Canada readjusts COVID-19 vaccine rollout to target frontline workers [Internet]. Global News. [cited 2021 Apr 15]. Available from: https://global news.ca/news/7751429/cda-covid-19-vaccination-frontline-workers/.

30. BC Centre for Disease Control. Public health statement on deferral of second dose of COVID-19 vaccine in BC [Internet]. [updated 2021 Mar 3; cited 2021 Apr 5]. Available from: http://www.bccdc.ca/Health-Info-Site/Documents/COVID-19_vaccine/Public_health_statement_deferred_second_dose.pdf.

31. Sonawane K, Troisi CL, Deshmukh AA. COVID-19 vaccination in the UK: Addressing vaccine hesitancy. *The Lancet Regional Health — Europe* [Internet]. 2021 Feb 1 [cited 2021 Apr 3];1. Available from: https://www.thelancet.com/journals/lanepe/article/PIIS2666-7762(20)30016-8/abstract.

32. Paul E, Steptoe A, Fancourt D. Attitudes towards vaccines and intention to vaccinate against COVID-19: Implications for public health communications. *The Lancet Regional Health — Europe*. 2021;1:100012.

33. Coronavirus (COVID-19) Vaccinations — Statistics and Research [Internet]. Our World in Data. [cited 2021 Apr 10]. Available from: https://ourworld indata.org/covid-vaccinations.

34. Rosen B, Waitzberg R, Israeli A. Israel's rapid rollout of vaccinations for COVID-19. *Israel Journal of Health Policy Research*. 2021;10(1):6.

35. McKee M, Rajan S. What can we learn from Israel's rapid roll out of COVID 19 vaccination? *Israel Journal of Health Policy Research*. 2021;10(1):5.

36. Glied S. Strategy drives implementation: COVID vaccination in Israel. *Israel Journal of Health Policy Research*. 2021;10:1–2.

37. Teerawattananon Y, Dabak SV. COVID vaccination logistics: Five steps to take now. *Nature*. 2020;587(7833):194–196.

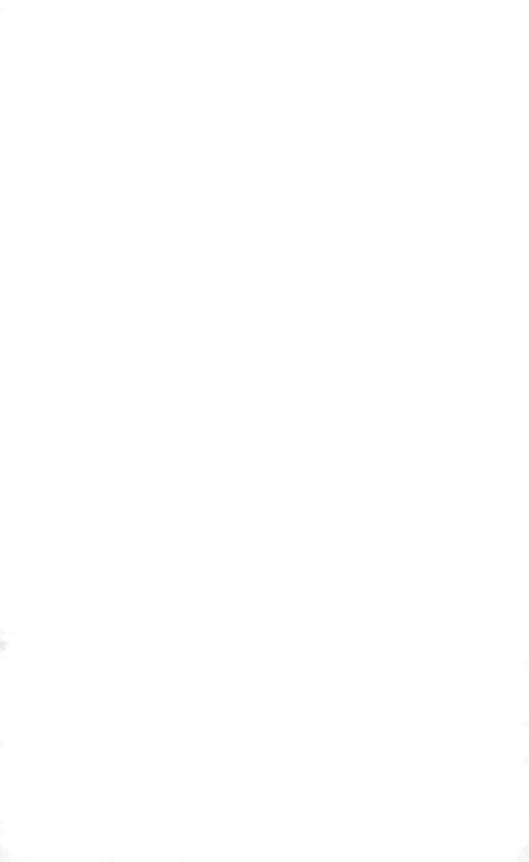

Chapter 15

COVID-19 Vaccine Safety

Marian Orhierhor and Julie A. Bettinger

*School of Population and Public Health, University of British Columbia,
Vancouver, Canada*

*Vaccine Evaluation Center, BC Children's Hospital Institute,
Vancouver, Canada*

Key Message

- The COVID-19 pandemic experience has led to the development of novel creative solutions in medicine. This includes the expedited production of vaccines using both old and new technology platforms.
- Vaccines were developed using a framework distinct from traditional vaccine development, rigorous safety assessments have been carried out in Phase 1, 2, 3 clinical trials and continue in post-marketing surveillance.
- Vaccines are among the most successful preventive and control measures for vaccine-preventable diseases, and safe COVID-19 vaccines will improve vaccine acceptability and uptake and will increase the feasibility of achieving herd immunity.
- Given the short period of clinical trials and paucity of data for the COVID-19 vaccines, the importance of active and passive post-marketing safety surveillance cannot be over-emphasised.
- Vaccine-safety surveillance systems will ensure immunisation safety and identify safer vaccines through detecting, reporting, investigating,

and responding to severe and rare adverse events, adverse events of special interests (AESI) and safety signals. This is also a vital consideration to provide data on the safety and effectiveness of the vaccines for immunocompromised individuals, pregnant and breastfeeding women, seniors living in congregate settings, and other populations who may be vulnerable to COVID-19 because of medical and socio-economic conditions but were not or under-represented in clinical trials.

• *Vaccine safety* is a global priority, and it remains an essential tool in decreasing vaccine hesitancy and achieving herd immunity.

1. Introduction

When SARS-Cov-2 was declared a pandemic by the WHO on March 11, 2020, effective treatments or vaccines were nonexistent; this caused widespread difficulties for healthcare systems worldwide.[1,2] The pandemic caused significant mortality and morbidity and exacerbated existing health, social and economic inequities. Additionally, the implementation of infection control measures such as social distancing, isolation and quarantine had adverse impacts on the economy of many countries.[3,4]

Taking into account these challenges, the development of effective treatments and vaccines was crucial. Starting December 2020, vaccines such as the Pfizer/BioNTech mRNA vaccine received emergency use authorization (EUA) from the WHO and other regulatory bodies such as Health Canada and the USA Food and Drug Administration (FDA).[5,6] This was indeed an appropriate measure to combat the pandemic; nonetheless, the accelerated production of the COVID-19 vaccines raised public concern about whether safety could be compromised in the rapid pursuit of vaccine immunity. While a reasonable question, the SARS-Cov-2 pandemic has occurred at a time when robust vaccine safety monitoring systems are in place. This chapter highlights some key considerations on vaccine safety, summarises the most up-to-date information on vaccine safety as of April 19th, 2021, and the local, international and global strategies to monitor vaccine safety.

All vaccines undergo rigorous testing in pre-clinical and clinical trials before they are approved for use to ensure their safety and efficacy, and the COVID-19 vaccines were no exception. Vaccine safety assessment

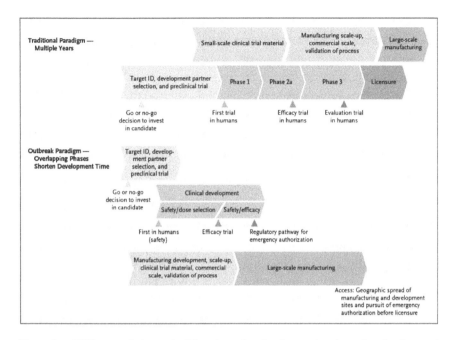

Figure 1: Differences between traditional vaccine development and vaccine development using a pandemic framework.[7]

occurs in **Phase 1**, **Phase 2**, **Phase 3** and **Phase 4 (post-market surveillance)** clinical trials, while efficacy is tested in Phase 2 and 3 and effectiveness in Phase 4. Nevertheless, developing a vaccine promptly during a pandemic requires that multiple stages be executed in parallel.[7] For instance, if a vaccine technology platform has been investigated in humans prior to the pandemic, phase 1 clinical trials may start in parallel with animal model testing.[7] Figure 1 from Lurie *et al.* illustrates the phases of vaccine development and how this framework differs in the context of traditional vaccine development and a pandemic.

1.1 *Factors enabling expedited COVID-19 vaccine development*

1. Lessons learned from previous epidemics of H1N1 influenza, Ebola, and Zika, spurred discourse on the need for vaccine technology

platforms that can be readily adapted to new pathogens.[7] With financial commitments from governmental and non-governmental organisations, vaccine and biotech companies have been investing in developing these platforms for investigational vaccines against viral prototype pathogens and epidemic pathogens on the priority list of the World Health Organization (WHO).[7] When the gene sequence of SARS-Cov-2 was released on January 12th, 2021, vaccine researchers who were developing vaccines for the Middle East Respiratory Syndrome began SARS-Cov-2 vaccine development immediately on some of these newer platforms.[1,7]

2. The DNA and mRNA vaccine platforms have been used for oncology vaccines and were investigated in clinical trials prior to the pandemic.[7,8] Consequently, there was human resource expertise in developing and manufacturing these vaccines with these platforms. This facilitated rapid development and testing. For example, Moderna launched Phase 1 clinical trials for their mRNA vaccine on March 16th, 2020, less than ten weeks after the first gene sequence was released.[7]

3. Vaccine production is an expensive process, and in the context of the COVID-19 pandemic, building production and supply capacity for novel vaccine technology platforms costs hundreds of millions of dollars. However, with the global pandemic, vaccine manufacturing plants have shifted from other vaccines to COVID-19 vaccine to enable more manufacturing capacity while new manufacturing plants are built.[7] Also, Pfizer and Moderna produced millions of vials of vaccine prior to regulatory approval in order to have vaccine supply available for distribution once approval was in place.

2. Pre-Clinical and Clinical Trials for the COVID-19 Vaccines

2.1 *Pre-clinical studies*

Laboratory studies examine the infectious agent, antigens, and the disease's epidemiology. Animal studies examine the safety of candidate vaccines in animals. Animals utilised for investigating the safety and efficacy of the COVID-19 vaccines include the Wistan han rats, mice, hamsters and Rhesus macaques.[9,10] These studies help to ascertain the absence of toxicities that would affect humans. The mRNA vaccines demonstrated protection in animal challenge experiments with no safety concerns, which then allowed for Phase 1 clinical studies in humans.[11,12]

2.2 Clinical studies

- Phase 1 — examine safety and usually enroll tens of volunteers. Essential questions that are answered include: Is the vaccine safe? What is a safe dose? What are the side effects?[13]
- Phase 2 — examine safety and efficacy and enroll hundreds of volunteers. Essential questions that are answered include: Is it safe in a larger group of number of people? What is the best dose and schedule in the target population? Does it work?[13]
- Phase 3 — examine efficacy and safety and enroll thousands of volunteers. Important questions that are answered in this phase include: Does the vaccine prevent disease? Is it safe? How well does it work? What are the side effects?[13]

2.3 Safety reports of the COVID-19 vaccines from clinical trials

Safety assessments for vaccines in clinical trials entail monitoring vital signs, solicited and unsolicited adverse events, solicited and unsolicited severe adverse events, medically attended adverse events, and laboratory investigations for any abnormalities. Adverse events are graded according to a severity score ranging from Grade 1–4. Grade 1 is mild, Grade 2 is moderate, Grade 3 is severe and Grade 4 is potentially life-threatening. Very common adverse events occur in greater than or equal to 10% of vaccine recipients, common adverse events occur in 1% to <10% of vaccine recipients, uncommon events occur in 0.1% to <1% of vaccine recipients and rare and very rare events occur in 0.01 to <0.1% and <0.01% of vaccine recipients, respectively.[14] Table 1 provides a snapshot

Table 1:   Summary of safety assessments of the COVID-19 vaccine types in clinical trials.

Vaccine type	Results of safety assessment in clinical trials
1. Whole Inactivated vaccines a) Sinovac (CoronaVac) b) Sinopharm-Beijing c) Sinopharm-Wuhan d) Covaxin (Bharat Biotech)	a) Sinovac — Phase 1 and 2 trials.[15,16] • Excluding events of headache and mucocutaneous eruption, which were a bit higher in the 6 μg group, the incidence of adverse events after each dose was not significantly different in the vaccine groups and placebo group. • Pain at the injection site and fever was common among all groups. • Adverse events were of mild to moderate severity and resolved after 48 hours. • Vaccine-related serious events were not reported. b) Sinopharm BBIBP-CorV — Phase 1 and 2 trials[17] • Pain at the injection site was very common among vaccine recipients and was higher among the 18–59 age group. • Fever was commonly reported among vaccine recipients. • Serious adverse events were not reported. • Adverse events were of mild to moderate severity and resolved after 48 hours. c) Bharat Biotech — Phase 2 trial[10] • Common solicited adverse events in the vaccine and placebo groups included injection site pain, headache, fatigue, fever, and nausea. • Solicited adverse events were mild or moderate in severity and frequently occurred after the first dose. • There was no significant difference in reported events in both the vaccine and placebo groups. • Vaccine-related serious events were not reported.
2. Protein Subunit a. Novavax	Phase 1–2 trials[18] • Common adverse events included fatigue, headache, malaise, tenderness, and joint pain. • Headache, fatigue, malaise tenderness, joint pain and fatigue were uncommon. • Reactogenicity was absent or was mild when present, after both the first and second doses, and was resolved between 2–7 days. • No serious adverse events or AESI were reported. • There was one unsolicited adverse event of mild cellulitis, which was deemed not associated with the vaccine.

3. Viral Vector
   a) Oxford-AstraZeneca
   b) Janssen
   c) Gameleya
      (Sputnik-V)
   d) CanSino

a) Oxford-AstraZeneca — Phase 3 trials[14,19]
   - Very common solicited adverse events included pain at the injection site, fatigue, headache, muscle pain, malaise, chills, feverishness, fever, joint pain, nausea, tenderness, warmth, bruising, redness, pruritus and swelling. However, most were mild or moderate in severity.
   - Fever, headache, and fatigue was very common after the administration of any dose of the vaccine.
   - Solicited adverse events were milder and less frequent after the second dose of the vaccine in all age groups.
   - Serious adverse events were reported in less than 1% of participants, and the rates were similar in both the vaccine and placebo group.
   - Two serious adverse events of Pyrexia and transverse myelitis were deemed related to the vaccine.

b) Janssen — Interim analysis of Phase 3 trials[20]
   - Very common solicited adverse events include injection site pain, headache, fatigue, myalgia and nausea.
   - A severe allergic reaction of anaphylaxis was reported in one vaccinated individual.
   - Serious adverse events of prolonged pain in the injected arm and severe generalised weakness, fever and headache were reported and were deemed to be associated with the vaccine.
   - There was one case of thromboembolic event in a vaccinated participant. Seizures and tinnitus occurred more in the vaccine group when compared to the placebo group. However, the causality of these events is yet to be determined.

c) Gameleya — Interim analysis of Phase 3 trials[21]
   - Common adverse events included flu-like illness, injection site reactions, headache and asthenia.
   - Adverse events were mainly of mild severity.
   - No vaccine-related serious adverse events were reported.

d) CanSino — Phase 2 trials[22]
   - Solicited adverse events were significantly higher in the vaccine groups when compared to the placebo group.
   - Very common solicited events included fatigue, fever, headache and injection site pain.
   - Pre-existing Ad5 immunity, older age, and being male were associated with lower fever incidence after doses were given.
   - No vaccine-related serious adverse events were reported.

(Continued)

Table 1: (*Continued*)

Vaccine type	Results of safety assessment in clinical trials
4. mRNA a) Pfizer-BioNTech b) Moderna	Pfizer-BioNTech and Moderna — Phase 3 trials[11,12,14] • Pain at the injection site, redness, fatigue, headache, muscle pain, chills, fever, joint pain, redness and swelling were common among vaccine recipients compared to the placebo groups. • Localised axillary swelling and tenderness was very common among vaccine recipients in the Moderna trial, and the severity increased after the second dose. • In the Pfizer trial, older age groups (>=56 years) experienced more severe and frequent systemic events when compared to younger age groups (16–55 years). • Severe systemic events were more frequent after the administration of the second dose. Fever was very common after the administration of the second dose. • Systemic adverse events were primarily mild or moderate in severity and resolved after a few days. • In the Moderna trial, two cases of facial swelling and one case of nausea and vomiting with headaches were considered associated with trial interventions. • Also, severe adverse events of 1 case of autonomic dysfunction, and 1 case of rheumatoid arthritis occurred in the vaccine group, and 5 cases of severe adverse events in the placebo group. These events were deemed to be associated with the trial. • In the Pfizer trial, proportions of severe adverse events were similar among the vaccine and placebo groups. One case each of shoulder injury and ventricular arrhythmia. They were considered associated with the study intervention by investigators. • Unsolicited severe adverse events of lymphadenopathy was recorded in 0.3% of participants, with a larger proportion belonging to the younger age group. 47 out of 64 of these events were considered related to the vaccine.

of the available safety evidence from clinical trials published in peer-reviewed journals and manufacturers press release.

2.4 *Reportable events*

The following events are monitored in Phase 1, 2 and 3 clinical trials and in post-marketing surveillance.

1. Adverse Events Following Immunisation (AEFI): The WHO defines an AEFI as "any untoward medical event that follows immunisation that does not necessarily have a causal relationship with the vaccine's usage".[2] This includes any "unintended sign, abnormal laboratory finding, symptom or disease".[2,26]
2. Serious Adverse Events: Events are classified as serious, if it results in expiration, its life-threatening, requires in-patient hospitalisation or prolongation of existing hospitalisation, results in disability or results in congenital defect.[2,26]
3. Medically Important Event: "As defined by the International Council on Harmonization, these events are not immediately life-threatening but would require medical interventions to prevent severe outcomes classified as serious adverse events".[27]
4. Adverse Events of Special Interests (AESI): The operational definition of an AESI is "a pre-specified medically significant event that has the potential to be casually associated with a vaccine product and requires special monitoring through an active process and warrants investigation by further studies".[2,26,27] Some examples of AESIs include thrombocytopenia, anosmia and ageusia, anaphylaxis, vaccine-associated enhanced diseases, and events that apply to particular populations, e.g. coronary artery disease in the elderly.[2,26,27] The Brighton Collaboration has drafted a standardised list and case definitions for AESIs that are of particular interest to the COVID vaccines, and countries can modify this list to reflect the epidemiology of their regions.[28]
5. Safety Signal: This is new information from one or more sources indicating a potential causal association between a vaccine and an event, or a set of related events previously unknown or incompletely

documented that have health implications.[2,27] For instance, if an AESI occurs more frequently in the vaccinated population than in the unvaccinated population.[2,27] To investigate causality, epidemiological, pathological or laboratory studies are employed.[29] The Global vaccine safety Initiative of the WHO aims to ensure that all safety signals are investigated, and appropriate public health action is taken.[29]

2.5 *Licensure: The final stage of approval*

The WHO provides authorisation for medical products. Regulatory bodies in various countries also provide authorisation before medical products such as drugs and vaccines can be used commercially. Some examples of regulatory organisations are The FDA (USA), the Medicines and Healthcare Products Regulatory Agency (MHRA) (United Kingdom), and the European Medicines Agency (European Union) and Health Canada. The same applies to Canada, as Canada's independent vaccine authorisation follows an in-depth review process. The review of all COVID-19 medications and vaccines is a priority, and more resources have been dedicated to this cause,[13] thus enabling a quicker review process. Vaccine manufacturers submit their applications through an interim order process to Health Canada.[13] The evidence from clinical trials is reviewed by an expert medical team of Health Canada's Biologic and Radiopharmaceutical Drugs Directorate (BRDD).[13] Approval is exclusively based on medical and scientific evidence, a risk-benefit analysis, and a review of the vaccine's safety, performance and conformity to manufacturing standards.[13] When a vaccine candidate meets the set standards, they are approved, purchased and distributed across Canada.[13] By law, manufacturing companies must provide Health Canada data on the safety, efficacy and quality of the vaccine for at least two years after approval, as active surveillance continues for all clinical trial participants.[13,23] Currently, the COVID-19 vaccines have EUA.[5,6] An EUA is a mechanism to facilitate the availability and use of medical countermeasures, including vaccines to diagnose, treat or prevent serious or life-threatening conditions during public health emergencies, especially in the case where there are no adequate, approved, and available alternatives.

3. Phase 4: Post-Marketing Surveillance

Post-marketing surveillance is undertaken after the vaccine is approved for use to monitor vaccine safety, quality, effectiveness and answers research questions that were not addressed in clinical trials.[2,23] The system ensures vaccine safety through detecting, reporting, investigating, and responding to adverse events. In Canada, the vaccine safety monitoring system involves health professionals, the provinces and territories, the Public Health Agency of Canada, Health Canada, vaccine manufacturers, and collaborations with other international regulators.[23,25] In Canada, all healthcare professionals are mandated by law to report AEFI to the Canadian Adverse Event Following Immunization Surveillance System (CAEFISS).[25]

3.1 *Objectives of COVID-19 vaccines post-marketing safety surveillance*

1. To detect safety signals occurring after vaccination.
2. To identify rare adverse events and events not detected in clinical trials.
3. To ascertain the risk and the risk factors in populations vaccinated with the vaccines.
4. To calculate the relative risk of an adverse event. This is done by comparing the risk of an adverse event in vaccinated individuals to unvaccinated individuals or individuals who received a comparator vaccine.
5. To monitor the rate of adverse events and the trends in adverse events over time.

3.2 *Types of vaccine safety surveillance systems*

1. Passive vaccine surveillance systems: This system collects information on all events which follow vaccination. They facilitate identifying potential safety signals for AEFIs that are unforeseen or unknown at the time of clinical trials.[26] Examples of this system include the Vaccine Adverse Event Reporting System (USA), and EudraVigilance (EU). In

Canada, there is The Canada Vigilance Program, which receives data from vaccine manufacturers, healthcare professionals and from members of the public who make direct reports.[23]

2. The WHO has the largest and most comprehensive data base on adverse reactions to medicines and vaccines. This global database called VigiBase collects Individual Case Safety Reports (ICSRs) of suspected adverse events of medicines, submitted by over 150 countries.[24]

3. Active Vaccine Surveillance Systems (AVSS): This system mitigates underreporting and collect complete and precise information about AEFIs and AESIs.[26] The size of the population from which the AEFI was detected is known, and the relative risk is calculated to determine if an association exists between an AEFI and the vaccine, which would require additional investigation.[26,30] Surveillance could be prospective or retrospective, and the methods used can be cohort event monitoring, sentinel surveillance, or data linkage of mobile health and electronic health records using case definitions.[26] Examples of this system include CDC's Vaccine Safety Datalink (USA), FDA Biologics Effectiveness and Safety System (USA), FDA BEST Sentinel Initiative (USA), Accelerated Development of Vaccine Benefit-Risk Collaboration in Europe (ADVANCE) (EU). In Canada, this is implemented by the Canadian National Vaccine Safety Network (Canvas-COVID)[31,32,33] and Canadian Immunization Monitoring Program Active (IMPACT), which is a pediatric hospital-based network, that closely monitors hospital admissions for AEFI.[25]

3.3 *Unreportable events*

These are events that are not reportable to the passive surveillance system because they were detected in the clinical trial and not serious and do not need further monitoring. These events do not pose a potential risk to the recipient's health. Events related to reactogenicity, e.g. pain at the injection site, redness, swelling.[25,26] Events related to the act of injection, e.g. anxiety about immunisations, or events related to pre-existing conditions.[25,26]

3.4 *What happens after adverse events are reported?*

Medical expert teams evaluate all serious events to determine if safety issues should be addressed. If safety issues are confirmed, action would be taken, which could encompass communicating any new risks to vaccine recipients and healthcare providers or changing the product's recommended use.[23]

3.5 *A case study of real-world application of vaccine post-marketing safety surveillance: Oxford/AstraZeneca*

The *ChAdOx1* vaccine (Oxford AstraZeneca) was authorised for use in adults 18 years and older in the United Kingdom and Europe in January 2021 and on February 26th, 2021, in Canada. As of March 2021, over 25 million doses of the AstraZeneca vaccine had been administered in UK and Europe.[34,35] By March 2021, 191 cases of blood coagulation disorders were reported both in studies before licensing and after vaccination rollout in Europe. These adverse events included disseminated intravascular coagulation (DIC), pulmonary embolism, and deep vein thrombosis, occurring within two weeks after vaccination.[34,35] Rare adverse events were also reported; this included 24 cases of splanchnic vein thrombosis, 62 cases of cerebral venous sinus thrombosis (CVST), 18 of which ended in death.[34] Following these initial signals, some countries-Denmark, Norway, Iceland, Bulgaria, Estonia, Lithuania, Luxembourg, halted *ChAdOx1* use pending investigation, while others such as Italy, Romania and Austria discontinued shots from a particular batch. Other countries such as France, Germany, Poland, and Nigeria continued vaccination roll-outs as regulators continued investigation.[35,36]

These events were considered a safety signal and were investigated by the UK's Medicines and Health Care Products Regulatory Agency and the Pharmacovigilance risk assessment committee (PRAC) of the European Medicine Agency.[34,35] After preliminary investigations on March 18th, 2021, it was concluded that the benefits of the vaccine continue to outweigh its risk, as the vaccine was not associated with an increase in the overall risk of blood clots in vaccinated individuals.[34,37] There was also no evidence of a specific problem related to a specific batch of the vaccine.[34,37]

However, the evidence suggests a plausible association between the vaccine and very rare and unique thromboembolic events in combination with thrombocytopenia.[38] This adverse event has been termed Vaccine-Induced Thrombotic Thrombocytopenia.[34,39,40] While originally an observation in women under 60, further cases were recorded across the age and sex spectrum.[34] Since these events are generally rare, it is difficult to estimate the background rate in those who have not had the vaccine; however, surveillance data on these rare events before SARS-Cov-2 showed a clear increase over expected with the vaccine.[34] For instance, by March 16th, 2021, an average of 1.35 cases of CVST might have been expected among people under 50 within 14 days of getting the vaccine; however, 12 cases of CVST were observed.[34]

The regulators have concluded unusual blood clots with low blood platelets should be listed as a rare side effect of the vaccine, and the product monograph was updated to include more information on these risks. PRAC has emphasised the need for prompt specialist medical care for vaccine recipients experiencing symptoms of blood clots and has provided guidance and information for healthcare professionals.[34,35]

In light of these findings, further investigations were carried out by vaccine manufacturers and regulators to determine specific risk factors and explanations on the mechanism of causality. By April 4th, 2021, 34 million people have received the vaccine, and EU has recorded 169 cases of CVST and 53 cases of sphlanic vein thrombosis.[34] Following these findings, Denmark and Norway has completely halted its use, Italy, France, Belgium, and the United Kingdom have included age restrictions in its use.[41] In Canada, cases continued to accrue after the first case reports. Most provinces offer the option of a second dose with an mRNA vaccine for those who received a viral vector vaccine as first dose. Health Canada has updated the AstraZeneca and COVISHIELD monograph to provide information on these events.[27,40]

4. COVID-19 Vaccine Safety for Populations

4.1 *COVID-19 vaccine contraindications at the date of writing*

The vaccines are not recommended in individuals with a history of anaphylactic reaction after a previous dose of the vaccine or individuals with a history of severe allergic reaction to any vaccine component; these individuals were excluded from clinical trials.[14] A potential allergen in the mRNA vaccine is Polyethylene glycol, tromethamine is found in the Moderna mRNA vaccine, and the AstraZeneca vaccine contains polysorbate80.[14] Labels and contraindications are constantly being updated based on experience and the readers should look to up to date guidance from their national regulator.

4.2 *COVID-19 vaccine safety for specific populations*

The following groups represent populations excluded from clinical trials or represented in small numbers. In most countries, these groups have been included in vaccine recommendations, with support from specialist bodies and variable advice about individual risk assessment.[14] As a result, information on safety and effectiveness is accruing quickly at the time of writing consent:

1. Immunosuppressed due to disease or treatment.
2. Individuals with an autoimmune condition.
3. Pregnant or breastfeeding women.
4. Children and adolescents 12–15 years of age.
5. Seniors living in congregate settings, e.g. Long term care homes.

Israel began a swift inoculation campaign with the Pfizer BioNTech mRNA vaccine and was thus one of the first countries to produce insight into the real-world effectiveness and safety of the vaccines. The Ministry of Health of Israel vaccinated adolescents between the ages of 12–16 with conditions such as obesity, diabetes, severe lung and heart disease, immunosuppression disorders and cancer; children of severely immunocompromised parents were also vaccinated.[42] Currently, no side effects have been recorded in this vaccinated group.[42] Since this time and supported by extended trial data from manufacturers, adolescents 12 and over are eligible for immunisation in most countries.

Preliminary results from the British Columbia Centre for Disease Control have answered some of the critical questions of the mRNA vaccine's effectiveness and safety in residents of long-term care homes[43] and older adults in the community. Surveillance data from December 2020–February 2021 show that taking a single dose of the mRNA vaccine reduced the risk of COVID-19 in long-term care residents and health workers by 80% within two-three weeks of getting vaccinated.[43]

NACI strongly recommends that clinical trials be undertaken to determine the safety and efficacy of the COVID vaccines in the populations highlighted above. Some of these trials are already underway; the University of Oxford announced that the AstraZeneca vaccine would be tested on individuals between the ages of 6–17, the Pfizer-BioNTech vaccine has been tested on individuals 12–50, and the Moderna vaccine for the age 12–18.[44–46] With the emergence of more transmissible variants of the SARS-Cov-2 virus, these populations are critical in reducing the R_0.

5. COVID-19 Vaccine Types and Adjuvants

Adjuvant are substances added to vaccines to increase the robustness of the body's humoral and/or cellular immune response.[47] There are currently no adjuvants in the mRNA vaccines and the adenovirus viral vector vaccines, but other vaccine candidates in clinical trials and candidates that have been approved make use of adjuvants. Table 2 summarises the vaccine types, adjuvants, safety concerns about the components and/or technology of these vaccines, and the current evidence from the COVID-19 vaccines and other produced vaccines.

5.1 *The administration of COVID-19 vaccine with other treatments*

In Canada, basic infection prevention precautions, including COVID-19 screening before and during patient visits, have been implemented to ensure that routine immunisation services and post-exposure prophylaxis (PEP) vaccinations for other vaccine-preventable diseases are not disrupted as a result of the pandemic.[14]

5.2 *Concomitant/simultaneous administration with other vaccines*

There is currently no data on the simultaneous administration of COVID-19 vaccines with other vaccines.[14] The National Advisory

Table 2: COVID-19 vaccine types, adjuvants and safety issues of concern.

Vaccine types	Adjuvants	Issue of concern	Current evidence
1. Whole inactivated vaccines a) Sinovac b) Sinopharm-Beijing c) Sinopharm-Wuhan d) Bharat Biotech	Aluminum Hydroxide in Sinovac and Sinopharm Algel-IMDG adjuvant in Bharat Biotech	i. Inactivation: Failure of the inactivation procedure would leave an active virus in the final vaccine product and cause vaccine-associated diseases.[48] ii. Adverse effects from adjuvants.	i. This vaccine technology platform is well studied and has been used for polio, seasonal influenza, and pertussis vaccines.[8,48] The β-propiolactone inactivating agent, commonly used for rabies vaccines and currently used for the COVID-vaccines, has the advantage of being hydrolyzed within hours to non-toxic products; hence the killed pathogenic organisms are unable to reproduce in the host cells, as such, they cannot cause disease.[8,48] ii. Aluminum salts are used for hepatitis A and B vaccines, HPV vaccine, and meningococcal vaccines. 50% of the aluminum is expelled from the body within 24 hrs, and 75% is eliminated within two weeks.[49] Currently, no adverse events related to adjuvants have been reported in clinical trials for the whole inactivated vaccines[15]

(*Continued*)

Table 2: *(Continued)*

Vaccine types	Adjuvants	Issue of concern	Current evidence
2. Protein subunit a) Novavax	Matrix-M™	Adverse effects from Matrix M adjuvants.	The Matrix M adjuvant has been evaluated in clinical trials in seasonal and pandemic influenza vaccines and has been found to have an acceptable safety profile.[50] In phase 1–2 trials of the Novavax vaccine, no serious or severe adverse events were recorded among those who received the vaccine with adjuvant, however, more reactogenicity was seen in this group, but this was mild in severity and was resolved after two days.[18]
3. Viral vector a) Oxford-AstraZeneca b) Janssen c) Gameleya d) CanSino	None present	Adenovirus viral vector: The possibility of the viral vector causing diseases.	This vaccine platform was used to produce the Ebola vaccine. Adenoviruses are common viruses in circulation in the environment; the viral vector is modified and cannot replicate in host cells, thus enable to cause diseases.[51,8]
4. mRNA a) Pfizer-BioNTech b) Moderna	None present	The RNA's timeframe in the host system and its effect on the host cell's nucleus. The effect of the lipid nanoparticles that encloses the RNA.	Current evidence suggests that the RNA does not enter the cell's nucleus or interact with the cell's nucleus or change and interact with the human DNA. RNA is not very stable, and it degrades quickly. The mRNA, the lipid nanoparticle and the spike protein are degraded or excreted within days to weeks after vaccination.[14]

Committee on Immunization has given the following recommendations to maximise the benefits of the COVID-19 vaccines and minimise any risk of harm or the false attribution of an AEFI to any of the vaccines.[14]

- No simultaneous administration with other live or inactivated vaccines unless these vaccines are required for PEP.
- There should be a waiting period of 28 days after a dose of a COVID-19 vaccine before administering another vaccine, except in the case where the other vaccine is needed for PEP.
- There should be a waiting period of 14 days after administering another vaccine before administering a COVID-19 vaccine.

5.3 *COVID-19 vaccines interactions with drugs, blood products, and human immunoglobulins*

Currently, there is insufficient evidence on the receipt of the products named above with COVID-19 vaccines.[14] Therefore, administration timing and the potential interactions or interferences between these products are unknown.[14] The NACI advises that there should be no simultaneous administration with monoclonal antibodies or convalescent plasma, and expert clinical opinion should be consulted on a case-by-case basis.[14]

6. Conclusion

Detecting safety signals for COVID-19 vaccines, demonstrates the timeliness and sensitivity of the safety surveillance systems described, and there is confidence that the systems are operating as intended.

COVID-19 vaccine safety is a global priority and recognising that the capacity for post-marketing surveillance differs across countries and is especially problematic for LMICs, there is a need for increased collaboration and support for LMICs to ensure their vaccine supply is safely monitored as well as in high income countries.

References

1. Wang H, Li X, Li T, Zhang S, Wang L, Wu X, *et al.* The genetic sequence, origin, and diagnosis of SARS-CoV-2 [Internet]. Vol. 39, European Journal

of Clinical Microbiology and Infectious Diseases. Springer Science and Business Media Deutschland GmbH; 2020 [cited 2021 Apr 17]. pp. 1629–35. Available from: /pmc/articles/PMC7180649/.

2. WHO. Covid-19 vaccines: Safety surveillance manual. 2020;1–232. Available from: https://apps.who.int/iris/bitstream/handle/10665/338400/9789240018280-eng.pdf?sequence=1&isAllowed=y&fbclid=IwAR12xpv3fjwzujV3CDd3Qq5ZgZEkk0ITpqtjK5XFO2b66ZJVEf1Bb6QICjM.

3. The Global Economic Outlook During the COVID-19 Pandemic: A Changed World [Internet]. [cited 2021 Apr 17]. Available from: https://www.worldbank.org/en/news/feature/2020/06/08/the-global-economic-outlook-during-the-covid-19-pandemic-a-changed-world.

4. Dhanda S, Osborne V, Lynn E, Shakir S. Postmarketing studies: Can they provide a safety net for COVID-19 vaccines in the UK? *BMJ Evidence-Based Med* [Internet]. 2020 Oct 21 [cited 2021 Apr 8];0. Available from: http://ebm.bmj.com/.

5. FDA Takes Key Action in Fight Against COVID-19 By Issuing Emergency Use Authorization for First COVID-19 Vaccine | FDA [Internet]. [cited 2021 Apr 17]. Available from: https://www.fda.gov/news-events/press-announcements/fda-takes-key-action-fight-against-covid-19-issuing-emergency-use-authorization-first-covid-19.

6. WHO issues its first emergency use validation for a COVID-19 vaccine and emphasizes need for equitable global access [Internet]. [cited 2021 Apr 17]. Available from: https://www.who.int/news/item/31-12-2020-who-issues-its-first-emergency-use-validation-for-a-covid-19-vaccine-and-emphasizes-need-for-equitable-global-access.

7. Lurie N, Saville M, Hatchett R, Halton J. Developing Covid-19 vaccines at pandemic speed. *New England Journal of Medicine* [Internet]. 2020 May 21 [cited 2021 Apr 4];382(21):1969–1973. Available from: http://www.nejm.org/doi/10.1056/NEJMp2005630.

8. Nelson KE. Infectious disease. *The Lancet*. 1936;228:815.

9. Gruber W. BNT162b2 Vaccine Candidate Against COVID-19 Senior Vice President Vaccine Clinical R&D Pfizer. 2020.

10. Ella R, Reddy S, Jogdand H, Sarangi V, Ganneru B, Prasad S, *et al.* Safety and immunogenicity of an inactivated SARS-CoV-2 vaccine, BBV152: Interim results from a double-blind, randomised, multicentre, phase 2 trial, and 3-month follow-up of a double-blind, randomised phase 1 trial. *Lancet Infectious Diseases* [Internet]. 2021 Mar [cited 2021 Apr 17];0(0). Available from: www.thelancet.com/infection.

11. Polack FP, Thomas SJ, Kitchin N, Absalon J, Gurtman A, Lockhart S, *et al.* Safety and efficacy of the BNT162b2 mRNA Covid-19 vaccine. *New England Journal of Medicine.* 2020;383(27):2603–2615.

12. Baden LR, El Sahly HM, Essink B, Kotloff K, Frey S, Novak R, *et al.* Efficacy and safety of the mRNA-1273 SARS-CoV-2 vaccine. *New England Journal of Medicine* [Internet]. 2021 Feb 4 [cited 2021 Mar 12];384(5):403–416. Available from: http://www.nejm.org/doi/10.1056/NEJMoa2035389.

13. Vaccine development and approval in Canada — Canada.ca [Internet]. [cited 2021 Mar 12]. Available from: https://www.canada.ca/en/health-canada/services/drugs-health-products/covid19-industry/drugs-vaccines-treatments/vaccines/development-approval-infographic.html.

14. Recommendations on the use of COVID-19 vaccines — Canada.ca [Internet]. [cited 2021 Mar 12]. Available from: https://www.canada.ca/en/public-health/services/immunization/national-advisory-committee-on-immunization-naci/recommendations-use-covid-19-vaccines.html.

15. Zhang Y, Zeng G, Pan H, Li C, Hu Y, Chu K, *et al.* Safety, tolerability, and immunogenicity of an inactivated SARS-CoV-2 vaccine in healthy adults aged 18–59 years: A randomised, double-blind, placebo-controlled, phase 1/2 clinical trial. *Lancet Infectious Diseases.* 2021;21(2):181–192.

16. Wu Z, Hu Y, Xu M, Chen Z, Yang W, Jiang Z, *et al.* Safety, tolerability, and immunogenicity of an inactivated SARS-CoV-2 vaccine (CoronaVac) in healthy adults aged 60 years and older: A randomised, double-blind, placebo-controlled, phase 1/2 clinical trial. *Lancet Infectious Diseases* [Internet]. 2021 [cited 2021 Apr 16];0(0). Available from: www.thelancet.com/infectionPublishedonline.

17. Xia S, Zhang Y, Wang Y, Wang H, Yang Y, Gao GF, *et al.* Safety and immunogenicity of an inactivated SARS-CoV-2 vaccine, BBIBP-CorV: A randomised, double-blind, placebo-controlled, phase 1/2 trial. *Lancet Infectious Diseases* [Internet]. 2021 Jan 1 [cited 2021 Apr 16];21(1):39–51. Available from: /pmc/articles/PMC7561304/.

18. Keech C, Albert G, Cho I, Robertson A, Reed P, Neal S, *et al.* Phase 1–2 trial of a SARS-CoV-2 recombinant spike protein nanoparticle vaccine. *New England Journal of Medicine* [Internet]. 2020 Dec 10 [cited 2021 Apr 17];383(24):2320–2332. Available from: http://www.nejm.org/doi/10.1056/NEJMoa2026920.

19. Emary KRW, Golubchik T, Aley PK, Ariani C V, Angus B, Bibi S, *et al.* Efficacy of ChAdOx1 nCoV-19 (AZD1222) vaccine against SARS-CoV-2 variant of concern 202012/01 (B.1.1.7): An exploratory analysis of a randomised

controlled trial. www.thelancet.com [Internet]. 2021 [cited 2021 Apr 19];397. Available from: https://doi.org/10.1016/.

20. Clinical Trial Data | Janssen COVID-19 Vaccine — HCP [Internet]. [cited 2021 Apr 17]. Available from: https://www.janssencovid19vaccine.com/hcp/clinical-trial-data.html.

21. Logunov DY, Dolzhikova IV, Shcheblyakov DV, Tukhvatulin AI, Zubkova OV, Dzharullaeva AS, *et al*. Safety and efficacy of an rAd26 and rAd5 vector-based heterologous prime-boost COVID-19 vaccine: An interim analysis of a randomised controlled phase 3 trial in Russia. *Lancet* [Internet]. 2021 Feb 20 [cited 2021 Apr 17];397(10275):671–681. Available from: https://covid19.

22. Zhu FC, Guan XH, Li YH, Huang JY, Jiang T, Hou LH, *et al*. Immunogenicity and safety of a recombinant adenovirus type-5-vectored COVID-19 vaccine in healthy adults aged 18 years or older: A randomised, double-blind, placebo-controlled, phase 2 trial. *Lancet* [Internet]. 2020 Aug 15 [cited 2021 Apr 17];396(10249):479–488. Available from: http://www.

23. Vaccines and treatments for COVID-19: Safety after authorization — Canada.ca [Internet]. [cited 2021 Apr 19]. Available from: https://www.canada.ca/en/public-health/services/diseases/2019-novel-coronavirus-infection/prevention-risks/covid-19-vaccine-treatment/safety-after-authorization.html.

24. UMC | VigiBase [Internet]. [cited 2021 Apr 18]. Available from: https://www.who-umc.org/vigibase/vigibase/.

25. Vaccine safety and pharmacovigilance: Canadian Immunization Guide — Canada.ca [Internet]. [cited 2021 Mar 12]. Available from: https://www.canada.ca/en/public-health/services/publications/healthy-living/canadian-immunization-guide-part-2-vaccine-safety/page-2-vaccine-safety.html.

26. COVID-19 Vaccines: Safety Surveillance Manual Module: Establishing active surveillance systems for adverse events of special interest during COVID-19 vaccine introduction.

27. COVID-19 vaccine safety: Weekly report on adverse effects following immunization — Canada.ca [Internet]. [cited 2021 Apr 19]. Available from: https://health-infobase.canada.ca/covid-19/vaccine-safety/.

28. COVID-19 — Brighton Collaboration [Internet]. [cited 2021 Mar 12]. Available from: https://brightoncollaboration.us/covid-19/.

29. Investigation of safety signals [Internet]. [cited 2021 Mar 8]. Available from: https://www.who.int/initiatives/the-global-vaccine-safety-initiative/investigation-of-safety-signals.

30. Chandler RE. Optimizing safety surveillance for COVID-19 vaccines. *Nature Review Immunology* [Internet]. [cited 2021 Apr 8]; Available from: https://www.vaccineconfidence.org/.

31. De Serres G, Gariepy MC, Coleman B, Rouleau I, McNeil S, Benoit M, *et al.* Short and long-term safety of the 2009 AS03-adjuvanted pandemic vaccine. *PLoS One.* [Research Support, Non-U.S. Gov't]. 2012;7(7):e38563.

32. Bettinger JA, Rouleau I, Gariepy MC, Bowie WR, Valiquette L, Vanderkooi OG, *et al.* Successful methodology for large-scale surveillance of severe events following influenza vaccination in Canada, 2011 and 2012. *Eurosurveillance.* [Research Support, Non-U.S. Gov't]. 2015;20(29):21189.

33. Bettinger JA, De Serres G, Valiquette L, Vanderkooi OG, Kellner JD, Coleman BL, *et al.* 2017/18 and 2018/19 seasonal influenza vaccine safety surveillance, Canadian National Vaccine Safety (CANVAS) Network. Euro surveillance: Bulletin Europeen sur les maladies transmissibles = European communicable disease bulletin. 2020 Jun; 25(22).

34. COVID-19 Vaccine AstraZeneca: Benefits still outweigh the risks despite possible link to rare blood clots with low blood platelets | European Medicines Agency [Internet]. [cited 2021 Apr 6]. Available from: https://www.ema.europa.eu/en/news/covid-19-vaccine-astrazeneca-benefits-still-outweigh-risks-despite-possible-link-rare-blood-clots.

35. Wise J. Covid-19: European countries suspend use of Oxford-AstraZeneca vaccine after reports of blood clots. [cited 2021 Apr 18]. Available from: http://dx.doi.org/10.1136/bmj.n699.

36. After reports of blood clots, some countries pause use of AstraZeneca Covid vaccine [Internet]. [cited 2021 Apr 6]. Available from: https://www.nbcnews.com/health/health-news/after-reports-blood-clots-some-countries-pause-use-astrazeneca-covid-n1260888.

37. Statement of the WHO Global Advisory Committee on Vaccine Safety (GACVS) COVID-19 subcommittee on safety signals related to the AstraZeneca COVID-19 vaccine [Internet]. [cited 2021 Apr 6]. Available from: https://www.who.int/news/item/19-03-2021-statement-of-the-who-global-advisory-committee-on-vaccine-safety-(gacvs)-covid-19-subcommittee-on-safety-signals-related-to-the-astrazeneca-covid-19-vaccine.

38. Meeting highlights from the Pharmacovigilance Risk Assessment Committee (PRAC) 6-9 April 2021 | European Medicines Agency [Internet]. [cited 2021 Apr 19]. Available from: https://www.ema.europa.eu/en/news/meeting-highlights-pharmacovigilance-risk-assessment-committee-prac-6-9-april-2021.

39. Pai M, Grill A, Ivers N, Maltsev A, Miller KJ, Razak F, *et al.* Vaccine induced prothrombotic immune thrombocytopenia (VIPIT) following AstraZeneca COVID-19 vaccination [Internet]. 2021 Mar [cited 2021 Apr 6]. Available from: https://covid19-sciencetable.ca/sciencebrief/vaccine-induced-

prothrombotic-immune-thrombocytopenia-vipit-following-astrazeneca-covid-19-vaccination.

40. AstraZeneca COVID-19 vaccine use in younger adults: NACI recommendation — Canada.ca [Internet]. [cited 2021 Apr 19]. Available from: https://www.canada.ca/en/public-health/services/immunization/national-advisory-committee-on-immunization-naci/rapid-response-recommended-use-astrazeneca-covid-19-vaccine-younger-adults.html.

41. Countries change tack on AstraZeneca vaccine despite EU call for unity | Euronews [Internet]. [cited 2021 Apr 19]. Available from: https://www.euronews.com/2021/04/07/countries-change-tack-on-astrazeneca-vaccine-despite-eu-call-for-unity.

42. No side effects seen in dozens of Israeli kids vaccinated due to risk factors. *The Times of Israel* [Internet]. [cited 2021 Mar 7]. Available from: https://www.timesofisrael.com/report-no-side-effects-in-dozens-of-israeli-kids-vaccinated-due-to-risk-factors/.

43. Early findings show the first vaccine dose reduced the risk of COVID-19 by 80 per cent or more [Internet]. [cited 2021 Mar 6]. Available from: http://www.bccdc.ca/about/news-stories/news-releases/2021/early-findings-show-the-first-vaccine-dose-reduced-the-risk-of-covid-19-by-80-per-cent-or-more.

44. Oxford University extends COVID-19 vaccine study to children | University of Oxford [Internet]. [cited 2021 Mar 6]. Available from: https://www.ox.ac.uk/news/2021-02-12-oxford-university-extends-covid-19-vaccine-study-children.

45. A Phase 3 Study to Evaluate the Safety, Tolerability, and Immunogenicity of Multiple Production Lots and Dose Levels of BNT162b2 Against COVID-19 in Healthy Participants — Full Text View — ClinicalTrials.gov [Internet]. [cited 2021 Mar 6]. Available from: https://www.clinicaltrials.gov/ct2/show/NCT04713553?term=pfizer&cond=Covid19&draw=2.

46. A Study to Evaluate the Safety, Reactogenicity, and Effectiveness of mRNA-1273 Vaccine in Adolescents 12 to <18 Years Old to Prevent COVID-19 — Full Text View — ClinicalTrials.gov [Internet]. [cited 2021 Mar 12]. Available from: https://clinicaltrials.gov/ct2/show/NCT04649151.

47. Di Pasquale A, Preiss S, Da Silva FT, Garçon N. Vaccine adjuvants: From 1920 to 2015 and beyond [Internet]. Vol. 3, Vaccines. MDPI AG; 2015 [cited 2021 Apr 6]. pp. 320–43. Available from: /pmc/articles/PMC4494348/.

48. Antiviral Immunity and Virus Vaccines. In: *Fenner's Veterinary Virology*. Elsevier; 2017. pp. 79–104.

49. Vaccine safety, concerns and possible side effects — Canada.ca [Internet]. [cited 2021 Mar 12]. Available from: https://www.canada.ca/en/public-health/services/vaccination-children/safety-concerns-side-effects.html.

50. Magnusson SE, Altenburg AF, Bengtsson KL, Bosman F, de Vries RD, Rimmelzwaan GF, *et al.* Matrix-M^{TM} adjuvant enhances immunogenicity of both protein- and modified vaccinia virus Ankara-based influenza vaccines in mice. *Immunology Research* [Internet]. 2018 Apr 28 [cited 2021 Apr 6]; 66(2):224–233. Available from: http://link.springer.com/10.1007/s12026-018-8991-x.

51. What you should know: AstraZeneca COVID-19 vaccine — Canada.ca [Internet]. [cited 2021 Mar 12]. Available from: https://www.canada.ca/en/health-canada/services/drugs-health-products/covid19-industry/drugs-vaccines-treatments/vaccines/astrazeneca.html.

Part 8

Public Engagement and Combating the Infodemic

Chapter 16

Public Engagement

Tania Bubela*, Katie Fenn[†,‡], Sally Greenwood[§],
Anne-Marie Nicol[¶], Beverly Pomeroy[‖,**], Harlan Pruden[‡],
Emily Rempel[¶], and Alice Virani[††,‡‡]

*Faculty of Health Sciences, Simon Fraser University,
Burnaby, Canada

†Provincial Health Service Authority,
Vancouver, Canada

‡BC Centre for Disease Control,
Vancouver, Canada

§Genome British Columbia,
Vancouver, Canada

¶Knowledge Translation (KT) Team, BC Centre for Disease Control,
Vancouver, Canada

‖BC Support Unit — Fraser Centre, Vancouver, Canada

**Department of Evaluation and Research, Fraser Health Authority,
Surrey, Canada

††Department of Medical Genetics, University of British Columbia,
Vancouver, Canada

‡‡Ethics Service, Provincial Health Service Authority of BC,
Clinical Support Building, Vancouver, Canada

Key Message

- Pillar two of the World Health Organization (WHO) COVID-19 Strategic Preparedness Response Plan addresses pandemic communications and community engagement.
- The WHO has identified an "infodemic" that parallels the COVID-19 pandemic, jeopardizes public health initiatives, and is caused by a confluence of technology, social media, and the spread of misinformation, either unintentionally or deliberately (disinformation).
- Related are conspiracy theories, which persist globally, even in the absence of evidence, to explain the causation of "big" events and place blame on a set of malevolent actors. Conspiratorial thinking is linked to lower levels of education, conservative political and religious affiliations, anxiety, powerlessness, and the need to feel part of a group which is unique or underappreciated compared to others.
- Strategies to combat misinformation, disinformation, and conspiracy theories target both individuals, including debunking and tools for critical thinking, and the structural level, including working with social media companies to combat spread.
- Trust in information and its sources are needed to build community resilience to the infodemic, especially in historically oppressed and excluded communities.
- The pandemic provides an opportunity to build or rebuild that trust through improved models for risk communication, grounded in meaningful community engagement and informed by decades of research into the psychology and sociology of risk.
- Evaluation of these models and their impact around the world will inform future preparedness and ongoing response activities.

1. Introduction

Risk communication and community engagement form Pillar 2 of the 2020 World Health Organization (WHO) COVID-19 Strategic Preparedness and Response Plan.[1] The Pillar addresses the substance and form of communications and a community-engaged approach. The latter requires active participation from diverse communities in the co-development of "responsive, empathic, transparent and consistent messaging in local languages" and dissemination "through trusted channels of communication, using community-based networks and key influencers".[1,2] This approach recognizes that "building capacity of local entities is essential to establish authority and trust".[1]

Risk communication is the "exchange of real-time information, advice and opinions between experts and people facing threats to their health, economic or social well-being".[3] Its goal is to "enable people at risk to make informed decisions to protect themselves and their loved ones".[3] However, many psycho-social and political factors, trust in experts and institutions, and the rise of digital and social media platforms may mitigate against effective risk communication.[4] Risk communication does not occur within an informational vacuum and must therefore account for circulating misinformation and disinformation. Misinformation refers to false or inaccurate information, while disinformation is developed with the intention to mislead and may be promulgated by state and non-state actors.

The degree to which misinformation about COVID-19 has been circulated, especially on social media, has led the WHO and other global organizations to draw attention to an "infodemic" that parallels the current pandemic. The infodemic sits at the confluence of technology, social media and information, caused by those with alternative agendas who may wittingly or unwittingly manipulate and amplify false or misleading information, jeopardizing public health initiatives to control the pandemic. Such manipulation has real-world physical and mental health impacts, may increase stigmatization, and may lead people not to observe public health measures and campaigns with proven population health benefits. In May 2020, the World Health Assembly called on WHO Member States to "develop and implement action plans to manage the infodemic".[5]

Here, we provide background and synthesize evidence on the challenges and opportunities inherent in risk communication grounded in community engagement for the COVID-19 and future pandemics. We discuss the evidence, if any, that supports the WHO Pillar 2 action recommendations (Table 1).[1]

Table 1: WHO Pillar 2 action recommendations.

Step 1	a. Implement national risk-communication and community engagement plan for COVID-19, including details of anticipated public health measures.
	b. Conduct rapid behaviour assessment to understand key target audience, perceptions, concerns, influencers and preferred communication channels.
	c. Prepare local messages and pre-test through a participatory process, specifically targeting key stakeholders and at-risk groups.
	d. Identify trusted community groups (local influencers such as community leaders, religious leaders, health workers, community volunteers) and local networks (women's groups, youth groups, business groups, traditional healers, etc.).
Step 2	a. Establish and utilize clearance processes for timely dissemination of messages and materials in local languages and adopt relevant communication channels.
	b. Engage with existing public health and community-based networks, media, local NGOs, schools, local governments and other sectors such as healthcare service providers, education sector, business, travel and food/agriculture sectors using a consistent mechanism of communication.
	c. Utilize two-way "channels" for community and public information sharing such as hotlines (text and talk), responsive social media such as U-Report where available, and radio shows, with systems to detect and rapidly respond to and counter misinformation.
	d. Establish large scale community engagement for social and behaviour change approaches to ensure preventive community and individual health and hygiene practices in line with the national public health containment recommendations.
Step 3	a. Systematically establish community information and feedback mechanisms including through: social media monitoring; community perceptions, knowledge, attitude and practice surveys; and direct dialogues and consultations.
	b. Ensure changes to community engagement approaches are based on evidence and needs, and ensure all engagement is culturally appropriate and empathetic.
	c. Document lessons learned to inform future preparedness and response activities.

2. Pandemic Communications

Risk communication is an intractive process for the exchange of information among stakeholders about potential, emerging or existing threats to human health or the environment. Risk communication practice is informed by the interdisciplinary field of risk communications, that incorporates psychology, sociology, decision science and communications.[6] Psychology helps us understand how individuals process uncertainty under a range of conditions and emotions; sociology enables understanding of the structures and informational networks that transmit information and build trust (or mistrust); decision science characterizes uncertainty and performance of complex systems; and communications explores how information is transmitted over diverse channels, interpreted by diverse audience, and how information affects beliefs, attitudes, and behaviours.[6]

In the context of a pandemic, the goal of pandemic communications is to encourage individual, community and societal behaviour change and acceptance for the uptake of public health measures to control the spread of the infectious agent. Public health measures include those that prevent or reduce its spread: wearing of masks and other personal protective equipment (PPE); hand-washing and hygiene; social/physical distancing, size of social groups, quarantine, stay-at home orders and occupancy limits; screening, diagnostic testing and contact-tracing; paid or unpaid sick-leave; and vaccination.[7] However, receptivity to communications about public health measures varies according to individual characteristics, such as age; race; sex; gender; socio-economic status; education level; scientific literacy; and social, political, cultural, and religious identity.[8–10]

During a pandemic, public health officials operate in a complex environment with increased time-pressures and communication frequency.[11] Simultaneously, there is a need for transparency in the presentation of evidence, balanced against privacy interests and the duty of confidentiality.[11] Communications need to present evolving information and associated uncertainty in ways that are effective and accessible to diverse audiences and offer practical advice for individual and collective action.[11,12] Communications need to account for differing risk factors and the ways in which individuals perceive and respond to risk.[13,14] For example, in the context of the COVID-19 pandemic, older adults are at greater risk for mortality[15] and may be motivated by considerations of self-protection, while younger adults may be motivated by fear of spreading the virus to vulnerable family members or concerns about socioeconomic or educational impacts.[12]

Further complicating pandemic communications is the diversity of communications platforms that range from traditional media to online content and social media. These communications channels are increasingly fragmented, attracting partisan audiences.[16] Low adherence to public health measures is linked to exposure to conservative media outlets, conservative political views, and low levels of trust in science and scientists. Conversely, liberal political views, exposure to mainstream news outlets and high confidence in science and scientists is linked to high adherence,[17,18] as is a collectivist ethos.[19] Information overload from social media use may negatively impact prevention behaviours by increasing the perception of their costs relative to their benefits.[20]

In this complex media environment, international organizations, such as the United Nations and World Health Organization, and national/ regional governments developed media strategies to communicate public health responses to the pandemic. These include the UN Coronavirus (COVID-19), WHO "myth busters" and United States Centers for Disease Control updates, dashboards, and news portals.[21] Organizations included daily or weekly briefings covered by traditional media, where politicians and public health officials presented pandemic data and measures to control the spread of the virus. In addition to traditional media, many governments and organizations developed social media strategies. For example, the Group of Seven world leaders used Twitter to provide informative (82.8%), morale-boosting (9.4%), and political (6.9%) content.[22]

3. Misinformation, Disinformation and Conspiracy Theories

Pandemic risk communications are complicated by the spread of misinformation and disinformation, particularly on social media. Misinformation is "information considered incorrect based on the best available evidence from relevant experts at the time",[23] while disinformation is the intentional spread of false information "to influence public opinion or obscure the truth".[24] The spread of both mis- and disinformation is a global phenomenon,[25,26] with lower-income countries having a higher prevalence of misinformation than higher-income countries,[27] as well as higher circulation rates.[28] Both strategies may also be used to sow distrust in institutions, including public health authorities, and their decision-making processes.

The spread of mis- and disinformation is a multifaceted phenomenon, amplified by, but not unique to, the COVID-19 pandemic. Contributing to the phenomenon are transformations in our media and information environments, increasing political partisanship, psycho-social factors in the way people select and process information, and even misaligned incentives in scientific systems.[29] The latter stems from the speed at which pandemic science has been prioritized; carried out; disseminated, sometimes without adequate peer-review on pre-print servers;[30] and reported on by researchers, institutions, and media.[18] High profile studies have been retracted due to methodological and other concerns only after informing clinical or public health practice and being endorsed by political leaders and celebrities. For example, initial studies on the clinical utility of the anti-malarial, suggested hydroxycholoroquine as a treatment for COVID-19.[18] Definitive evidence now exists that hydroxychloroquine has no clinical benefit in treating hospitalized COVID-19 patients,[31] despite being promoted by high-profile individuals, such as Elon Musk and former President Donald Trump.[32] The story of Vitamin D followed a similar arc.[33] In another example, a pre-print allegedly written by an Indonesian academic has been used more than 100,000 times; cited in academic articles, including in the *British Medical Journal*; downloaded; mentioned in social media posts; and shared, despite the author having no academic profile and the purported hospital where the study took place not being a COVID treatment centre.

Individual ability to identify mis- and disinformation depends on information processing and motivation to engage with falsehoods combined with an individual's social networks and information ecologies.[34] Heightened anxiety, in the context of a pandemic or other stressors, may lead individuals to increase their screen time and share information in online environments.[35,36] Susceptibility to mis- and disinformation is exacerbated by incomplete or biased science education.[34] It may also be influenced by demographic characteristics. For example, older adults who rely on social media had greater levels of anxiety, and the contradictory information encountered on these platforms caused confusion.[37]

Mis- and disinformation about COVID-19 are amplified on social media platforms because of the number of users (over 3 billion),[36] the ease and speed with which information can be shared,[21,38] and the increased digital screen time that derives from isolation and anxiety.[36]. Social media have shifted the prominence of discourse from scientific experts;[39] they have blurred the provenance of information, as individuals motivated by personal or family connection to the information share it with their social networks.[38] Such sharing reinforces social connections, which, in turn, override critical judgement as to the credibility of the information and its source.[38]

Of greatest concern, misinformation spreads more rapidly on social media than science-based or fact-based evidence.[40–45] Misinformation targets vaccination[46] and other public health measures, such as mask wearing.[47] Social media concerns about mask-wearing are dominated by arguments on constitutional rights/freedom of choice and fear-inducing narratives about population control, big pharma, fake news and pandemic denial.[47] Misinformation has been identified on a variety of social media platforms, including WeChat, Twitter, Facebook, Instagram, Pinterest, Tencent, Whatsapp, YouTube, and TikTok[46,48] and GoFundMe, a crowd-funding platform.[49] Campaigns on the latter platform aim to develop interventions, including dietary supplements and so-called immune system boosters, as well as a range of complementary and alternative and other unproven medical interventions. Many make claims of therapeutic efficacy and prophylaxis.[49] On Twitter, misinformation focused tweets were more negative than informational tweets.[50]

The spread of misinformation on social media is further amplified by Internet trolls and bots: "a troll is an actor who uses social media to start arguments, upset people, and sow confusion among users by circulating inflammatory and often false information online. Many trolls are actually bots — automated accounts pretending to be humans — which can be programmed to spread false and misleading stories rapidly through online social networks".[48] Trolls and bots are prevalent on social media platforms such as Twitter, Facebook and YouTube.[41,48] Their business model relies on the "click" patterns of users and the gaming of social media algorithms that lead users to click through to content similar to that previously consumed. The algorithms progressively narrow the range of topics and information, which, in the case of misinformation, may lead users to ever more extreme views. The amount of misinformation on the Internet has "multiplied rapidly through the rising influence of dark money, funds of unknown provenance that sponsor trolls and bots to sow confusion and create distrust".[48] However, commercial interests may also use misinformation to lead users to marketable products purported to be treatments or preventive measures for the virus, such as nutritional supplements and immune-system boosters.[51]

Closely related to the spread of mis- and disinformation is conspiratorial thinking, which is more likely to emerge during societal crises.[26] Conspiracy theories are persistent, even in the absence of evidence and explain the causation of "big" events blamed on a set of malevolent conspirators.[52] The rise of political populism feeds conspiratorial thinking. Populist leaders such as former President Donald Trump and Brazil's President Jair Bolsonaro characterize their political movements as a struggle of the virtuous populace against corrupt, establishment elites, including scientists and academic institutions.[53,54] Science-related populism manifests around strongly politicized topics such as climate change and vaccination or alternative world views on nutrition or homeopathy.[54]

Conspiratorial thinking is global,[55] with confirmatory studies in China,[56-58] Japan,[59] Australia and New Zealand,[60,61] France,[58] Spain,[62] the United States,[63] and Brazil.[64] In the United States, the majority of 3,019 adults surveyed believed in at least one conspiracy theory about the SARS-CoV-2 virus, including that: it was intentionally created, it was accidentally released by China, it is a bioweapon, it was intentionally created to harm President Trump, it is a hoax, it has had its seriousness exaggerated by the media to harm President Trump, Democrats are refusing to administer tests to harm President Trump, it is spread by 5G Technology, Bill Gates is creating a tracking device for COVID-19 vaccines, and that it was intentionally created to reduce world population.[65] Eighty-five percent of those surveyed believed in more than one of these conspiracy theories, 60% believed in three or more, and 30% believed at least six.[65]

The author concluded that "interchangeability of these beliefs may make attempts to debunk them by tackling each one individually akin to a futile game of whack-a-mole".[65]

Other theories on conspiratorial thinking link it to individual attempts to explain significant events by finding patterns and constructing meaning where none exist and making causal inferences.[66] It is linked to lower levels of education, conservative political and religious affiliations, anxiety, powerlessness, and the need to feel part of a group which is unique or underappreciated compared to others.[52] Conspiracy theories are consequential, as they raise skepticism in government recommendations and actions[66] and reject scientific authority and knowledge generated using scientific methods.[60] With respect to public health measures, conspiracy theorists reject claims about natural phenomena, such as human disease and immunity and ameliorative causes of action, such as vaccination.[60] Indeed, belief in conspiracy theories predict vaccine hesitancy.[55] Conspiracy theorists are more likely to "like" and share related posts on social media (Facebook and Twitter) than debunkers of those theories.[52]

Conspiracy theories premised on blaming another group have broader societal consequences.[66] For example, right-wing populist, Australian politician, Pauline Hanson, has used the COVID-19 crisis to bolster her racist immigration agenda on social media.[67] The pandemic has given rise to a wave of racist sentiment, in particular, anti-Asian racism, promulgated on social media around the world.[68,69]

Ironically, one of the SARS-CoV-2 origin beliefs that has to date been labelled a conspiracy theory is being reconsidered by experts.[70] In May 2020, the *Washington Post*'s Fact Checker team reported that the "balance of the scientific evidence strongly supports the conclusion that the new coronavirus emerged from nature." A joint report by the World Health Organization and China, released in February 2021, said a lab escape of the virus was "extremely unlikely." But by late March 2021, the WHO Director-General stated at the Member State Briefing that: "Although the team has concluded that a laboratory leak is the least likely hypothesis, this requires further investigation, potentially with additional missions involving specialist experts".[71] In late May 2021, a group of 18 pre-eminent scientists published a letter in the journal *Science* saying a new investigation is needed, because "theories of accidental release from a lab and zoonotic spillover both remain viable".[72] The scientists call for independent, transparent, and ongoing research into the origins of the SARS-CoV-2 virus, but the claims fall short of condoning deliberate genetic manipulation of viruses, bioweapons development, or deliberate release of a known human pathogen. Any laboratory leak would have been due to mishandling and breaches of biosafety protocols of a naturally occurring Coronavirus, sampled from wildlife populations, likely bats. Nevertheless, political considerations by the WHO and other leaders early in the pandemic, which resisted criticism of China and its lack of transparency about the origins of the virus, may feed a prevalent conspiracy theory, further reducing public trust in public health authorities.

4. Strategies to Combat Misinformation, Disinformation and Conspiracy Theories

Since conspiracy theories are often multilayered and nebulous, they are resistant to disconfirmation.[66] The better strategy may be to address the political and psychological needs that give rise to conspiratorial thinking, including: "situationally induced uncertainty, powerlessness, and concomitant anxiety".[65] Suggested strategies aim to help individuals identify and evaluate information and prevent exposure of individuals to mis- and dis-information at a structural level.[41] In this section, we first discuss strategies that target individuals, followed by a discussion of work at the structural level.

4.1 *Individual-level strategies*

Combating the Infodemic is a critical public health priority, and numerous authors have synthesized evidence that support concrete recommendations for a two-pronged approach to correct or debunk misinformation and to bolster individual and community resilience to misinformation.[51] Evidence suggests that both strategies have some positive effect, and strategies in support of the former include: using facts; providing clear, straightforward and shareable content; using trustworthy and independent sources; emphasizing scientific consensus where it exists, while recognizing that scientific knowledge evolves over time and may shift such consensus; being authentic and maintaining a civil tone;[73] using narratives rather than relying on numeric data; emphasizing gaps and flaws in the logic of the misinformation; making the facts the hook, not the misinformation; and focusing messages on the general public, not the hard-core believer or conspiracy theorist.[51] Further, promoting collectivist messages "we are all in this together" may also reduce susceptibility to misinformation.[66] This works because those with a collectivist world-view are more likely to comply with public health measures than.[66]

Debunking has largely been in the purview of fact-checking organizations, including international and national public health authorities, traditional media, and independent groups, such as the #ScienceUpFirst initiative in Canada.[74] The latter is a social media movement developed by a team of over 7,000 independent scientists, healthcare providers, and science communicators, who have come together to stop the spread of misinformation and provide shareable, verified information on social media — Twitter, Instagram and Facebook.

While such debunking initiatives are laudable, they are unlikely to be effective in isolation. These initiatives have the overwhelming hurdle the complex factors driving COVID-19 misinformation sharing, including "emotions, distrust, cognitive biases, racism and xenophobia".[69] Cognitive biases include confirmation bias, which encourages individuals to seek out information that supports preconceived opinions and beliefs, while ignoring contrary evidence and disconfirmation bias, which leads individuals to apply greater scrutiny to contrary arguments and evidence.[69] Further, the nature of scientific evidence, which is generally presented probabilistically, is counter-productive to the "confidence heuristic", namely those promulgating misinformation are free to express themselves with greater certainty, which can be interpreted as accuracy or knowledge,[69] thereby placing credible sources of information at a disadvantage. Further, information that elicits strong emotions, such as fear, anxiety, and sadness, are more likely to be shared.[44]

These limitations highlight the importance of the second strategy, which depends on providing people with the tools to become critical consumers of information.[51] These "pre-bunking" strategies include the teaching of critical thinking skills and media-literacy.[51,52] There is also need for improved understanding of incremental, iterative, and evolving scientific processes,[26,69] and improved health literacy, which makes people critical seekers and utilizers of health information.[75] "Inoculating" people with factual information on vaccines, for example, has decreased vaccine hesitancy, but only prior to conspiracy theories becoming established.[76] Individuals might be encouraged to think about the kinds of information they share on social media. This includes illuminating the credibility of disinformation agents by exposing their financial, political, and other interests. Finally, trusted actors have a role in these educational strategies for health misinformation, and their role is discussed further below.

4.2 *Strategies at the structural level*

Strategies at the structural level include working with social media companies to combat the spread of misinformation.[21] Google, for example has created a multi-lingual alert on COVID-19 and raised the profile of the WHO and its social media accounts in public searches. Amazon has restricted and removed advertisements that contain false claims about PPE, and Facebook, YouTube, Microsoft, and Twitter have placed restrictions and warnings on pandemic content and plan to remove scientifically disproven claims. Most notably, former US president Donald Trump has been permanently banned by Twitter and suspended by Facebook for two years. Such platforms have also banned or suspended individuals who spread disinformation. Similarly, medical and scientific publishers have fast-tracked peer-review and increased transparency by making their pandemic content open access. Pre-print servers have added warnings to articles to remind readers that these have not yet undergone peer-review.

Other recommendations include the verification of the accounts of public health personnel on social media platforms to enable the public to verify the credibility of the material and its source, promote the posts of public health and medical professionals, and monitor user engagement with information on social media platforms.[21] Initiatives focused on the latter lead to mechanisms for social media surveillance, which may even help predict waves of the pandemic and potential hotspots through the tracking symptom-related keywords.[77–79] Surveillance may also track public sentiment, responsiveness to public health messaging,[80,81] vaccine intention and anti-vaccination rhetoric.[82] Finally, it is clear that mental health plays a role in the promulgation of misinformation and trust in information and institutions, and public health authorities and governments need to invest in programs that help people cope with stress, anxiety, and fear.[21,83]

5. Pandemic Communications and Community Trust

5.1 *Trust*

Trust in information and its sources, such as the WHO,[84] is needed to build community resilience in the face of pandemic threats.[85,86] Trust positively influences people's willingness to adopt public health measures.[87] Trust in authorities can mitigate complexity in the face of information overload and support decision-making.[87] It is essential when people lack the knowledge to directly evaluate the risks and benefits of a technology or action.[87] However, trust is fragile — it is created slowly, and once it is lost, it takes a long time to rebuild.[4]

Historically oppressed and excluded communities, such as Indigenous,[88] Black and Hispanic communities, have low levels of trust in public health authorities.[85] These same communities are now being asked to trust the structures that have led to disproportionate health and economic impacts of COVID-19.[89,90] Even prior to the pandemic, lower levels of trust in healthcare systems derive from: historical experience of medical exploitation, unconsented experimentation, social and economic marginalization, systemic racism and discriminatory practices by healthcare providers, trauma and violence, lack of access, and language and logistical barriers. Logistical barriers include Black–White disparities in access to vaccination sites in the United States.[91,92] As a result of trust deficits, vaccine hesitancy are higher amongst Black and Hispanic Americans[93] and Black residents of the United Kingdom.[94]

The global rollout of COVID-19 vaccines will only be successful in ending the pandemic if high numbers of people are vaccinated. This will only be achieved if "cultural, socioeconomic and political barriers that lead to mistrust and hinder uptake of vaccines" can be overcome.[94] It is clear that social learning — learning by observing the behaviour of others — will play a role in adherence to vaccination and other public health measures.[7] Communication about expectations and prioritization schedules will need to be carefully disseminated to avoid trust-destroying events, especially in communities that are distrustful of healthcare professionals and other authorities.[95] Vaccine hesitancy may derive from concerns about safety, suspicions about the political and economic forces that drove vaccine development, a lack of knowledge about vaccines, lack of liability of pharmaceutical companies for adverse events, and confusing messages from public health leaders.[96] However, they may also derive from broken social contracts between governments and populations whose health needs have not been well-served to-date.[94] Communications should, therefore, be field-tested and account for country-level variation in vaccine hesitancy,[97] individual preferences and the characteristics of available vaccines.[98] Broad community engagement, discussed below, will be essential to communications initiatives for vaccines and other public health measures.

5.2 *The role of influencers*

Community trust in pandemic communications may be augmented if messages are delivered from a trusted source or community influencer. Influencers may be cultural, political or religious leaders, celebrities and social media influencers, or trusted healthcare providers.

5.2.1 *Clinicians and patient organizations*

Clinicians maintain a high level of public trust and are central in sharing trustworthy health information during clinical encounters.[99,100] Increasingly, clinicians are engaging in awkward conversations about misinformation and likely require further support and training to do so.[38] Simple advice for clinicians is to listen and demonstrate humility in not over-stating certainty while explaining facts, patience and compassion in discussion. In engaging in conversation with patients, it is important for clinicians to acknowledge their perspectives and lived experience.[39] While time consuming, building trust is key, which includes transparency with respect to conflicts of interest.[39] Clinicians can also help support the mental health effects of COVID-19, including that which is due to anxiety from excessive media exposure.[101] Beyond clinical encounters, some clinicians have developed social media profiles and large followings to spread validated information.[102] Not limited to social media, Dr. Terri Aldred, avTl'Azt'En, mixed European and Métis Cree clinician was featured in a televised public service announcement/commercial and on roadside billboards in British Columbia. Patient organizations similarly have roles to play amongst their constituent membership, which comprises individuals at greater risk due to co-morbidities. Patient organizations have substantial online and social media presence, as well as patient-engagement mechanisms.

5.2.2 *Social media influencers and other celebrities*

Social media influencers are "digital first personalities" whose success depends on likeability, trending topics, visibility, sensationalism to attract followers and sustain an advertising revenue.[103] A variety of governments, including Finland, Japan and Indonesia have enlisted the assistance of influencers as disseminators of information on social media, especially among younger audiences.[103] More traditional celebrities are highly influential in that their actions and decisions may be watched and emulated by wide audiences. They may use their celebrity to market products, some of questionable health benefit such as Gwyneth Paltrow's Goop brand.[104] Celebrity social media posts are liked and circulated at a rate that far exceeds politicians and public health officials.[105] Some celebrities have shared their COVID-19 experiences, such as actor, Tom Hanks, and one study indicated a stronger willingness to engage in prevention behaviours in response.[106]

5.2.3 *Religious leaders*

Religion is part of the world view and lifestyle of many people. Religious leaders are trusted gatekeepers to communities of faith and can play a vital role in the context of COVID-19.[107] Some faith communities, especially in the United States, are part of the misinformation problem, claiming epistemic and cultural authority that undermines science-informed public health measures.[108] In British Columbia, Evangelical church leaders in the hardest-hit health region have continued to advocate for and conduct large, in-person services, even in the face of repeated fines.[109] However, the work of other faith leaders is central to healthcare responses and meeting community-wide needs.[110] Such leaders can mobilize assistance and resources to meet gaps in social services and provide a pastoral role of reassurance and comfort.[110] Religious leaders can play an active role in promoting vaccination initiatives, especially in diaspora communities that may be difficult to reach because of language, cultural and socio-economic barriers. For example, in British Columbia, with the support of leadership, public health officials in the Fraser Health Authority actively met community members in their significant spaces, targeting vaccination registration events at gurdwaras, mosques, and temples.

5.2.4 *Community leaders*

Other community leaders, such as teachers and leaders of sports and youth clubs, can also play key roles in supporting public health measures and modeling protective behaviours, including vaccination. For example, in British Columbia, Canada, educators have played a critical role in dispelling social anxiety about COVID-19 spread in classroom settings, while practicing public health measures. Their daily interactions with families and students to promote the safety of the school setting was arguably the crux of keeping public schools and daycares open and operating.

In British Columbia, the region served by the Fraser Health Authority had the highest number of COVID-19 cases in British Columbia. It was important, therefore, to work with community leaders to understand barriers to accessing health information and vaccination. Initiatives that emerged in tandem with municipal and community groups included supports for isolating families, such as food and transportation to testing sites.

In Canada, for example, the Morning Star Lab based at the University of Saskatchewan and the British Columbia Centre for Disease Control's COVID-19 Indigenous Knowledge Translation Working Group engaged with Indigenous Elders and other community/thought leaders to develop COVID-19 prevention and vaccination messages. The Elders, who attended for the first wave of vaccinations specifically for Elders, were offered these resources to take back to their communities.

5.3 *The form of communication*

Different people interpret risk in different ways, making the form of communication important. Lessons from cognitive psychology suggest the humans comprehend risks both experientially and analytically. The former is intuitive, fast, automatic, and unconscious; the latter is relatively slow, requiring effort and conscious control to apply logic and algorithmic and normative rules.[111] The experiential system relies on "images and associations, linked by experience to emotion and affect and operates interdependently with the system for rational analysis.[111] Both systems are prone to systematic errors, many identified in the seminal work of Kahneman and Tversky, including: strong emotions, like fear and hatred occasion departures from rationalityaffect heuristic); perceptions of potential losses loom larger than gains (prospect theory); optimism in estimating personal risk relative to average risk (optimism bias); and the ease with which an instance or example of an occurrence can be brought to mind (availability heuristic).[112] Understanding how individuals interpret risk probabilities, therefore, informs the structure and form of communications.[113]

Effective communications need to account for human emotion and the ways emotions are generated.[114] For example, presenting risks as frequencies (one in a hundred people) as opposed to probabilities (1%) can facilitate a mental image of the risk and a corresponding emotional response.[114] Because processing of such numerical information depends on individual numeracy, communication can be improved by presenting qualitative distinctions, or the gist of the risk. This is benefited by the use of meaningful messages and visual displays,[115] including tabular and graphical formats.[113] Shareable infographics from credible sources can improve communications.[23] When communicating using visual media, however, it is important to minimize discrepancies in audio and visual content.[116] Public health spokespeople can lose control of their verbal message, if accompanying visual content focuses on negative or fear-inducing images, such as body-bags, emergency rooms, and long vaccination lineups.[116]

5.4 *Strategies: Public engagement*

It is essential for pandemic communicators to understand whether social media and other messages are effectively meeting the needs of specific populations.[117] For example, women and younger older adults were more likely to search for and share information about COVID-19 than men and their older counterparts.[118] Racial and gender differences in vaccine intention clearly point to the need to tailor campaigns based on gender and race.[119] The global nature of the pandemic requires consideration of communications in all countries, including those that have regional, cultural, linguistic and ethnic diversity, and high burdens of poverty and COVID-19.[120] Previous experience with public health emergencies and vaccination campaigns highlights the need to tailor health promotion messages for different racial minorities. For example, in the United States for traditionally underserved Black, Hispanic and Native communities.[121] and those who face intersecting disadvantages, such as Black women.[91] Another example is the set of COVID-19 Informational Media Content and Infographics in over twenty South Asian languages.[122] Three South Asian Women from the UK, USA and Canada created the resource the help of a network of student from over 53 countries to address misinformation, reduce panic, and provide free, accessible, shareable, and accurate content. The content was developed with the guidance and advice of the WHO, the US CDCP.

While targeting messages to specific groups poses challenges for communicators, these challenges may be mitigated through effective models of community engagement.[85] This is especially true for hardly reached special populations, including those with who are neuro diverse or differently abled or who face language or cultural barriers, lack of access to communications channels, distrust in healthcare providers or systems based on historical oppression and structural/individual racism, or psycho–social–political biases that shape reactions to pandemic communications.[85] For example, the BCCDC COVID-19 Indigenous Knowledge Translation Working Group was established with 65% Indigenous membership, of whom some are embedded in their traditional lands and home communities. The leadership of the Working Group is shared by one Indigenous and a non-Indigenous person. With this structure, this Working

Group, becomes a site of engagement while it supports content development and dissemination of new COVID-19 resources.

It is imperative for public health communicators to involve communities in the collection and dissemination of information.[123] Communities are not homogeneous. An effective communications strategy is built on a process of co-design that engenders trust by engaging communities in the development of clear and tailored messages delivered via appropriate spokespeople via appropriate channels.[94,124] Such engagement enables diverse local voices to be heard. It best addresses the social determinants of health and rights "within dynamics of relational power and inequality".[125] Public engagement models may be most effective when deployed upstream, beginning societal dialogue about potential issues prior to formal decision-making processes.[126]

However, care needs to be taken that engagement processes are participatory and do not entrench existing privilege and power structures.[126] In developing pandemic communications strategies, it is essential to understand the life experiences of community members, which may include the recognition of past trauma and resiliency. Accounting for trauma and resiliency suggests approaches that empower individuals, provide choice and account for preferences, maximize collaboration among community members and public health professionals, ensure physically and emotionally safe spaces for dialogue among community members and public health professionals, and build trust by creating clear expectations.[127,128]

For example, the British Columbia Centre for Disease Control (BCCDC) established a knowledge translation user engagement network, which orchestrated rapid response surveys with a pre-screened and pre-pared subset of heterogeneous communities. The surveys informed knowledge translation product development in response to the evolving public health measures or interventions. Broader ongoing population health level surveys (Misinformation in Health and COVID-speaks) informed the localization of inequities in the Provincial response, and, as a result, where resources and community engagement needed to be focused.

An inclusive, co-creation model for pandemic communication delineates the distinction between risk communication or a top-down strategy for crisis management to a model of knowledge translation. Best practices for knowledge translation engage stakeholders and rightsholders in adapting knowledge to local contexts, which include trauma and resilience; assessing barriers to its use; and evaluating outcomes.[129] Indeed, it is encouraging that the rich and evolving literature reviewed in the Chapter instantiates the WHO evaluation recommendation to "document lessons learned to inform future preparedness and response activities".

6. Conclusion

The COVID-19 pandemic has brought into sharp relief concerns about media and political environments. Public health officials have been combating not only a pandemic, but also a parallel Infodemic. There will likely be a political and regulatory reckoning for the forces that have created the informational environment that has jeopardized public health measures to bring the pandemic under control. The pandemic has brought into sharp relief the social inequities within our health systems and the lack of trust in public health authorities. The pandemic now provides an opportunity to build or rebuild that trust through improved models for risk communication, grounded in meaningful community engagement and informed by decades of research into the psychology and sociology of risk. Evaluation of these models and their impact around the world will inform future preparedness and ongoing response activities.

References

1. Organization WH. COVID-19 Strategic Preparedness and Response Plan: Operational Planning Guidelines to Support Country Preparedness and Response. Geneva, Switzerland, 2020.
2. Wu JH, John SD. The ethics of COVID-19 risk communication. *Journal of General Internal Medicine*. 2021;36(4):1092–1093.
3. Organization WH. Risk Communication: General Information on Risk Communication 2021. Available from: https://www.who.int/risk-communication/background/en/.
4. Slovic P. Trust, emotion, sex, politics, and science: Surveying the risk-assessment battlefield. *Risk Analysis*. 1999;19(4):689–701.

5. COVID-19 response, (19 May 2020).

6. Fischhoff B, Scheufele DA. The science of science communication III. *Proceedings of the National Academy of Sciences of the United States of America*. 2019;116(16):7632–7633.

7. Majid U, Wasim A, Bakshi S, Truong J. Knowledge, (mis-)conceptions, risk perception, and behavior change during pandemics: A scoping review of 149 studies. *Public Understanding of Science*. 2020;29(8):777–799.

8. Wood S, Schulman K. Beyond politics — promoting Covid-19 vaccination in the United States. *New England Journal of Medicine*. 2021;384(7):e23.

9. Weisberg DS, Landrum AR, Hamilton J, Weisbert M. Knowledge about the nature of science increases public acceptance of science regardless of identity factors. *Public Understanding of Science*. 2020;30(2):120–38.

10. Lang R, Benham JL, Atabati O, Hollis A, Tombe T, Shaffer B, *et al.* Attitudes, behaviours and barriers to public health measures for COVID-19: A survey to inform public health messaging. *BMC Public Health*. 2021;21(1).

11. Lasser J, Ahne V, Heiler G, Klimek P, Metzler H, Reisch T, *et al.* Complexity, transparency and time pressure: Practical insights into science communication in times of crisis. *Journal of Science Communication*. 2020;19(05): N01.

12. Noar SM, Austin L. (Mis)communicating about COVID-19: Insights from Health and Crisis Communication. *Health Communication*. 2020; 35(14):1735–9.

13. Sandman PM. Crisis communication best practices: Some quibbles and additions. *Journal of Applied Communication Research*. 2006;34(3): 257–262.

14. Sandman PM, Lanard J. Crisis communication: Guidelines for action: American Industrial Hygiene Association; 2004. Available from: www. psandman.com/handouts/AIHA-DVD.htm.

15. Sharma A. Estimating older adult mortality from COVID-19. *The Journals of Gerontology: Series B*. 2021;76(3):e68–e74.

16. Hopp T, Ferrucci P. A Spherical rendering of deviant information resilience. *Journalism & Mass Communication Quarterly*. 2020;97(2):492–508.

17. Bekalu MA, Dhawan D, McCloud R, Pinnamaneni R, Viswanath K. Adherence to COVID-19 mitigation measures among American adults: The need for consistent and unified messaging. *Health Education Research*. 2021;36(2):178–191.

18. Caulfield T, Bubela T, Kimmelman J, Ravitsky V, Blais JM. Let's do better: Public representations of COVID-19 science. *FACETS*. 2021;6:403–423.

19. Huang F, Ding H, Liu Z, Wu P, Zhu M, Li A, *et al*. How fear and collectivism influence public's preventive intention towards COVID-19 infection: A study based on big data from the social media. *BMC Public Health*. 2020;20(1).
20. Farooq A, Laato S, Islam AKMN, Isoaho J. Understanding the impact of information sources on COVID-19 related preventive measures in Finland. *Technology in Society*. 2021;65.
21. Mheidly N, Fares J. Leveraging media and health communication strategies to overcome the COVID-19 infodemic. *Journal of Public Health Policy*. 2020;41(4):410–420.
22. Rufai SR, Bunce C. World leaders' usage of Twitter in response to the COVID-19 pandemic: A content analysis. *Journal of Public Health*. 2020;42(3):510–516.
23. Vraga EK, Bode L. Addressing COVID-19 misinformation on social media preemptively and responsively. *Emerging Infectious Diseases*. 2021;27(2): 396–403.
24. Merriam-Webster. Merriam-Webster. The Real Story of 'Disinformation'.
25. Adekoya CO, Fasae JK. Social media and the spread of COVID-19 infodemic. *Global Knowledge, Memory and Communication*. 2021.
26. Agley J, Xiao Y. Misinformation about COVID-19: Evidence for differential latent profiles and a strong association with trust in science. *BMC Public Health*. 2021;21(1).
27. Cha M, Cha C, Singh K, Lima G, Ahn YY, Kulshrestha J, *et al*. Prevalence of misinformation and factchecks on the COVID-19 pandemic in 35 countries: Observational infodemiology study. *JMIR Hum Factors*. 2021;8(1).
28. Nsoesie EO, Cesare N, Muller M, Ozonoff A. COVID-19 misinformation spread in eight countries: Exponential growth modeling study. *Journal of Medical Internet Research*. 2020;22(12):e24425.
29. Scheufele DA, Hoffman AJ, Neeley L, Reid CM. Misinformation about science in the public sphere. *Proceedings of the National Academy of Sciences of the United States of America*. 2021;118(15).
30. Fraser N, Brierley L, Dey G, Polka JK, Pálfy M, Nanni F, *et al*. The evolving role of preprints in the dissemination of COVID-19 research and their impact on the science communication landscape. *PLoS Biology*. 2021;19(4).
31. Gould S, Norris SL. Contested effects and chaotic policies: the 2020 story of (hydroxy) chloroquine for treating COVID-19. *The Cochrane Database of Systematic Reviews*. 2021;3:ED000151.

32. Liu M, Caputi TL, Dredze M, Kesselheim AS, Ayers JW. Internet searches for unproven COVID-19 therapies in the United States. *JAMA Internal Medicine*. 2020;180(8):1116–8.

33. Henrina J, Lim MA, Pranata R. COVID-19 and misinformation: How an infodemic fuelled the prominence of vitamin D. *British Journal of Nutrition*. 2021;125(3):359–60.

34. Scheufele DA, Krause NM. Science audiences, misinformation, and fake news. *Proceedings of the National Academy of Sciences*. 2019;116(16): 7662–7669.

35. Freiling I, Krause NM, Scheufele DA, Brossard D. Believing and sharing misinformation, fact-checks, and accurate information on social media: The role of anxiety during COVID-19. *New Media and Society*. 2021.

36. Banerjee D, Meena KS. COVID-19 as an "infodemic" in public health: Critical role of the social media. *Frontiers in Public Health*. 2021;9.

37. Chun Wong FH, Liu T, Yi Leung DK, Zhang AY, Hong Au WS, Kwok WW, *et al.* Consuming information related to COVID-19 on social media among older adults and its association with anxiety, social trust in information, and COVID-safe behaviors: Cross-sectional telephone survey. *Journal of Medical Internet Research*. 2021;23(2).

38. Abbasi J. COVID-19 conspiracies and beyond: how physicians can deal with patients' misinformation. *JAMA — Journal of the American Medical Association*. 2021;325(3):208–10.

39. Baker DW. Trust in health care in the time of COVID-19. *JAMA — Journal of the American Medical Association*. 2020;324(23):2373–2375.

40. Lewandowsky S, Ecker UKH, Seifert CM, Schwarz N, Cook J. Misinformation and its correction. *Psychological Science in the Public Interest*. 2012;13(3):106–31.

41. Lazer DMJ, Baum MA, Benkler Y, Berinsky AJ, Greenhill KM, Menczer F, *et al.* The science of fake news. *Science*. 2018;359(6380):1094–1096.

42. Del Vicario M, Bessi A, Zollo F, Petroni F, Scala A, Caldarelli G, *et al.* The spreading of misinformation online. *Proceedings of the National Academy of Sciences*. 2016;113(3):554–549.

43. Pulido CM, Villarejo-Carballido B, Redondo-Sama G, Gómez A. COVID-19 infodemic: More retweets for science-based information on coronavirus than for false information. *International Sociology*. 2020;35(4):377–392.

44. Vosoughi S, Roy D, Aral S. The spread of true and false news online. *Science*. 2018;359(6380):1146–1151.

45. Obiała J, Obiała K, Mańczak M, Owoc J, Olszewski R. COVID-19 misinformation: Accuracy of articles about coronavirus prevention mostly shared on social media. *Health Policy and Technology*. 2021;10(1): 182–186.

46. Basch CH, Meleo-Erwin Z, Fera J, Jaime C, Basch CE. A global pandemic in the time of viral memes: COVID-19 vaccine misinformation and disinformation on TikTok. *Human Vaccines and Immunotherapeutics*. 2021.

47. Al-Ramahi M, Elnoshokaty A, El-Gayar O, Nasralah T, Wahbeh A. Public discourse against masks in the COVID-19 Era: Infodemiology study of twitter data. *JMIR Public Health Surveillance*. 2021;7(4).

48. Iyengar S, Massey DS. Scientific communication in a post-truth society. *Proceedings of the National Academy of Sciences*. 2019;116(16): 7656–7661.

49. Snyder J, Zenone M, Caulfield T. Crowdfunding campaigns and COVID-19 misinformation. *American Journal of Public Health*. 2021;111(4):739–742.

50. Gerts D, Shelley CD, Parikh N, Pitts T, Ross CW, Fairchild G, *et al.* "Thought I'd share first" and other conspiracy theory tweets from the COVID-19 infodemic: Exploratory study. *JMIR Public Health Surveillance*. 2021;7(4).

51. Caulfield T. Does Debunking Work? Correcting COVID-19 Misinformation on Social Media. In: *Vulnerable: The Law, Policy and Ethics of COVID-19*. Flood CM, MacDonnell V, Philpott J (eds.). Ottawa: University of Ottawa Press, 2020, pp. 183–200.

52. Lewandowsky S, Cook J. The Conspiracy Theory Handbook Bristol: University of Bristol, 2020. Available from: https://www.climatechange communication.org/wp-content/uploads/2020/03/ConspiracyTheory Handbook.pdf.

53. Calvo E, Ventura T. Will I Get COVID-19? Partisanship, social media frames, and perceptions of health risk in Brazil. *Latin American Politics and Society*. 2021;63(1):1–26.

54. Mede NG, Schafer MS. Science-related populism: Conceptualizing populist demands toward science. *Public Understanding of Science*. 2020;29(5): 473–491.

55. Hornsey MJ, Chapman CM, Alvarez B, Bentley S, Salvador Casara BG, Crimston CR, *et al.* To what extent are conspiracy theorists concerned for self versus others? A COVID-19 test case. *European Journal of Social Psychology*. 2021.

56. Zou W, Tang L. What do we believe in? Rumors and processing strategies during the COVID-19 outbreak in China. *Public Understanding of Science.* 2021;30(2):153–168.

57. Su Y, Lee DKL, Xiao X, Li W, Shu W. Who endorses conspiracy theories? A moderated mediation model of Chinese and international social media use, media skepticism, need for cognition, and COVID-19 conspiracy theory endorsement in China. *Computers in Human Behavior.* 2021;120.

58. Schück S, Foulquié P, Mebarki A, Faviez C, Khadhar M, Texier N, *et al.* Concerns discussed on chinese and french social media during the COVID-19 lockdown: Comparative infodemiology study based on topic modeling. *JMIR Formative Research.* 2021;5(4).

59. Cato S, Iida T, Ishida K, Ito A, Katsumata H, McElwain KM, *et al.* The bright and dark sides of social media usage during the COVID-19 pandemic: Survey evidence from Japan. *International Journal of Disaster Risk Reduction.* 2021;54.

60. Marques MD, Kerr JR, Williams MN, Ling M, McLennan J. Associations between conspiracism and the rejection of scientific innovations. *Public Understanding of Science.* 2021;0-000:1–14.

61. Pickles K, Cvejic E, Nickel B, Copp T, Bonner C, Leask J, *et al.* COVID-19 misinformation trends in Australia: Prospective longitudinal national survey. *Journal of Medical Internet Research.* 2021;23(1).

62. Fernández-Torres MJ, Almansa-Martínez A, Chamizo-Sánchez R. Infodemic and fake news in spain during the COVID-19 pandemic. *International Journal of Environmental Research and Public Health.* 2021;18(4):1–13.

63. Xiao X, Borah P, Su Y. The dangers of blind trust: Examining the interplay among social media news use, misinformation identification, and news trust of conspiracy beliefs. *Public Understanding of Science.* 2021; 0-000:1–16.

64. Cardoso CRB, Fernandes APM, Santos IKFM. What happens in brazil? A pandemic of misinformation that culminates in an endless disease burden. *Revista da Sociedade Brasileira de Medicina Tropical.* 2021;54:1–2.

65. Miller JM. Do COVID-19 conspiracy theory beliefs form a monological belief system? Canadian *Journal of Political Science.* 2020;53(2): 319–326.

66. Douglas KM. COVID-19 conspiracy theories. *Group Processes and Intergroup Relations.* 2021;24(2):270–275.

67. Sengul K. Never let a good crisis go to waste: Pauline Hanson's exploitation of COVID-19 on Facebook. *Media International Australia.* 2021;178(1): 101–105.

68. Jang H, Rempel E, Roth D, Carenini G, Janjua NZ. Tracking COVID-19 discourse on twitter in North America: Infodemiology study using topic modeling and aspect-based sentiment analysis. *Journal of Medical Internet Research.* 2021;23(2).

69. Chou WYS, Gaysynsky A, Vanderpool RC. The COVID-19 misinfodemic: moving beyond fact-checking. *Health Education and Behavior.* 2021; 48(1):9–13.

70. Kessler G. Timeline: How the Wuhan lab-leak theory suddenly became credible. Washington Post, May 25, 2021.

71. WHO Director-General's remarks at the Member State Briefing on the report of the international team studying the origins of SARS-CoV-2 [press release]. March 31, 2021.

72. Bloom JD, Chan YA, Baric RS, Bjorkman PJ, Cobey S, Deverman BE, *et al.* Investigate the origins of COVID-19. *Science.* 2021;372(6543):694–.

73. Tully M, Bode L, Vraga EK. Mobilizing users: Does exposure to misinformation and its correction affect users' responses to a health misinformation post? *Social Media + Society.* 2020;6(4):2056305120978377.

74. First SU. Together Against Misinformation 2021. Available from: https://www.scienceupfirst.com/.

75. Jordan JE, Buchbinder R, Osborne RH. Conceptualising health literacy from the patient perspective. *Patient Education and Counseling.* 2010; 79(1):36–42.

76. Jolley D, Douglas KM. Prevention is better than cure: Addressing anti-vaccine conspiracy theories. *Journal of Applied Social Psychology.* 2017;47(8):459–69.

77. Cuomo RE, Purushothaman V, Li J, Cai M, Mackey TK. A longitudinal and geospatial analysis of COVID-19 tweets during the early outbreak period in the United States. *BMC Public Health.* 2021;21(1).

78. Yousefinaghani S, Dara R, Mubareka S, Sharif S. Prediction of COVID-19 waves using social media and Google search: A case study of the US and Canada. *Frontiers in Public Health.* 2021;9.

79. Su Y, Venkat A, Yadav Y, Puglisi LB, Fodeh SJ. Twitter-based analysis reveals differential COVID-19 concerns across areas with socioeconomic disparities. *Computers in Biology and Medicine.* 2021;132.

80. Crocamo C, Viviani M, Famiglini L, Bartoli F, Pasi G, Carrà G. Surveilling COVID-19 emotional contagion on twitter by sentiment analysis. *European Psychiatry*. 2021;64(1):1–21.
81. Ugarte DA, Cumberland WG, Flores L, Young SD. Public attitudes about COVID-19 in response to President Trump's social media posts. *JAMA Netw Open*. 2021;4(2):e210101.
82. Pullan S, Dey M. Vaccine hesitancy and anti-vaccination in the time of COVID-19: A Google trends analysis. *Vaccine*. 2021;39(14):1877–1881.
83. De Coninck D, Frissen T, Matthijs K, d'Haenens L, Lits G, Champagne-Poirier O, *et al*. Beliefs in conspiracy theories and misinformation about COVID-19: Comparative perspectives on the role of anxiety, depression and exposure to and trust in information sources. *Frontiers in Psychology*. 2021;12.
84. Varghese NE, Sabat I, Neumann-Böhme S, Schreyögg J, Stargardt T, Torbica A, *et al*. Risk communication during COVID-19: A descriptive study on familiarity with, adherence to and trust in the WHO preventive measures. *PloS One*. 2021;16(4 April 2021).
85. Crouse Quinn S. Crisis and emergency risk communication in a pandemic: A model for building capacity and resilience of minority communities. *Health Promotion Practice*. 2008;9(4 Suppl):18S–25S.
86. Paton D, Parkes B, Daly M, Smith L. Fighting the flu: Developing sustained community resilience and preparedness. *Health Promotion Practice*. 2008;9(4 Suppl):45S–53S.
87. Siegrist M, Zingg A. The role of public trust during pandemics: Implications for crisis communication. *European Psychologist*. 2014;19(1):23–32.
88. Vogel L. Broken trust drives native health disparities. *CMAJ: Canadian Medical Association Journal = Journal de l'Association Medicale Canadienne*. 2015.
89. Laurencin CT. Addressing justified vaccine hesitancy in the black community. *Journal of Racial and Ethnic Health Disparities*. 2021;8(3):543–546.
90. Mylan S, Hardman C. COVID-19, cults, and the anti-vax movement. *The Lancet*. 2021;397(10280):1181.
91. Burger AE, Reither EN, Mamelund SE, Lim S. Black-white disparities in 2009 H1N1 vaccination among adults in the United States: A cautionary tale for the COVID-19 pandemic. *Vaccine*. 2021;39(6):943–951.
92. Volpp KG, Loewenstein G, Buttenheim AM. Behaviorally informed strategies for a national COVID-19 vaccine promotion program. *JAMA: The Journal of the American Medical Association*. 2020.
93. Khubchandani J, Sharma S, Price JH, Wiblishauser MJ, Sharma M, Webb FJ. COVID-19 vaccination hesitancy in the United States: A rapid national assessment. *Journal of Community Health*. 2021;46(2):270–277.

94. Burgess RA, Osborne RH, Yongabi KA, Greenhalgh T, Gurdasani D, Kang G, *et al.* The COVID-19 vaccines rush: Participatory community engagement matters more than ever. *Lancet.* 2021;397(10268):8–10.

95. Warren GW, Lofstedt R. COVID-19 vaccine rollout risk communication strategies in Europe: A rapid response. *Journal of Risk Research.* 2021.

96. Griffith J, Marani H, Monkman H. COVID-19 vaccine hesitancy in Canada: Content analysis of tweets using the theoretical domains framework. *Journal of Medical Internet Research.* 2021;23(4).

97. Sallam M. Covid-19 vaccine hesitancy worldwide: A concise systematic review of vaccine acceptance rates. *Vaccines.* 2021;9(2):1–15.

98. Verger P, Peretti-Watel P. Understanding the determinants of acceptance of COVID-19 vaccines: A challenge in a fast-moving situation. *Lancet Public Health.* 2021;6(4):e195–e196.

99. Arora VM, Madison S, Simpson L. Addressing Medical Misinformation in the Patient-Clinician Relationship. *JAMA: The Journal of the American Medical Association.* 2020;324(23):2367.

100. Kowal SP, Jardine CG, Bubela TM. "If they tell me to get it, I'll get it. If they don't…": Immunization decision-making processes of immigrant mothers. *Canadian Journal of Public Health.* 2015;106(4):e230–e235.

101. Looi JCL, Allison S, Bastiampillai T, Maguire PA. Clinical update on managing media exposure and misinformation during COVID-19: Recommendations for governments and healthcare professionals. *Australasian Psychiatry.* 2021;29(1):22–25.

102. Malecki KMC, Keating JA, Safdar N. Crisis communication and public perception of COVID-19 risk in the era of social media. *Clinical Infectious Diseases.* 2021;72(4):697–702.

103. Abidin C, Lee J, Barbetta T, Miao WS. Influencers and COVID-19: Reviewing key issues in press coverage across Australia, China, Japan, and South Korea. *Media International Australia.* 2021;178(1):114–135.

104. Caulfield T. Is Gwynneth Paltrow wrong about everything? when celebrity culture and science clash. Toronto, Ontario: Penguin Canada, 2015.

105. Kamiński M, Szymańska C, Nowak JK. Whose tweets on COVID-19 gain the most attention: Celebrities, political, or scientific authorities? *Cyberpsychology Behaviour, and Social Networking.* 2021;24(2):123–128.

106. Myrick JG, Willoughby JF. The "celebrity canary in the coal mine for the coronavirus": An examination of a theoretical model of celebrity illness disclosure effects. *Social Science and Medicine.* 2021;279.

107. Barmania S, Reiss MJ. Health promotion perspectives on the COVID-19 pandemic: The importance of religion. *Global Health Promotion.* 2021; 28(1):15–22.

108. Perry SL, Baker JO, Bruggs JB. Ignorance of culture war? Christian nationalism and scientific literacy. *Public Understanding of Science*. 2021; 0-000:1–17.

109. Weichel A. Church fined $2,300 for violating COVID-19 restrictions in Kelowna: RCMP. *CTV News*. May 26, 2021.

110. Levin J. The faith community and the SARS-CoV-2 outbreak: Part of the problem or part of the solution? *Journal of Religion and Health*. 2020; 59(5):2215–2228.

111. Slovic P, Finucane ML, Peters E, Macgregor DG. Risk as analysis and risk as feelings: Some thoughts about affect, reason, risk, and rationality. *Risk Analysis*. 2004;24(2):311–322.

112. Kahneman D. Thinking, Fast And Slow (1st Edn). New York: Farrar, Straus and Giroux, 2013, p. 499.

113. Bodemar N, Gaissmaier W. Risk Perception. 2015 2021/05/17. In: *The SAGE Handbook of Risk Communication* [Internet]. Thousand Oaks, Thousand Oaks, California: SAGE Publications, Inc., pp. 10–23. Available from: https://sk.sagepub.com/reference/the-sage-handbook-of-risk-communication.

114. Dickert S, Vastfjall D, M'auro R, Slovic P. The Feeling of Risk: Implications for Risk Perception and Communication. 2015 2021/05/17. In: *The SAGE Handbook of Risk Communication* [Internet]. Thousand Oaks, Thousand Oaks, California: SAGE Publications, Inc., pp. 41–54. Available from: https://sk.sagepub.com/reference/the-sage-handbook-of-risk-communication.

115. Brust-Renck PG, Reyna VF, Corbin JC, Royer CE, Weldon RB. The Role of Numeracy in Risk Communication. 2015 2021/05/17. In: *The SAGE Handbook of Risk Communication* [Internet]. Thousand Oaks, Thousand Oaks, California: SAGE Publications, Inc., pp. 134–45. Available from: https://sk.sagepub.com/reference/the-sage-handbook-of-risk-communication.

116. Luth W, Jardine C, Bubela T. When pictures waste a thousand words: Analysis of the 2009 H1N1 pandemic on television news. *PloS One*. 2013;8(5):e64070.

117. Murthy BP, Leblanc TT, Vagi SJ, Avchen RN. Going viral: The 3rs of social media messaging during public health emergencies. *Health Security*. 2021;19(1):75–81.

118. Campos-Castillo C. Gender divides in engagement with COVID-19 information on the internet among U.S. older adults. *The Journals of Gerontology: Series B*. 2021;76(3):e104–e110.

119. Latkin C, Dayton LA, Yi G, Konstantopoulos A, Park J, Maulsby C, *et al.* COVID-19 vaccine intentions in the United States, a social-ecological framework. *Vaccine.* 2021;39(16):2288–2294.

120. Ataguba OA, Ataguba JE. Social determinants of health: The role of effective communication in the COVID-19 pandemic in developing countries. *Global Health Action.* 2020;13(1).

121. Shafiq M, Elharake JA, Malik AA, McFadden SM, Aguolu OG, Omer SB. COVID-19 sources of information, knowledge, and preventive behaviors among the US adult population. *Journal of Public Health Management and Practice.* 2021;27(3):278–284.

122. Asian HS. Hello south Asians 2020. Available from: https://hellosouth-asians.com/.

123. Myers N. Information sharing and community resilience: Toward a whole community approach to surveillance and combatting the "infodemic". *World Med Health Policy.* 2021.

124. Hyland-Wood B, Gardner J, Leask J, Ecker UKH. Toward effective government communication strategies in the era of COVID-19. *Humanity and Social Science Communication.* 2021;8(1).

125. Loewenson R, Colvin CJ, Szabzon F, Das S, Khanna R, Coelho VSP, *et al.* Beyond command and control: A rapid review of meaningful community-engaged responses to COVID-19. *Global Public Health.* 2021.

126. Besley JC. Public Engagement in Risk-Related Decision Making. 2015 2021/05/17. In: *The SAGE Handbook of Risk Communication* [Internet]. Thousand Oaks, Thousand Oaks, California: SAGE Publications, Inc., pp. 317–329. Available from: https://sk.sagepub.com/reference/the-sage-handbook-of-risk-communication.

127. Urquhart C, Jasiura F. *Trauma-Informed Practice Guide.* Vancouver: BC Provincial Mental Health and Substance Use Planning Council, 2013.

128. Menschner C, Maul A. *Key Ingredients for Successful Trauma-Informed Care Implementation,* 2016.

129. Manns BJ. *Evidence-Based Decision Making 5: Knowledge Translation and the Knowledge to Action Cycle.* Methods in Molecular Biology: Humana Press Inc., 2021, pp. 467–482.

Part 9

Epilogue

Chapter 17

Preventing the Next Pandemic

Ali Okhowat[*,†,‡]

*School of Population and Public Health, University of British Columbia,
Vancouver, Canada*

†*Department of Family Practice, Faculty of Medicine,
University of British Columbia,
Vancouver, Canada*

‡*Division of Global Health, Faculty of Medicine,
University of British Columbia, Vancouver, Canada*

"We, Leaders of G20 and other states, in the presence of the Heads of international and regional organisations .... Underline that sustained investments in global health, towards achieving Universal Health Coverage with primary healthcare at its centre, One Health, and preparedness and resilience, are broad social and macro-economic investments in global public goods, and that the cost of inaction is orders of magnitude greater."

— *Rome Declaration*, EU Global Health Summit, 21 May 2021[1]

COVID-19 has devastated societies at a scale and scope of disruption that defies simple statistics. Nevertheless, three statistics from the pandemic's first year provide us a glimpse into its crushing consequences:

- As of April 28, 2021, three million people had died across 223 countries, territories and areas.

- At the height of the pandemic in 2020, 90% of school-age children were absent from school due to pandemic-related attendance disruptions.
- By the end of 2021, the pandemic's economic effects are expected to have led to lost economic output totalling $10 trillion.

Our international system, measured in megatons and gigawatts, struggled to defend itself against a threat measured in nanometers and microliters. While exceedingly complex in effect, the causative factors that allowed a cluster of symptoms to morph into an epidemic then accelerate exponentially to become a pandemic were comparatively simple. These have been succinctly documented in the reports by Independent Panel on Pandemic Preparedness and Response, quotes of which have been extracted below to preface the elaboration of three key shortcomings.

1. Learning from the Current Pandemic

"Pandemic preparedness planning is a core function of governments and of the international system and must be overseen at the highest level. It is not a responsibility of the health sector alone."

— Independent Panel on Pandemic Preparedness and Response[2]

First, prevention (and by extension, preparation) was never prioritised at the level needed to combat a pathogen with pandemic potential. From SARS, H1N1 and MERS to Ebola, Zika and other disease outbreaks, health security had always been top of mind for countries but never for the world as a whole. Case in point, the voluntary Joint External Evaluations of the International Health Regulations (IHR) (2005) were meant to, in part, identify how prepared countries were to address the introduction of a highly infectious pathogen. Countries scores and their breakdowns were recorded within the Global Health Security Index (GHSI). However, a review of age-standardised COVID-19 deaths per hundred thousand people in the 50 days following the date of the first death in that country showed that countries' GHSI rankings did not predict their performance in responding to COVID-19 (see Figure 1). Going back to earlier initiatives, the 2001 Global Health Security Initiative, adoption of the IHR in 2005

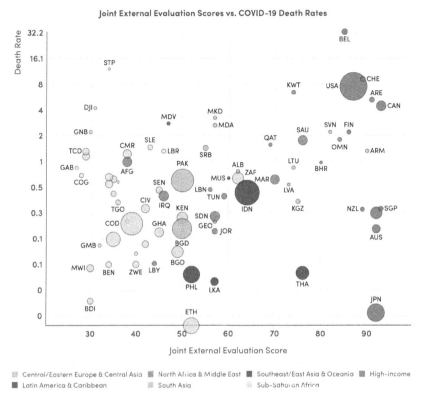

Figure 1: Age-standardised COVID-19 deaths per hundred thousand people in the 50 days following the date of the first death in that country versus countries' Global Health Security Index scores following voluntary Joint External Evaluation per IHR (2005).

and the US-led Global Health Security Agenda in 2014 were among the more significant attempts of the past two decades in bringing about an attempt at coordinated prevention and response. Despite these initiatives and more than 16 reports by 11 high-level panels since the 2009 H1N1 influenza pandemic, the majority of recommendations were never implemented, and national-level pandemic preparedness plans remained vastly underfunded or neglected. Case in point, Canada's vaunted Global Public Health Intelligence Network was shut down in May 2019, only a few months before early signals of the emergence of SARS-CoV-2 would emerge.

> "The [global infectious hazard] alert system does not operate with sufficient speed when faced with a fast-moving respiratory pathogen ... the legally binding IHR (2005) are a conservative instrument as currently constructed and serve to constrain rather than facilitate rapid action ... and the precautionary principle was not applied to the early alert evidence when it should have been."
>
> — Independent Panel on Pandemic Preparedness and Response[3]

Second, global and national surveillance and alert systems were underpowered to match the exponential spread of SARS-CoV-2. This was compounded by a lack of precautionary leadership at all levels to stem the rising tide of cases. Throughout the pandemic's early period, the rapidity of information generation through open source data collection and collaborative assessments of epidemiological trends contrasted with the slow and deliberate steps of the IHR and related instruments at the national and regional levels.[4] This is painfully apparent when we look to the rapid increase in cases during the "lost" month of February 2020, where inaction, denial and complacency marked most countries' responses to the threat of COVID's spread. It was not until March 2021 — after an official pandemic had been declared by the WHO and local spread had been well documented — that most countries activated their emergency management systems and implemented their public health and social measures in earnest.

> "The Panel notes that COVID-19 has been a pandemic of inequalities and inequities. Those with less social protection were more likely to have pre-existing health conditions that made them more vulnerable to COVID-19, and they were often also more exposed to the virus owing to the nature of their work and their living conditions. When exposed to COVID-19, a lack of social protection prevented vulnerable and sick people from staying at home because of the risk of a loss of income."
>
> — Independent Panel on Pandemic Preparedness and Response[5]

Third, no matter how well countries initially responded to the virus, the vast majority were unable to sustain the response through the punctuated onslaught of rising cases and hospitalisations. As a prolonged crisis, COVID-19 tested the limits of health systems and workers in responding to health needs, stressed the economic and social protections — if they were adequately present — of governments in responding to challenges to peoples' livelihoods and exposed or widened trust deficits that were present between people and their institutions and leaders. Supply shortages in personal protective equipment, diagnostics and therapeutics hindered the ability of health systems to respond consistently to the ebb and flow of local epidemics. Vaccine nationalism and the hoarding of critical supplies similarly prolonged what could have been localised outbreaks and instead allowed them to spread unchecked.

2. Preventing the Next Pandemic

It is fitting that the title of this volume, *Intelligence and Intervention,* alludes to what we know and have done. Yet similar to the press conference announcing the first global conference on COVID-19, the purpose of this book is to shine a light on what we know, as well as to help chart a course in framing the questions that remain unanswered and the lessons we should glean from a year of action — and inaction.

Will we ever be able to reach herd immunity against COVID-19? How long will our immunity last? Will COVID-19 be a seasonal challenge that we'll have to prepare for, much like we do for influenza? How will the rise of COVID-19 variants influence our approach to diagnostics, therapeutics and vaccines? How can we best tackle the equity-related faults that have been laid bare throughout the pandemic? And most importantly, how can we prevent the next pandemic in a manner that balances what we could come to know from our science and solutions with how we could know it in a world of fragile freedoms?

Since the start of pandemic, numerous initiatives have been launched at the sub-national, national, and international levels aimed at enhancing knowledge, improving coordination, and strengthening responsiveness and recovery — not only against COVID-19 but all infectious hazards. The leadup to the World Health Assembly and G20 Global Health Summit in May 2021 saw a dizzying array of initiatives and partnerships announced relating to pandemic preparedness and response. These included the launch of the Global Pandemic Radar in the UK, the Germany-based WHO Hub for Pandemic and Epidemic Intelligence, and the first WHO BioHub Facility (as part of the WHO BioHub System) in Geneva. Renewed calls for solidarity emerged through the establishment of new councils and expert panels, such as the WHO Council on the Economics of Health for All, the COVID-19 Global Research and Innovation Forum, and the One Health High-Level Expert Panel, as well as countries' decisions to support temporary waivers on intellectual property rights for COVID-19 vaccines.

Despite this seeming progress, the world bore witness to countless tragedies that occurred as countries and leaders were slow to respond to the threat of COVID-19's spread or resurgence. Public health and social measures were relaxed prematurely, health resources and workforces were mismanaged, manufacturing capacity for diagnostics, therapeutics and vaccines were highly concentrated or fragmented, and supply chains screeched to a halt or could not overcome critical bottlenecks.

As we make a "Sprint to September" to vaccinate 10% of the people in every country, we are reminded that most health emergencies — whether borne of infectious hazards, natural or technological disasters, or conflict — are lengthened less by their biology than by misaligned incentives that promote an "us versus them" mentality. This is nowhere more true than in the context of pandemics. Vaccine nationalism and the hoarding of essential health supplies has led to a tragedy of the health commons the likes of which was readily cautioned against, yet we are nevertheless surprised by. In order to prevent such an occurrence, we've distilled insights from several recent publications — including the reports of the Independent Panel on Pandemic Preparedness and Response, the Independent Oversight and Advisory Committee for the WHO Health Emergencies Programme, and the Review Committee on the Functioning of the IHR (2005) during the COVID-19 Response — among others, into five lessons below that we must heed if we ever hope to ensure that this pandemic will be the last.

2.1 *Prioritise pandemic preparedness as a top political and leadership priority*

Preparing for the next pandemic begins now. This must be done through a transformed, coordinated, and global pandemic preparedness and response system involving countries, technical agencies, and multilateral organisations. The highest levels of political leadership, including the UN Secretary-General and Heads of States, must lead this new system through a whole-of-government and whole-of-system approach that does not treat this cause as one alone for the health system to fight. The economic and social consequences of the pandemic have it made this all too clear. A Pandemic Framework Convention that would be complementary to the IHR, with fit-for-purpose policies and processes, would allow for concrete commitments by governments and clarify responsibilities they have in interacting with international organisations. Whether a Global Health Threats Council or related body is formed under the direction of the United Nations General Assembly, a body that sits at the highest levels of political discourse is needed to monitor progress towards a post-pandemic future, allocate resources appropriately and enforce accountability measures through regular reports.

2.2 *Establish a new global pandemic surveillance system*

The speed of a digital-first surveillance system must be matched with the processes of a validation and alerts system. Modern-day systems that monitor human health concerns must be merged with animal and environmental health surveillance systems to create a true One Health surveillance system that is always connected, coordinated and quick to respond. Yet improved technology and information merging is only part of the solution. Currently, the gears of government and official signoffs prevent the rapid transmission of this information or stifle its communication. This is partly due to the fact that there are significant disadvantages for a country to signal the detection of a cluster of cases or an outbreak. This new surveillance system must therefore be aligned with incentives that promote rapid alerts and validation assessments.

In addition to strengthening surveillance, risk assessment and information sharing protocols needs to be dramatically improved. The ability of a surveillance system to independently and rapidly verify a signal, assess its risk, and report back to concerned parties is paramount in ensuring its effectiveness. Standard forms and information sharing protocols should be developed to structure the rapid exchange of information in follow up to an investigation into a possible hazard. With an empowered

WHO, events with information in the public domain deemed to be of significant risk (and for which an adequate response is not received in reply to a WHO verification request) should be communicated publicly and acknowledged as unverified.

2.3 *Launch a pandemic supply chain platform*

The key in launching a supply chain platform is to create a structure that allows for equitable access to its outputs. While the Access to COVID-19 Tools Accelerator and the COVID-19 Supply Chain System provide a valuable model, there are as many lessons to learn from their weaknesses as there are of their strengths. A fit-for-purpose pandemic supply chain platform must be pre-negotiated and built on principles of inclusivity with metrics of success that measure how quickly the right supplies were delivered to those in need. Ensuring that such a platform has the right governance, financing, technologies and horizon scanning functions is paramount. Related to what is shared on the platform is how it is shared. The platform should have clear priorities for its membership on the commitments for technology transfer and voluntary licensing, especially where there has been the involvement of public financing of research and development.

2.4 *Institute rapid and sustained financing mechanisms for pandemic preparedness and response*

Global public goods, such as an effective pandemic response system, must be funded regularly and rapidly. This requires predictable funding that meets three criteria: regular payment, rapid response and long-term focus. First, it must be delivered at predictable times and in sufficient amounts to support the activities and resources required by the system. Bilateral arrangements through official development assistance programs and the relatively short-term commitments of multilateral financing institutions are not sufficient. Second, there must be a mechanism for rapid increases in funding to counter an emerging threat. A fit-for-purpose financing program for pandemics would acknowledge that unpredictable developments in the identification of a potential pathogen or progression of an outbreak require a coordinated response that may need to be scaled up with little time to wait for responses to official appeals. Lastly, the focus of such a fund should be inherently long-term, with annual contributions by State Parties and commitments of a minimum of 10 years.

2.5 *Empower a focused, independent and fully funded World Health Organization*

WHO's annual budget is equivalent to that of some hospital systems or cities' health budgets. Not only is its annual funding paltry in comparison; in addition, the quality of funding is lacking. Agreements that restrict the use of funds to specific projects or programs prevent the WHO, at times, from utilising the funding that it has efficiently, effectively and equitably. A recommendation by the Independent Panel to restrict the WHO's Director-General's term of office to a non-renewable term of seven years is one that should be seriously considered as a means to the independence of the office. While political capital has been used effectively since WHO's inception as a means of health diplomacy, ample evidence exists to suggest that it has also hindered prompt action and response, especially in time-sensitive situations of health emergencies.

3. Preparing for a Post-Pandemic World

With the outbreak of Ebola in West Africa, public health practitioners have become accustomed to declarations of the end of an outbreak only to be followed by the start of another a short while later. At some point in the — hopefully near — future, the COVID-19 pandemic will be declared over. New measures, initiatives and organisations will be put in place to support the call to never again allow an infectious disease to spread so mercilessly. Yet the statement that opens this chapter challenges our policy makers and public health practitioners to ponder what that new world with its renewed appreciation for global public goods will look like. Our investments in Universal Health Coverage, One Health and preparedness and resilience systems will be built on the corpus of evidence we have to know what has worked and how it might be improved the next time around.

While subsequent volumes will address those pillars not covered in this book — namely those on surveillance and disease control and institutional and governance-related factors — the science and solutions explored in this book have hopefully instilled a modicum of hope and strengthened a sense of solidarity in showing how we cannot overcome COVID-19 and future infectious hazards like it anywhere if it is not defeated everywhere. With new institutions, policies and regulations in place, it is hoped that we'll never again need to make the impossible choices that the pandemic forced upon us. Yet if we've learned anything from this experience it must be that no matter how foolproof we deem our systems to be, we must prepare for the worst and hope for the very best in us to emerge if it happens.

References

1. Rome Declaration. European Union Global Health Summit, 21 May 2021. Available from: https://global-health-summit.europa.eu/rome-declaration_en [Accessed 22 May 2021].
2. COVID-19: Make it the last pandemic. Independent Panel on Pandemic Preparedness and Response. Toronto, Canada. May 2021, p. 20. https://theindependentpanel.org/wp-content/uploads/2021/05/COVID-19-Make-it-the-Last-Pandemic_final.pdf [Accessed 21 May 2021].
3. COVID-19: Make it the last pandemic. Independent Panel on Pandemic Preparedness and Response. Toronto, Canada. May 2021, p. 26. https://theindependentpanel.org/wp-content/uploads/2021/05/COVID-19-Make-it-the-Last-Pandemic_final.pdf [Accessed 21 May 2021].
4. Review committee on the functioning of the international health regulations 2005. Report by the Review Committee on the Functioning of the International Health Regulations (2005) during the COVID-19 Response. https://cdn.who.int/media/docs/default-source/documents/emergencies/a74_9add1-en.pdf?sfvrsn=d5d22fdf_1&download=true [Accessed 01 May 2021].
5. COVID-19: Make it the last pandemic. Independent Panel on Pandemic Preparedness and Response. Toronto, Canada, May 2021, p. 43. https://theindependentpanel.org/wp-content/uploads/2021/05/COVID-19-Make-it-the-Last-Pandemic_final.pdf [Accessed 21 May 2021].

Index

World Scientific Series in Global Health Economics and Public Policy

(Continued from page ii)

World Scientific Series in Global Health Economics and Public Policy

(Continued from page ii)

CPSIA information can be obtained
at www.ICGtesting.com
Printed in the USA
JSHW040159030422
24286JS00001B/6